SE

Intelligent Control in Biomedicine

Intelligent Control in Biomedicine

edited by

D.A. Linkens

*Department of Automatic Control
and Systems Engineering
University of Sheffield*

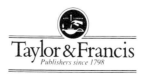

UK   Taylor & Francis Ltd, 4 John St, London WC1N 2ET

USA Taylor & Francis Inc., 1900 Frost Road, Suite 101, Bristol PA 19007

Copyright © Taylor & Francis Ltd 1994

All rights reserved. No part of this publication may be reproduced, stored in a retrieval system, or transmitted, in any form or by any means, electronic, electrostatic, magnetic tape, mechanical, photocopying, recording or otherwise, without the prior permission of the copyright owner and the publisher.

British Library Cataloguing in Publication Data

A catalogue record for this book is available from the British Library

ISBN 0-7484-0115-6

Cover design by Amanda Barragry

Typeset in Great Britain by Keyword Publishing Services
Printed in Great Britain by Burgess Science Press, Basingstoke
on paper which has a specified pH value on final paper
manufacture of not less than 7.5 and is therefore 'acid free'.

Contents

Series Introduction		vii
Preface		ix
Contributors		xii
Chapter 1	Introduction to intelligent control paradigms and system modelling D.A. Linkens	1
Chapter 2	A real-time expert system for anaesthesia validated in clinical trials S.G. Greenhow	19
Chapter 3	Generalized predictive control (GPC) in the operating theatre M. Mahfouf	37
Chapter 4	A comparative study of generalized predictive control (GPC) and intelligent self-organizing fuzzy logic control (SOFLC) for multivariable anaesthesia M. Mahfouf and M.F. Abbod	79
Chapter 5	Hierarchical supervisory self-organizing fuzzy control for muscle relaxation anaesthesia M.F. Abbod	133
Chapter 6	Hierarchical fuzzy modelling and fault detection for muscle relaxation anaesthesia J.S. Shieh	175
Chapter 7	Unified fuzzy reasoning and blood pressure management Junhong Nie	203
Chapter 8	Learning-based fuzzy and neural control for blood pressure management Junhong Nie	235

Contents

Chapter 9 Self-organizing fuzzy-neural control for blood pressure management   265
Junhong Nie

Chapter 10 Neural network control for unconsciousness anaesthesia   291
H.U. Rehman

Chapter 11 Genetic algorithms in the control of anaesthesia   321
H. Okla Nyongesa

Chapter 12 Multifaceted knowledge representation and acquisition applied to the modelling of the cardiovascular system   361
E. Tanyi

Chapter 13 Automated qualitative model abduction based on bond graphs   385
S. Xia

Chapter 14 Epilogue   407
D.A. Linkens

Index   417

Series Introduction

Control Systems has a long and distinguished tradition stretching back to nineteenth-century dynamics and stability theory. Its establishment as a major engineering discipline in the 1950s arose, essentially, from Second World War driven work on frequency response methods by, amongst others, Nyquist, Bode and Wiener. The intervening 40 years has seen quite unparalleled developments in the underlying theory with applications ranging from the ubiquitous PID controller widely encountered in the process industries through to high-performance/fidelity controllers typical of aerospace applications. This development has been increasingly underpinned by the rapid developments in the, essentially enabling, technology of computing software and hardware.

This view of mathematically model-based systems and control as a mature discipline masks relatively new and rapid developments in the general area of robust control. Here intense research effort is being directed to the development of high-performance controllers which (at least) are robust to specified classes of plant uncertainty. One measure of this effort is the fact that, after a relatively short period of work, 'near world' tests of classes of robust controllers have been undertaken in the aerospace industry. Again, this work is supported by computing hardware and software developments, such as the toolboxes available within numerous commercially marketed controller design/simulation packages.

Recently, there has been increasing interest in the use of so-called intelligent control techniques such as fuzzy logic and neural networks. Basically, these rely on learning (in a prescribed manner) the input-output behaviour of the plant to be controlled. Already, it is clear that there is little to be gained by applying these techniques to cases where mature mathematical model-based approaches yield high-performance control. Instead, their role is (in general terms) almost certainly going to lie in areas where the processes encountered are ill-defined, complex, nonlinear, time-varying and stochastic. A detailed evaluation of their (relative) potential awaits the appearance of a rigorous supporting base (underlying theory and implementation architectures for example) the essential elements of which are beginning to appear in learned journals and conferences.

Elements of control and systems theory/engineering are increasingly finding use outside traditional numerical processing environments. One such general area in which there is increasing interest is intelligent command and control systems which are central, for example, to innovative manufacturing and the management of advanced transportation systems. Another is discrete event systems which mix numeric and logic decision making.

It is in response to these exciting new developments that the present book series on Systems and Control was conceived. It will publish high-quality research texts and reference works in the diverse areas which systems and control now includes. In addition to basic theory, experimental and/or applications studies are welcome, as are expository texts where theory, verification and applications come together to provide a unifying coverage of a particular topic or topics.

The book series itself arose out of the seminal text: the 1992 centenary first English translation of Lyapunov's memoir *On the General Problem of the Stability of Motion* by A.T. Fuller, and was followed by the 1994 publication of *Advances in Intelligent Control* by C.J. Harris. The current volume in the series is *Intelligent Control in Biomedicine* by D.A. Linkens. Forthcoming titles in the series include *True Digital Control* by P.C. Young, A. Chotai and W. Tych, *Sliding-Mode Control* by V. Utkin and *A Knowledge-Based Approach to Systems Control* by G.K.H. Pang.

E. Rogers
J. O'Reilly

Preface

This book emanates from a series of research studies undertaken over recent years into the application of advanced control strategies in the area of computer-assisted drug administration. The main area of interest has been high-dependency units in health care, comprising operating theatres and intensive care units. The particular spheres of decision support have been those of anaesthesia and blood pressure management. Within the field of anaesthesia, research studies have been undertaken for both muscle relaxation (i.e. drug-induced paralysis) and unconsciousness (i.e. drug-induced hypnosis). The third of the 'triad' of responsibilities which the anaesthetist manages is pain relief (i.e. analgesia), but this is not addressed in the contributions in this book. It is, however, under active research consideration.

The introductory chapter of the book gives an overview of what intelligent control is currently considered to comprise. It gives some basic definitions and thoughts on 'intelligence' and 'systems', then proceeds with brief chronologies and concepts of the main paradigms which are currently being considered within the remit of intelligent systems.

Chapter 2 is concerned with the development and clinical validation of a real-time expert system for advice on drug administration for unconsciousness. Since there is no single measurement variable for determining depth of anaesthesia (DOA), a number of clinical signs and on-line monitored physiological variables are combined into a multi-sensor fusion system. The emphasis is on the knowledge acquisition problem, the need for good human computer interface (HCI) and extensive clinical trials to validate the large knowledge-base.

In contrast to DOA, muscle relaxation (MR) can be quantified using stimulated twitch responses of the hand. Since good measurements are available on-line, new methods of quantitative control can be used. Thus, in Chapter 3 generalized predictive control (GPC) is applied to MR, with validation and evaluation in a series of clinical trials. GPC is a popular form of model-based predictive control (MBPC), which has had considerable exposure in industrial settings in recent years.

To provide a comparison between modern quantitative and qualitative advanced control strategies, Chapter 4 describes studies using GPC and fuzzy logic control (FLC) on a multivariable anaesthesia model which provides for simultaneous control of DOA and MR. The model has been elicited in collaboration with Dr A.J. Asbury at the Western Infirmary,

Glasgow, UK, who has been our anaesthetist co-investigator in many parts of the work described in this book. In this chapter, the studies include an investigation into the ability of the algorithms to be self adapting: a key element in an intelligent system. Not surprisingly, it is found that better control is achievable when a good model is available (as for GPC), than when only a crude model is assumed (as for FLC).

Beyond the requirements for regulatory control there is the common need for fault detection and diagnosis to determine the integrity of a closed-loop system. This is particularly important in safety-critical applications such as the biomedical systems considered here. Chapter 5 considers fault detection for MR using fuzzy logic as the underlying methodology. Faults considered include instrumentation defects, actuator faults and changes in system (i.e. patient) dynamics.

Fuzzy logic is again the theme of Chapter 6, allied to MR. However, the basic component in the hierarchical fault management system becomes a fuzzy model of the process (i.e. the patient). In this chapter, a method for self-elicitation of the MR fuzzy model is described. This hierarchical architecture is currently being used to extend the techniques into DOA, as well as MR.

The area of application changes to that of blood pressure management in Chapters 7, 8 and 9. The theme is multivariable drug management, with a number of increasingly ambitious aims being pursued. Chapter 7 lays down a framework for a generic, unified approach to approximate reasoning. This attempts to co-ordinate the many suggested algorithms for fuzzy reasoning, and to give guidelines for choices of algebraic operators and parameters. It also casts the algorithms into an expert system framework, dealing with uncertain data measurements. In Chapter 8, fuzzy and neural network ideas are linked in a synergetic manner within the context of learning systems based on a type of model reference adaptive control (MRAC). In Chapter 9, these concepts are extended to include the possibility of control strategies which self-organize their own structures, again based on a neural network (NN) architecture.

Neural networks are again the theme of Chapter 10, which uses them in the context of unconsciousness anaesthesia. Initially the NN is made to replicate the RESAC expert system controller of Chapter 2. From there, extensions are made to include NN models of patient dynamics and to perform simulation studies of closed-loop behaviour using total NN controller/patient models. These NN models are compared with equivalent structures developed via standard regression methods (both linear and nonlinear). The NN approach was found to out-perform the regression methods.

A major difficulty with fuzzy control is the elicitation of good knowledge-bases on which the control inference is based. In Chapter 11, genetic algorithms (GAs) are used to produce optimized values for the rules, membership functions and scaling factors for fuzzy control of multivariable anaesthesia (see also Chapter 4). These are the major design features for FLC, and GAs are shown to be capable of producing optimized values for these factors in either off-line or on-line architectures.

The final two chapters concentrate on modelling aspects of intelligence allied to biomedicine, rather than control. In Chapter 12, an artificial intelligence (AI) approach is used to develop an object-oriented modelling and simulation environment called KEMS (knowledge-based environment for modelling and simulation). Although initially developed for industrial processes, it also has various applications, including those of biomedicine. It has an intelligent front-end for knowledge capture, called KAM (knowledge acquisition module).

Qualitative reasoning (QR) has been considered for a range of applied science applications, but exhibits certain disadvantages such as the generation of many spurious solutions. In Chapter 13, bond graphs (BG) are introduced as a sound, formal modelling language to which QR is attached as the underlying simulation and reasoning methodology. Again, this was introduced originally for engineering applications, but has clear advantages in life science modelling.

Some tentative conclusions and suggestions for the way forward are given in the Epilogue. These reflect the editor's views, and not necessarily the thoughts of the other contributors!

All of the contributors to the book have worked with the Editor's research group on modelling and control in biomedicine, either as research fellows or research students. It is a pleasure to acknowledge their many contributions in this work, and to record their enthusiasm, diligence and hard work in their research studies and in the production of this book.

Thanks are also due to the UK Engineering & Physical Sciences Research Council and the Leverhulme Trust who have funded some of the research projects which are described in the book.

Contributors

Dr M.F. Abbod	Department of Automatic Control & Systems Engineering, The University of Sheffield, Mappin Street, PO Box 600, Sheffield S1 4DU, UK
Dr S.G. Greenhow	242 Northridge Way, Chaulden, Hemel Hempstead, Herts, HP1 2AS, UK
Prof. D.A. Linkens	Department of Automatic Control & Systems Engineering, The University of Sheffield, Mappin Street, PO Box 600, Sheffield S1 4DU, UK
Dr M. Mahfouf	Department of Automatic Control & Systems Engineering, The University of Sheffield, Mappin Street, PO Box 600, Sheffield S1 4DU, UK
Dr J. Nie	Department of Electrical Engineering, National University of Singapore, 10 Kent Ridge Road, Singapore 0511
Dr H.O. Nyongesa	Department of Automatic Control & Systems Engineering, The University of Sheffield, Mappin Street, PO Box 600, Sheffield S1 4DU, UK
Dr H. Rehman	SSS Dallah Albaraka, PO Box 430, Jeddah 21411, Saudi Arabia
Mr J.S. Shieh	Department of Automatic Control & Systems Engineering, The University of Sheffield, Mappin Street, PO Box 600, Sheffield S1 4DU, UK
Dr E. Tanyi	Department of Electrical Engineering, National Polytechnic Institute, University of Yaounde, BP 8390 Yaounde, Cameroon Republic, West Africa
Dr S. Xia	School of Computing & Mathematical Sciences, De Montfort University, Hammerwood Gate, Kents Hill, Milton Keynes, MK7 6HP, UK

Chapter 1
Introduction to intelligent control paradigms and system modelling

D. A. Linkens

In recent years there has been a move away from sporadic interest in artificial intelligence (AI) concepts by a small number of systems engineers to a worldwide passion for intelligent control, utilizing all of the tools that have been developed in the field of AI. This book is devoted to the use of intelligent system techniques in biomedicine and has been written as a result of the following factors:

- a personal interest dating from the time when expert systems were introduced into medicine a decade ago
- a burgeoning, but lagging, industrial interest
- the specialization of certain engineering laboratories in 'intelligent systems engineering'
- learned society journals devoted to the subject
- worldwide interest in the field, including a large influence from South East Asia, especially China and Japan
- widespread dissatisfaction with 'quantitative-led' engineering, with a recognized need for a qualitative dimension.

To set the scene we will attempt to give some concise definitions of the words used to describe the content of this book.

Definitions are always important in attempting to communicate ideas, and the following abbreviated suggestions cover the major concepts underlying the subject addressed in this book.

- *Intelligence*
  The ability to understand or reason (logically) and to learn or adapt.

- *System*
  An assembly of interacting elements (simple or complex: human or machine) which interacts with an environment (defined set of boundaries).

- *Engineering*
  An iterative process of top-down specification, design, implementation, commissioning and maintenance of a real-world system that satisfies, in a near optimal way, a defined goal.

Since much control systems design is model-based, it is appropriate to consider what we mean by *model* in the context of this research work. A taxonomy of system models could be divided into a number of branches. It is presupposed that we are concerned here with *mathematical models*, rather than *physical models*, although the latter have played an important part in industrial control engineering design.

Another sub-division could be made between *dynamic* and *static* models. Static models embody algebraic relationships, and many process plant models are of this nature, partly because of the difficulty of obtaining adequate dynamic data for the process. Thus, in chemical processes, static models involve the calculation of steady-state heat and material balances. These models are often used for optimization purposes, and are part of a hierarchical decomposition of the design problem, whereby the static model provides the 'set-points' for dynamic sub-processes lower down the hierarchy.

Dynamic models for control purposes may be classified as *single-variable* or *multivariable*. The number of inputs and outputs determines whether the system is single-variable or multivariable. Classical control design techniques have been largely successful in single-variable systems, whereas modern designs for multivariable systems have been much slower to gain ground. They have been mostly successful in aerospace systems, the key reason being the availability of good dynamic models, small noise corruption in measurements, and not many inaccessible variables. One of the attractions of intelligent system design for biomedicine is the possibility of producing multivariable system control without the need for extensive dynamic models of the process—something which is often impossible in the life sciences. It should be noted that a single-variable system may have a very complicated mathematical model (i.e. transfer function) between input and output. The main difficulty in the multivariable case is that of interaction between variables, and the related matter of sensitivity to faults in particular channels.

Modelling usually involves the use of computer simulation, often facilitated through special high-level languages. Conventionally, dynamic system simulations are either *continuous* (i.e. governed by differential equations) or *discrete* (i.e. event-triggered). Discrete system modelling and simulation is very important in the manufacturing industry. In this field there are currently not the same theoretical bases for analysis and design as for continuous systems, although derivatives of Petri net theory show some promise of providing design methodologies. As a result, simulation has been slow to develop for discrete systems. However, it is now recognized that modelling and simulation, coupled to computer-based animation, offers great scope for assisting conceptual design and management decision-making.

Continuous system models can be further sub-divided into those governed by ordinary differential and partial differential equations. The former arise from systems which can be represented via '*lumped*' components (e.g. blood flow in arteries and veins) and those of a '*distributed*' nature (e.g. flow in the branching airways of the respiratory system. The lumped representation is often an approximation, but since control design and computer simulation concentrates on ordinary differential equations, this is the format on which we shall focus attention in the following chapters.

Dynamic models may be either linear or non-linear. Nearly all the control design methods are based on linear systems, whereas in the real world most systems are non-linear! This anomaly is due to the vast difficulty that non-linear dynamics present to theoretical analysis. The most common approach is to linearize a system around a number of operating points (i.e. steady-state conditions), and design a number of appropriate controllers, or conversely find one robust controller that can cater for all conditions. Intelligent control offers an attractive alternative since fuzzy logic and neural networks naturally cater for non-linear system dynamics.

A final branch in a modelling taxonomy could be between *quantitative* (i.e. numeric) and *qualitative* (i.e. symbolic) models. Until recently the emphasis had been on quantitative mathematical models, since they offer a powerful 'language' of explanation, together with techniques for analysis and design, but in the last few years, interest has blossomed in qualitative reasoning, mainly from the artificial intelligence fraternity. Although the subject has not yet reached a degree of maturity, it is founded on the obvious notion that humans make decisions based on conceptual models which are imprecise and based on linguistic rather than numerical abstractions. It should be noted that the world 'abstraction' is used here to denote the essential nature of modelling which involves a simplification of real-world entities, rather than a process of vague thinking! The distinction between numeric and symbolic reasoning is illustrated by well-known probability theory and 'possibility' theory introduced by Zadeh in his notion of 'fuzzy logic'. The merging of qualitative and quantitative modalities offers fascinating prospects for improved understanding and control in the life sciences.

Mathematical models are commonly used in science to 'describe' a real system, or even to 'explain' an experimentally observable phenomenon. A 'description' provides an aggregated mathematical formulation, whereas an 'explanation' decomposes the phenomenon into more elementary relationships or laws which are already known. In the physical sciences, molecular models are commonly feasible, providing explanatory functions, whereas in the life sciences aggregated models are the norm and provide descriptive powers. In control engineering the model is utilized for design purposes, for which the model formulation should be 'good enough' to satisfy the performance objectives of the overall system (the principle of *parsimony*). In other words, using a quotation which originates from the realm of science, but which is equally relevant to engineering, 'Everything should be made as simple as possible, but no simpler' (Albert Einstein). Since we shall be considering certain complex systems and structures, it is well to remember this axiom and constantly recognize the elegance of simplicity in engineering design.

The complexity of a dynamic model used bears a strong relationship to the sophistication of the controller design, and this in turn is often strongly coupled to the 'tightness' of performance specified for the overall system. At the lowest level of modelling (and the strongest degree of abstraction) all that is required in the model is a knowledge of the gain and its sign for the system (i.e. does a positive input produce a positive output, or *vice versa*?). Intuitive control design then produces a simple proportional controller which hopefully gives a stable, albeit low-performance, system. Most human-centred control systems for decision making proceed initially along these lines, until more is learnt about the system (i.e. its dynamic model) via experience (i.e. experimental data). It is interesting to note that the technique of self-organizing fuzzy logic control (SOFLC) utilizes a similar approach whereby the controller rules are successively refined by probing the system with simple inputs and observing the output performance. This technique has been used on many industrial processes, and more recently for on-line drug infusion (Chapters 4 and 5).

Returning to the theme of intelligent control, a number of methodologies are currently being studied actively, both in industry and academia. These methodologies include: fuzzy logic, expert systems, neural networks, genetic algorithms, and qualitative reasoning.

To illustrate how these methodologies can interact and be applied extensively in a particular discipline, the following projects represent the editor's research group's attempts to investigate the use of intelligent system concepts in biomedicine, mostly in the realm of anaesthesia:

- *Intelligent modelling*
  Fuzzy modelling of unconsciousness.

- *Intelligent regulation*
  Fuzzy control for relaxation and hypnosis: automatic knowledge acquisition for relaxation (rules, scaling factors, membership functions).

Introduction to intelligent control paradigms and system modelling   5

- *Intelligent adaptation*
  Generalized predictive control; self-organizing fuzzy logic control; fuzzy/neural network/model reference adaptive control synergy for blood pressure.

- *Intelligent fault diagnosis*
  Supervisory control; generalized predictive control; self-organizing fuzzy logic control.

- *Intelligent signal processing*
  Audio evoked responses (AER) for assessment of hypnosis.

An important point to note is that although these methodologies have been developed initially in isolation, it is gradually being realized that the concepts may be merged to provide an integrated approach to design and analysis of complex systems. In these projects it is clear that there are

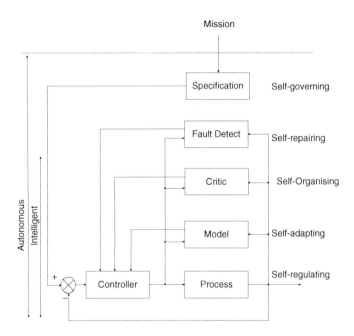

Physical systems have UNCERTAINTY

Figure 1.1 Autonomous control systems.

differing levels of structural complexity involved, ranging from a narrowly focused design aim in modelling studies to ambitious multilayer architectures necessary for intelligent fault detection and repair. What is clear is that if we are to move towards the realization of autonomous systems that can provide their own mechanisms for task planning and mission achievement within noise-contaminated and unreliable environments, we shall have to utilize a range of qualitative as well as quantitative methodologies. The architectural levels and components necessary to move from low-level self-regulating systems to high-level self-governing (i.e. autonomous) systems are shown in Figure 1.1 for the realm of the physical world. In such an environment, we are often confronted with massive uncertainties, and each level of the hierarchy attempts to reduce the effects of this via manipulations on the controller.

In providing now a highly condensed summary of the main intelligent system methodologies (i.e. 'paradigms' in fashionable artificial intelligence jargon), I hope to demonstrate some common themes behind the chronological development of the subject. The two main themes are those of the 'development decades' for maturity of a sub-discipline from its inception to its consumer utilization, and the gradual recognition of weaknesses and how they can be accommodated or alleviated in well-engineered products.

This is clearly demonstrated in the historical emergence of fuzzy logic control.

1.1 Fuzzy logic control

1.1.1 Fuzzy logic chronology

1965	Zadeh	Fuzzy set theory
1975	Mamdani and Assilian	Fuzzy control (steam engine)
1977	Ostergaard	Cement kiln control
1985	Togai, Watanabe	Fuzzy chip
1989	Sugeno	LIFE project, MITI, Japan
1990s	Japan/Germany	High-volume consumer products; car systems, e.g. Mitsubishi Gallant with six fuzzy computers
1990s	Harris, Linkens, etc.	Fuzzy/neural synergy.

1.1.2 Fuzzy logic features

- Can reason with imprecise data
- Leads to 'soft computing'
- Seventh generation computer?

Introduction to intelligent control paradigms and system modelling 7

- Concept of 'machine IQ'
- Copes with non-linear, complex, unknown processes
- Knowledge acquisition problem
- Link with neural networks and self-organizing systems
- Parameter selection problem
- Link with genetic algorithms
- Lack of stability theory

Of the five methods described in this chapter, fuzzy logic has the longest history. It stems from the theoretical work of Zadeh (1965), who proposed the use of fuzzy logic to mimic the human capacity of effective reasoning with imprecise information. The practical application of fuzzy control a decade later stems from the seminal work of Mamdani and Assilian (1975) who demonstrated its use on a laboratory steam boiler/engine combination. Since that time there have been many examples of the use of fuzzy control, surveys being given in Tong (1977), and Sugeno (1985). Two decades on there is a large resurgence of interest in the area throughout the world, with particular emphasis in low-cost consumer products in Japan, and automotive products in Germany.

The self-organizing aspects of fuzzy control stem from the work of Procyck and Mamdani (1979). This work has been extended and applied in aerospace systems (Daley and Gill, 1986) and biomedicine (Linkens and Hasnain, 1991, and Chapters 4 and 5 of this book).

A number of issues relating to the performance and success of fuzzy logic control have been identified, and are currently the subject of considerable research. These issues are: choice of algorithms for fuzzy reasoning; method of defuzzification; choice of membership functions for system variables; selection of scale factors for variables; extraction of a suitable rule-base; and selection of variables for the rule-base knowledge.

With the vast amount of attention that has been given to fuzzy logic theory, it is not surprising that many different algebraic operators have been proposed for fuzzy inference mechanisms. In an attempt to quantify and compare these numerous approaches, we have proposed a generalized framework for the theory of approximate reasoning (Linkens and Nie, 1992a, and Chapter 7 of this book). This has the capability of embedding all of the algebraic operators proposed, and also of including the concepts of uncertainty as commonly used in the expert system branch of AI. In seeking to evaluate the various architectures and algorithms for fuzzy systems, it is necessary to have suitable performance measures and indices for comparison purposes. The most commonly cited and utilized methods of defuzzification are those 'mean of maximum' (MOM) and 'centre of area' (COA). To evaluate the above techniques a multivariable simulation of a blood pressure system has been used (Linkens and Nie, 1992b, and Chapter 7 of this book). This comprises a dual-input drug regime (sodium nitroprusside and dopamine) for controlling mean arterial pressure (*MAP*) and cardiac output (*CO*) for humans in post-operative intensive care. This model is a challenging one since it incorporates strong cross-coupling. In the cited paper, numerous fuzzy algebraic operators and the two methods of defuzzification have been evaluated on the blood pressure model. It was found that most of the combination of methods succeeded in controlling the model, but the best performance was obtained overall, considering noise contamination and model uncertainty, using '*mmm*', '*ppm*' and '*ppc*' combinations. The first letter refers to an AND operator ('m' for minimum, and 'p' for algebraic), the second letter refers to the IF . . . THEN operator ('m' for minimum, and 'p' for algebraic), while the third letter refers to the defuzzification method ('m' for MOM, and 'c' for COA). In these experiments the rule-base was hand-crafted after the incorporation of a de-coupling pre-compensator to facilitate the rule acquisition.

The choice of membership function for the system variables (usually error, error-rate and output) requires selection of membership shape and location within the universe of discourse. In the work presented in Chapters 7–9 a triangular shape has been assumed throughout. This has the advantage that only two parameters are required to determine the membership function, these being the centre point value and the width of the base. An investigation into the automatic optimization of these parameters will be given in Chapter 11 on genetic algorithms. Numerous experimental studies have shown that triangular membership functions provide good, if not optimum, performance in a wide range of applications.

Determination of suitable scale factors for fuzzified variables has often been recognized as a matter of heuristic choice based on the particular application. In an attempt to provide a simple rule-base for initial selection of scale factors an extensive series of studies has been conducted on simulations and real-time experiments on anaesthetic and fluid-flow examples (Linkens and Abbod, 1992). The heuristics obtained provide initial selection of scale factors, which subsequently can be refined to give improved performance.

The selection of a suitable rule-base represents a major hurdle to the use of fuzzy logic control. The self-organizing method already referred to relies on an updating process driven by performance indices relating to a pre-defined reference model behaviour. An alternative approach is considered by Linkens and Nie (1993a, and Chapter 8 of this book) which constructs separated and decoupled rule-bases for multivariable systems incorporating time delays. This uses a reference model, a learning algorithm and a rule-base formation mechanism. Three learning algorithms have been studied and shown to be convergent under mild assumptions. The robustness of this rule-extraction approach to noise contamination, process mismatch and learning gains is considered in a companion paper (Linkens and Nie, 1993b).

All direct control strategies require some form of on-line monitoring to cater for faults and unusual operating conditions. This leads to the concept of supervisory SOFLC (Linkens and Abbod, 1993, and Chapter 5 of this book). In this work an architecture has been developed which provides for the on-line selection of design parameters for SOFLC (e.g. scale-factors), fault detection and recoverable operation (akin to self-repairing systems). This architecture has been implemented using a transputer-based platform and validated on electro-mechanical and biomedical systems. Similar concepts are also being used for hierarchical fuzzy modelling as described in Chapter 6.

1.2 Expert systems

1.2.1 Expert systems chronology

1965	Dendral	Molecular structures
1972	MYCIN (Shortliffe)	Anti-bacterial therapy advisor
1973	Prospector	Geological prospecting (found a mine!)
1970s		Considerable medical interest
1980s		Considerable industrial interest, some medical interest, e.g. RESAC anaesthesia advisor

1.2.2 Expert systems features

- Can reason with uncertainty, e.g. Pearl's causal probability networks
- Knowledge acquisition problem
- Explanation (key part of definition) difficult but better than neural networks
- Slow using functional languages.

A similar timescale of development as that for fuzzy control can be seen for expert systems, although with different results.

The applications to which expert systems have been exposed have embodied far greater complexity than that originally considered for fuzzy control. After all, the major hypothesis was that we should be able to encode human experience dealing with tasks requiring high intelligence and massive training (e.g. the anti-bacterial advisor system of MYCIN). Perhaps it should have been obvious that a superficial 'look-alike' approach to artificial intelligence would be beguiling but deceptive. Thus, the familiar scene of initial enthusiasm and exaggerated claims followed by a period of disillusionment has been demonstrated clearly in this field of endeavour. Doubtless, sanity will prevail and the real benefits and particular niches will be established in future years and the embodiment of expert systems will become commonplace in manufactured 'smart' instruments, actuators and controllers. Whether we shall see the incorporation of the elusive concept of 'deep knowledge' into complex advisory systems in the future is less clear.

In this book a description is given of an extensive expert system which has been developed for advice in anaesthesia. It is called RESAC (see Chapter 2) and required detailed knowledge elicitation and clinical trials to develop an adequate rule-base. Also, it gives much attention to the human computer interface (HCI) aspects, particularly within an operating theatre environment. This case study illustrates many of the common features relating to the development of a medium size expert system, operating in real-time.

Within the field of expert systems, there has been much research (and contention!) about how to incorporate uncertainty into the reasoning strategies. Several strands have developed, notably Shortliffe's measures of belief used in the early expert system (MYCIN), Bayesian subjective reasoning, Dempster–Shafer theory, and Pearl's evidential reasoning. For an overview and collected papers in this heavily researched topic, the reader is referred to Shafer and Pearl (1990). The RESAC inference engine used Bayesian subjective reasoning which has been embodied in many other expert systems.

Expert system techniques have also been utilized in the development of a computer-based modelling and simulation environment as described in Chapter 12.

1.3 Neural networks

1.3.1 Neural networks chronology (associative memories)

1943	McCulloch and Pitts	Neuron model
1962	Rosenblatt	Perceptron
1969	Minsky and Pappert	Challenge the perceptron
1986	Rumelhart, etc.	Multilayer perceptron
1990	Narendra	NN in control
1990s	Kosko; Linkens; Harris, etc.	Considerable industrial interest; some medical interest; synergy with fuzzy systems.

The theme of neural networks has a longer history than the two previous paradigms, albeit with very long gaps in its development. From the simple definition of 'intelligence' and its intuitive usage in everyday parlance it is obvious that mankind will always be fascinated with the inner workings of the brain. The enormous complexity of the neuronal structure of the brain will always remain a source of wonder and scientific investigation. Whether engineering will be able to capitalize on the knowledge elicited from these studies remains to be seen. Certainly, as a source of intellectual challenge and possible funding the artificial neural network (ANN) reigns supreme at present. The danger of claim and counter-claim is well illustrated in the concept of the 'perceptron' introduced by Rosenblatt in 1962. Its seminal contribution was severely challenged in 1969 when Minsky demonstrated its inability to deal with a simple 'exclusive–or' logic component. This had the effect of deflating interest in the ANN for almost two decades, before the generalization of the perceptron was introduced.

This has led to a burgeoning and intense interest in the multilayer perceptron (MLP) or back-propagation neural network (BNN) for almost every conceivable manifestation of modelling, control and signal processing. It has promised to be the all-pervasive engineering mathematician's tool for answering the pressing problem of endemic non-linearity in the real world. Such inflated hopes and aspirations are obviously in for a shock. Already we know of the limitations of the MLP and its inefficiency in processing and convergence. Hence the search is on for better structures and improved algorithms. Doubtless we shall see the inevitable phase of rapprochement into introspection, analytic consolidation, hardware embodiments and hopefully) commercialization of useful products by engineers.

A survey of some strands in neural-network control can be found in Hunt *et al.* (1992). In this book we shall concentrate on the relationship and synergy between fuzzy logic and neural networks. It has been demonstrated by Linkens and Nie (1994), and in Chapter 8 of this book, that the two key issues in fuzzy-rule-based systems, i.e. knowledge representation and associated approximate reasoning, can be handled effectively by BNN, providing a functional mapping between the two approaches. The underlying principles relating to generalization have been demonstrated via a small linguistic problem and a realistic problem of multivariable blood pressure control. This latter example requires a BNN with 26 inputs, 13 outputs and a total of 2013 weights and thresholds. The rule-base used in this study had been hand-crafted via a decentralized control strategy, referred to in the previous section.

In the absence of an existing rule-base or expert/teacher, a control knowledge-base must be directly constructed from the environment. A learning strategy similar to that used for fuzzy rule-base elicitation in the previous section is described in Linkens and Nie (1992c). The basic idea is first to derive required control signals and then to extract a set of training examples. Thus the whole process consists of four stages: on-line learning, off-line extracting, off-line training, and on-line application. The architecture includes a reference model, a learning algorithm and a short-term memory. It has been implemented successfully on the blood pressure model. The rules extracted from the above learning procedure may be used for explanation purposes, thus off-setting the possible criticism of BNN, which does not provide a clear insight into the reasoning mechanism.

The BNN approach is not really self-learning since its structure is predetermined. In an alternative strategy (Nie and Linkens, 1994, and Chapter 9 of this book), a simplified fuzzy control algorithm is structurally mapped into a counter propagation network (CPN) such that the control knowledge is explicitly represented in the form of connection weights of the nets. Then assuming that no control rules (or equivalently no hidden units in the CPN) exist at the beginning, the rule-base is gradually self-organized and self-constructed on-line, and is in turn used as a basis for carrying out approximate reasoning. The CPN consists of an input layer, a hidden Kohonen layer, and a Grossberg output layer. The number of units in the Kohonen layer are self-organized and establish the IF part of the corresponding rule-base. The weights in the Grossberg layer are self-learned, providing the THEN part of the rule-base. Again, the correspondence with a fuzzy rule-base facilitates explanation features for the intelligent control architecture.

In Chapter 10, neural networks for controllers and patient models are developed for measurement and decision-making relating to depth of anaesthesia.

1.4 Genetic algorithms

1.4.1 Genetic algorithms chronology

1975	Holland	'Adaptation in natural & artificial systems'
1989	Goldberg	'Genetic algorithms'
1990s		Burgeoning interest:
		multi-objective optimization
		non-linear control
		system identification
		design
		fuzzy parameters

1.4.2 Genetic algorithms features

- Global, not local minima
- Computing hyper-intensive
- Mostly off-line
- Synergy with fuzzy systems for design
- Can be parallelized

Perhaps the most recent and topical strand amongst the intelligent paradigms is that of genetic algorithms (GAs). The major motivation for the interest in GAs is the well-known limitation of quantitative optimization algorithms in that they often settle at a local rather than a global optimum. Since optimization is at the heart of nearly all decision-making processes, from low-level regulation to high-level autonomy, it is not surprising that the biologically motivated GA which lays claim to searching for global optima should be receiving so much current interest. Again, one expects to see a merging of this methodology with the other intelligent techniques in attempts to capitalize on the key advantages and to minimize the major limitations. GAs are exploratory adaptive search and optimization procedures that have been designed on the principles of natural population genetics (Holland, 1975). There are four main differences between the working of GAs and other optimization techniques:

(a) GAs work on a coding of the parameters, instead of the parameters themselves.
(b) GAs function by maintaining a population of trial structures (chromosomes), which represent a set of control points evaluated for usefulness to the system. Each trial structure has associated with it a fitness value that determines the viability of the structure.
(c) GAs use an objective function assessment, or feedback from an interacting environment, called pay-off or reward, to guide the search.
(d) GAs use probabilistic rules to make decisions.

A simple GA has three operators called *reproduction*, *crossover* and *mutation*. Reproduction is a process in which a new generation of population is formed by randomly selecting strings from an existing population, according to their fitness. This process results in individuals with higher fitness values obtaining one or more copies in the next generation whilst lower fitness individuals may have none; a "survival of the fittest" test. Crossover is the most dominant operator in the GA, responsible for producing new trials. Under this recombination scheme, two strings are selected to produce new offspring by exchanging portions of their structures. The offspring will then replace weaker individuals in the population. Crossover serves two complementary functions. First, it provides new points for further testing within the existing 'sub-spaces' (represented by the parents). Secondly, it introduces representative members of 'sub-spaces' not already existing (through offspring). Mutation is a secondary operator, and is applied with a very low probability of occurrence, typically less than 0.01. Its operation is to alter the value of a random position in a string. When used in this way, together with reproduction and crossover operators, mutation acts as an insurance against total loss of any bit value in a particular position in the population.

There are two issues to be considered in applying GAs to learn fuzzy control rules (Linkens and Nyongesa, 1992, and Chapter 11 of this book). First is the coding of the structures that represent the rules to be learnt. A genetic rule structure is a coding of the membership functions of the conditions and action of a rule. In this study the membership functions have been allowed to have a triangular (isosceles) shape. Hence, the parameters that need to be learned by the GA can be selected to be the position of the peak of the triangle and the width of its base.

The second consideration in designing the GA is the process of evaluating the rule structures (classifiers). Normally the GA evaluates the population structures using an objective function that returns a measure of each classifier's performance. In the case where the interacting environment is a dynamic process, the evaluation can only be based on the performance of the controller in driving the response of the process towards convergence on the desired state, which is made more difficult when the characteristics of the controlled process are not known to the GA. Two types of performance measure are generally available; a global criterion, for example integral square error (ISE), indicates the overall performance of the controller over a response trajectory; a local criterion on the other hand measures the performance of the controller over the neighbourhood of a few process states. One problem with the global measure is the difficulty in relating it to the actions which contributed to its achievement. For this reason a local performance measure has been preferred, which enables credit assignment to individual actions at each instant.

Usually, a GA is operated in batch mode, submitting all structures in a population to evaluation and then assigning new strengths using an objective function. In applying the GA to the control of an unmodelled dynamic process there are a number of constraints:

(a) There is no objective function assessment available, but the system relies on noisy performance feedback from an unknown environment.
(b) There is a limitation on the amount of computation that can be done between sampling instants.
(c) The GA must provide an appropriate control structure at each sample instant.

In such a case, an incremental GA, in which only one classifier from a population is evaluated in each time interval, has been preferred. Thus, from each population, a classifier is selected if it matches ('fires') the current input conditions. Then, during credit assignment, reward or punishment is spread over the neighbourhood of classifiers that fire the previous condition and which are responsible for the current performance measure, regardless of whether they existed in the population or not. The amount of reward given to each classifier depends on its weight (a matching factor), the 'value' of its action and the objective assessment received from the environment. Classifiers selected for evaluation are decoded into fuzzy rules, which are

Introduction to intelligent control paradigms and system modelling 15

then composed into a deterministic action—a weighted mean of all fired rules—using the compositional rule of inference. The above techniques have been applied to anaesthesia for both single-variable and multivariable control (see Chapter 11).

1.5 Qualitative reasoning

1.5.1 Qualitative reasoning chronology

    1980   Naive physics
    1980s Qualitative reasoning:
            constraint-based (QSIM) (Kuipers)
            component-based (De Kleer)
            process-based (Forbus)
    1990s Scale-up?
            Fuzzy synergy (FuSIM) (Leitch)
            Bond graph synergy (QREMS) (Linkens).

1.5.2 Qualitative reasoning features

- Can reason imprecisely, but not uncertainly
- Mimics human-type reasoning
- Gives 'spurious' results (need 'clever' filters)
- Problem of 'scale-up'
- Too many competing ideas

'Qualitative reasoning' (QR) has a recent history, motivated again, however, by the realization that humans can reason very successfully in a qualitative manner about subjects which we commonly attempt to analyse in complicated quantitative ways—hence the introduction of the 'naive physics' strand to artificial intelligence research. Although introduced at a scientific level, there have been attempts recently to introduce qualitative modelling and control into the engineering field. What is clear is that other strands of intelligent systems will have to be linked synergetically into this field if it is to develop significantly (e.g. the incorporation of fuzzy logic into QR by Leitch and co-workers). An apparently very different technique to QR is that of bond graphs which have been used for modelling and analysis of engineering dynamic systems. Each approach has strengths and weaknesses, and in an attempt to merge the relative strengths Linkens and co-workers have been attempting to integrate the methods to provide an integrated qualitative bond-graph environment (see also Chapter 12 of this book).

In this work an attempt is being made to develop a modern systems theory using computer-aided automation of the modelling process and model transformation (Linkens et al., 1991, and Chapter 13 of this book). In this approach, a physical system can be modelled at a high level automatically from its structure, and general properties about the system can be concluded. Gradually given more information, this high-level model can be articulated into a more detailed model, and properties in more detail can be analysed. This process starts with a structural system and ends with a numerical behaviour model of the system. These processes are being automated through examining what intermediate models are involved, how they are generated and what conclusions can be reached about the properties of the physical system at each stage. One of the main advantages of this approach is that analyses at multiple levels can be conducted (Linkens et al., 1993). A prototype system has been implemented in PROLOG. A schematic description of a physical system is used as an input to the prototype system. The bond-graph model of the physical system is then produced from the structural information through conceptual reasoning (Xia et al., 1993). Causalities are assigned into the bond graph and using this causal bond-graph model, a qualitative behaviour of the system is derived through simulation of the qualitative model. In addition, the environment enables model validation to be performed, together with provision of explanations of system behaviour. The techniques are clearly applicable to areas of fault-diagnosis as well as modelling, where structural changes requiring self-learning concepts are necessary.

All of the above intelligent systems paradigms have been under investigation in recent years by a research group in Sheffield in the context of biomedical systems research. As seen from the references in this chapter, these wide-ranging studies will be examined in detail in the following chapters contributed by the individual researchers.

In the descriptions given so far little reference has been made to model-based control design methods. The book would be incomplete without reference to the use of advanced quantitative control algorithms in biomedical control systems. Chapter 3 describes the successful application of generalized predictive control (GPC) to muscle relaxation anaesthesia. Of further interest is a comparative study between GPC and fuzzy logic control using a realistic non-linear multivariable model for anaesthesia (Chapter 4).

For further detailed studies in intelligent control, the reader is referred to works by Harris et al. (1993), Brown and Harris (1994) and White and Sofge (1992).

References

Brown, M. and Harris, C.R., 1994, *Neuro Fuzzy Adaptive Modelling and Control*, London: Taylor and Francis.

Daley, S. and Gill, K.F., 1986, A design study of a self-organising fuzzy logic controller, *Proceedings of the Institution of Mechanical Engineers*, **200**, 59–69.
Harris, C.J., Brown, M. and Moore, C., 1993, *Intelligent Control, Aspects of Fuzzy Logic and Neural Networks*, London: World Scientific Association.
Holland, J.H., 1975, *Adaption in Natural and Artificial Systems*, Reading, MA, Addison-Wesley.
Hunt, K.J., Shabaro, D., Zbikowski, R. and Gawthrop, P.J., 1992, Neural networks for control systems—a survey, *Automatica*, **28**, 1083–112.
Linkens, D.A. and Abbod, M.F., 1992, Self-organising fuzzy control and the selection of its scaling factors, *Transactions of the Institute of Measurement and Control*, **14**, 114–25.
Linkens, D.A. and Abbod, M.F., 1993, Supervisory intelligent control using a fuzzy logic hierarchy, *Transactions of the Institute of Measurement and Control*, **15**, 112–32.
Linkens, D.A., Bennett, S. and Xia, S., 1991, 'Qualitative reasoning and applications to dynamic systems: a bond graph approach', IMACS Int. Workshop on Qualitative Reasoning and Decision Support Systems, Toulouse, March.
Linkens, D.A. and Hasnain, S.B., 1991, Self-organising fuzzy logic control and applications to muscle-relaxant anaesthesia, *Proceedings of the IEE*, Pt.D, **138**, 274–84.
Linkens, D.A. and Nie, J., 1992a, A unified real-time approximate reasoning approach for use in intelligent control, Pt.1: theoretical developments, *International Journal of Control*, **56**, 347–63.
Linkens, D.A. and Nie, J., 1992b, A unified real-time approximate reasoning approach for use in intelligent control, Pt.2: application to multivariable blood pressure control, *International Journal of Control*, **56**, 365–97.
Linkens, D.A. and Nie, J., 1992c, Neural network-based approximate reasoning: principles and implementation, *International Journal of Control*, **56**, 399–413.
Linkens, D.A. and Nie, J., 1993a, Constructing rule-bases for multivariable fuzzy control by self-learning, Pt.1: system structure and learning algorithms, *International Journal of Systems Science*, **24**, 111–28.
Linkens, D.A. and Nie, J., 1993b, Constructing rule-bases for multivariable fuzzy control by self-learning, Pt.2: rule-base formation and blood pressure control application, *International Journal of Systems Science*, **24**, 129–58.
Linkens, D.A. and Nie, J., 1994, Back-propagation neural network-based fuzzy controller with self-learning teacher, *International Journal of Control*, in press.
Linkens, D.A. and Nyongesa, H.O., 1992, 'Real-time acquisition of fuzzy rules using genetic algorithms', presentation at the IFAC International Symposium on AI real-time control, Delft.
Linkens, D.A., Xia, S. and Bennett, S., 1993, 'A computer-aided qualitative modelling and analysis environment using unified principles (QREMS)', presentation at the International Conference on Bond Graphs for Modelling and Simulation, San Diego, January.
Mamdani, E.H. and Assilian, S., 1975, An experiment in linguistic synthesis with a fuzzy logic controller, *International Journal of Man-Machine Studies*, **7**, 1–13.
Nie, J. and Linkens, D.A., 1994, Fast self-learning multivariable fuzzy controller constructed from a modified CPN network, *International Journal of Control*, in press.
Procyck, T.J. and Mamdani, E.H., 1979, A linguistic self-organising process controller, *Automatica*, **15**, 15–30.
Rosenblatt, F., 1962, *Principles of Neurodynamics*, New York: Spartan Books.
Shafer, G. and Pearl, J., 1990, *Readings in Uncertain Reasonings*, San Mateo, California: Morgan Kaufmann.

Sugeno, M. (Ed.), 1985, An introductory survey of fuzzy control, *Information Science*, **36**, 59–83.

Tong, R.M., 1977, A control engineering review of fuzzy systems, *Automatica*, **13**, 559–69.

White, D.A. and Sofge, D.A., 1992, Handbook of intelligent control: neural, fuzzy & adaptive approaches, New York: van Nostrand–Reinhold.

Xia, S., Linkens, D.A. and Bennett, S., 1993, Automatic modelling and analysis of dynamic physical systems using qualitative reasoning and bond graphs, *IEE International Systems Engineering Journal*, Autumn, 201–12.

Zadeh, L.A., 1965, Fuzzy sets, *Information and Control*, **8**, 338–53.

Chapter 2
A real-time expert system for anaesthesia validated in clinical trials

S. G. Greenhow

2.1 Introduction

One important aspect of anaesthetists' work is the maintenance of an adequate level of unconsciousness in their patients by controlling the depth of anaesthesia during the surgical procedure. The required depth of anaesthesia varies with the amount of noxious stimulation supplied, and is assessed by observing multiple clinical signs. The clinical signs are responses to the surgical procedure by the autonomic nervous system. Multiple signs are required as no single measurement can be used to reliably determine the depth of anaesthesia.

These clinical signs consist of both objective measurements such as the patient's heart rate, and subjective indicators, such as the degree to which the patient is sweating. Numerous factors influence these signs rendering many potential signs too unreliable to be of any use. For instance, pupil diameter is rendered useless as a clinical sign if opiates are administered as the pupils will constrict. Clinical conditions such as anoxia, i.e. a lack of oxygen in the blood stream, can influence several clinical signs at once, as it can cause dilation of pupils, vomiting, rigidity of muscles, and increased blood pressure. Even environmental factors have to be taken into account, for instance the temperature of the operating room can influence the importance of sweating as a clinical sign.

Numerous attempts have been made to control the depth of anaesthesia by automated means. These attempts have been reviewed in a variety of papers, the earliest comprehensive review being conducted by Chilcoat

(1980). Various subsequent reviews have been conducted, for instance Kraft and Lees (1984), Westenskow (1984) and Greenhow *et al.* (1992). For a control system to be acceptable in the clinical situation the responses of the system must be as similar as possible to that of an anaesthetist. Hence both the closeness and speed of reaching the given targets for the outputs are less important than supplying a smooth but safe anaesthetic. Suitable warning messages must also be displayed at appropriate times. As anaesthetists consider multiple clinical signs, a control system should also attempt to consider several signs. However, different anaesthetists interpret the importance of a given clinical sign in different ways. As mentioned earlier, different operation types will require different anaesthetic regimes, and hence an automatic control system should be able to cope with a wide range of operating conditions. Ideally a control system should be able to 'know' about relevant medical conditions and their impact on anaesthesia. The paper by Schils *et al.* (1987) summarizes the problems of computerized control.

To deal with these requirements an expert system called RESAC (real-time expert system for advice and control) was produced. RESAC made use of eight clinical signs, as well as various patient parameters such as age and sex. RESAC also made use of information concerning drugs used during the operation. Due to the huge mass of medical conditions that could affect the anaesthetic state only two parameters were used to deal with the patient's medical condition, namely a generalized index of patient condition (called the ASA classification) and whether the patient was a heavy drinker. RESAC has been validated in a variety of different types of operation, with the selected patients deliberately not being standardized to replicate as far as possible routine surgical conditions. However, patients with known adverse medical conditions were excluded.

RESAC is a backward-chaining rule-based expert system shell which deals with both numerical and non-numerical facts. A variety of rule types are used to establish relations between the facts, information being freely transferred between the numerical and non-numerical facts (and vice versa). Fuzzy logic and Bayesian inference are used to cope with conflicting and uncertain evidence. The Bayesian inference was modified by the addition of the concept of 'Relevance'. Relevance was introduced to deal with the change in relative importance of a clinical sign due to certain circumstances, or even to remove entirely the effect of a clinical sign. For instance, during certain phases of heart surgery both blood pressure and heart rate would be ignored as indicators of depth of anaesthesia.

To reduce the data input required, RESAC was able to obtain some information from an on-line source (i.e. a Dinamap monitor that provides heart rate and blood pressure data). Due to the real-time nature of the problem, the program was written in 'C' rather than an AI-based language. The Atari range of computers was chosen as they provided a cheap platform with Digital Research's windowing environment called GEM. The RS-232 port on the Atari was used to communicate with the Dinamap instrument. The following section describes in detail the knowledge representation language used by RESAC.

2.2 Model representation in RESAC

The facts concerning the problem domain can be considered to be either numerical or non-numerical in nature. The non-numerical facts, which are referred to as Hypothesis elements, have a prior probability which is set in the range zero to one, and a relevance expressed as a certainty factor (CF). RESAC expresses CF values in the range −500 to +500, where a CF of −500 means the belief in the item is false, zero is uncertain, and +500 true. During a model run the inference engine attempts to determine the value of the posterior probability. Hypothesis elements are further divided into 'Goals' and 'Assertions'. The system attempts to evaluate all the Goals, whilst Assertions are only evaluated if required to determine the value of a Goal.

The numerical facts are stored as 'Object' elements. These Objects have an allowed range, and a default value. The inference engine attempts to determine the current value of the Object. If the Object is to obtain its value from the on-line source then an appropriate 'Monitor' code would be set.

The 'Results' element allows RESAC to display textual information. For meaningful messages the value of 'Hypothesis' elements are converted into an appropriate string, for instance 'fairly true', 'totally false', etc. An associated 'Provided' clause is used to control the activation of a Result element. This consists of an expression that must evaluate to a CF. For the element to fire the CF must be greater than uncertain. Both arithmetic and fuzzy logic operators can be used to make up the expression. For instance the following is a legal Provided clause '((EffectOpiate $\times$ 1.6) $\leq$ 0.0) and (not First-Time)'.

Relations between facts are established by using three possible 'Rule' elements, namely 'Plausible', 'Logical' and 'Arithmetic' rule types. Facts can also be determined directly from the anaesthetist by asking questions. The model representation language supports two element types of question, namely question elements and multi-choice question elements. The activation of a rule or question can be controlled by an associated Provided clause.

The logical rules (Gaschnig, 1982), otherwise known as 'if . . . then' rules, allow evidence to be combined using the fuzzy set operators. The template of this type of rule is:

    if   Expression
    then   H   LS LN.

The 'Expression' follows the same rules as in the Provided clause, thus numeric and non-numeric items can contribute to the value of the expression. This value is then used to update the posterior probability (or the Relevance posterior probability) of the Hypothesis element H. The LS and LN values are referred to as the rule strength.

A Plausible rule allows multiple items of evidence to contribute using Bayes' theorem to a Hypothesis element. In general it is expressed as:

'H depends on
Y_1 LS_1 LN_1
. . .   .
Y_n LS_n LN_n'

Each item of evidence is used to produce an 'effective LS', which is combined with others to determine the posterior probability of H. Note this rule cannot be used to establish the Relevance of the element.

The Arithmetic rule is used mainly to calculate the values for numeric elements. The template of the rule is:

X is Expression.

This rule can also be used to determine the posterior probabilities of Hypothesis elements, but the rule directly assigns the value of Expression to the Hypothesis element without any modification by a rule strength. This rule cannot be used to establish the Relevance of a Hypothesis element. An example of this rule used to establish a numeric value for the Object TargetSap is 'TargetSap is (108 + age)/2'.

To obtain information from the anaesthetist various question types are used. The standard Question element asks the anaesthetist to answer a question, the result being assigned to a single Object or Hypothesis element. The format of the question depends upon the type of element that the question provides an answer for, and various flags associated with the question, these flags being used to select the appropriate question form. The question forms are described in the user-interface section. If the Question element supplies a value for a Hypothesis element then the question can also be used to determine the Relevance of the Hypothesis element.

The multiple-choice question element supplies a value to one or more Hypothesis elements. The question is supplied as a list of possible scenarios, the associated question form is shown in the user-interface section. The question can be set to provide Relevance values for all the Hypothesis elements if so desired.

Both types of Question element have various modes of operation which alter the behaviour of the question element. The normal mode is where the system will show the question form the first time it is encountered. In subsequent model iterations the system will not re-display the question form, but will use the 'current value' of the question element, unless it detects a change in the underlying model that might make the current answer invalid. However, the user can at any time cause the question to be re-asked, and thus supply a new value. To do this the system maintains a list of questions that the user can fire. This list can be examined at any time. To reduce time spent searching for any given question the list is divided up into four separate sub-lists (Clinical signs, Relevance, Drugs and Misc).

A variant on the normal question is to force the appearance of the question form every time it can fire, with the Provided clause used to prevent the question appearing all the time. Some questions must only be asked once, for instance the age of the patient will not change during the operation, but the Question should continue to provide the same answer to the inference system when fired, such questions are referred to as 'static' questions.

For certain conditions control of a question via the Provided clause would not be appropriate, for instance with transitory facts such as an injection of a drug being given. To deal with this a Question element can be marked with the 'Ignore' condition. This has the effect of causing the question to fail to fire if the system attempts to display the form (with the exception of the first time the question element is evaluated). Thus only the user can cause the question to be fired, by explicitly re-invoking the question.

2.3 Inference process in RESAC

On 'compilation' of a knowledge base, RESAC produces an acyclic directed graph (referred to as the network). A graph structure consists of a set of nodes, with arcs interlinking them. The direction of travel along an arc is fixed. An acyclic directed graph constrains the structure so that beginning at any arbitrary node, regardless of the path taken thereafter, a return to the initial node is impossible (Van Wyk, 1988). This structure thus supports either backward or forward chaining (depending upon the imposed direction along the arc), backward chaining being chosen for RESAC. Circularities must be prevented from occurring in the graph as they would make the structure become non-directed, and hence generate segments of model code that would never terminate. Probabilities are propagated throughout the network by using Bayes' theorem as the model is evaluated. Approximately every minute RESAC re-evaluates the network, starting with the Goal elements in the model. After evaluating all the Goals the Result elements are evaluated, and during this phase the conclusions drawn by the system are displayed. This process is then repeated. As mentioned in the previous section, as far as possible RESAC avoids repeatedly re-asking the same question, so that for most iterations the system will not need to directly ask any questions.

Using the Model representation language described in the previous section a model was built that would determine the depth of anaesthesia, and suggest suitable control actions to acquire and then maintain the correct depth. On running the model, it would initially be in a pre-anaesthetic state where as many of the patient details as possible would be supplied. When required the anaesthetist would inform the system that the operation had begun. The advice output by RESAC depends on the underlying model, but the following information is always given:

- The anaesthetic state of the patient, expressed as a belief in any of the three states 'anaesthetic is light', 'anaesthetic is OK', and 'anaesthetic is deep'. Only states greater than uncertain are reported.
- Dosage of volatile anaesthetic agent to be supplied (0–5%).

In order for RESAC to be able to handle uncertain evidence (such as when the system asks a question like 'How certain are you that the patient is sweating?') the concept of certainty is used. Thus the answer from a question will be returned as a CF, which is then mapped into the posterior probability by the following (Alty and Coombs, 1984):

IF$(C:(E:E') \geq 0)$:

$$P(E:E') = P(E) + \frac{C(E:E')}{\text{MaxCert}} \times (1 - P(E))$$

IF less than 0:

$$P(E:E') = P(E) + \frac{C(E:E')}{\text{MaxCert}} \times P(E)$$

where $C(E:E')$ is the supplied certainty factor and MaxCert is the maximum certainty factor. The term $P(E)$ is the prior probability of evidence. The equations to determine $P(E:E')$ can be rearranged so that a certainty value is generated when both prior and posterior probabilities are known. This allows RESAC to display the belief in Hypothesis elements in 'certainty factors', which can also be converted into meaningful textual strings.

The posterior probability of a Hypothesis H ($P(H:E')$) must be determined, where $P(H:E')$ is the probability of Hypothesis being true given the evidence E. This is given by the following equation (Alty and Coombs, 1984):

$$P(H|E') = P(H)|-E) + \frac{(P(H) - P(H)|-E))}{P(E)} \times P(E|E')$$

For :
$$.0 \leq P(E|E') \leq P(E)$$

$$P(H|E') = P(H) + \frac{(PH|E) - P(H)}{1 - P(E)} \times (P(E|E') - P(E))$$

For :
$$P(E) \leqslant P(E|E') \leqslant 1$$

The terms $P(H|-E)$ and $P(H|E)$ are not known. To determine them, further equations must be used. The next equation shows how the probability of Hypothesis given no evidence, i.e. $P(H|-E)$, is determined (Duda et al., 1980):

$$P(H|-E) = \frac{LN \times P(H)}{(LN - 1) \times P(H) + 1}.$$

The term LN is referred to as the necessary factor, and it is a floating point value greater than or equal to zero. Note that it is frequently more convenient to work with the odds rather than the probabilities, and hence the equation becomes:

$$O(H|-E) = LN \times O(H).$$

To calculate the probability of H given E, i.e. $P(H|E)$, the following equation is used:

$$P(H|E) = \frac{LS \times P(H)}{(LS - 1) \times P(H) + 1}$$

where the likelihood ratio (LS) must be a number very much greater than one. As in the determination of $O(H|-E)$, $P(H|E)$ can be expressed in terms of odds:

$$O(H|E) = LS \times O(H)$$

Both LS and LN are usually obtained from the domain expert. Since some of the equations are being expressed in the odds form, the following two equations show how odds and probabilities can be converted from one form to the other. To convert odds to probability:

$$P = \frac{O}{O + 1}$$

and the reciprocal function is given by:

$$O = \frac{P}{1 - P}.$$

Assuming that contributing evidence is independent, a single general updating formula can be used. This uses the 'effective LS' (λ') for all contributing items (Duda et al., 1980):

$$O(H|E'_1 \ldots E'_n) = \left[\prod_{i=1}^{n} \lambda'_i\right] O(H).$$

To determine the ith 'effective LS' the following equation is used:

$$\lambda_i = O(H|E'_i)/O(H).$$

The term $O(H|E'_i)$ comes from $P(H|E'_i)$ and the term $O(H)$ comes from $P(H)$. Finally to determine $P(H|E')$, the value obtained for $O(H|E'_1 \ldots E'_n)$ is converted via the odds to a probability equation. Note that if there is no contributing evidence, then RESAC will set the posterior probability to the prior probability. The Hypothesis will then have a certainty value of uncertain.

The determination of Relevance is almost identical to that of determining certainty of a Hypothesis element. The Relevance of an item is determined before calculating the posterior probability. The only difference concerns the treatment when no evidence contributes to the determination of the Relevance of a Hypothesis element. In this situation it would be undesirable to set Relevance posterior probability to the Relevance prior probability, since the effect would be to make Relevance go to uncertain. A better default in this case is to make the posterior probability go to the maximum value, giving a Relevance of true. Note that for all Relevance values the prior probability is set to 0.5. The effect of Relevance (Rel in CF units) on $P(H|E')$ is given by:

$$P(H|E') = P(H) + \frac{(P(H|E') - P(H))}{\text{MaxCert}} \times \text{Rel}.$$

Thus if the Hypothesis's Relevance is totally true (Rel = MaxCert) posterior probability will not be affected. As Relevance becomes less true, the effect will be to reduce posterior probability. The effect of Relevance cannot make the posterior probability go less than the prior probability, hence Relevance values from false to uncertain have the same effect on posterior probability (i.e. $P(H|E') = P(H)$).

2.4 User interface

The use of a graphical user interface for RESAC was vital for the success of the system, since during an operation an anaesthetist may have little time to

A real-time expert system for anaesthesia validated in clinical trials 27

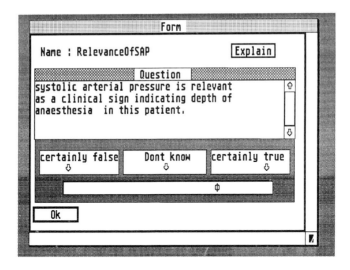

Figure 2.1 *Slider question form.*

maintain the state of the knowledge base. As expert systems determine many facts from the user of the system by asking questions, how easy it is to answer questions has a big impact on the acceptability of such a system. RESAC uses a series of question forms (see Figures 2.1–2.4) to ask questions. The only question form requiring the use of the keyboard is the Numeric question form (Figure 2.3), the other forms being driven by a mouse. Questions requiring the Numeric form tend to be static in nature, such as asking the patient's weight, or will only occur a few times during an operation, for instance asking for the amount of morphine given. Hence, for the majority of the time the mouse is the only input device required to drive RESAC.

At any time during the model run, the anaesthetist is able to inform RESAC of various events such as alteration in a clinical sign, administration of a drug etc. To do this the anaesthetist selects the appropriate question form from one of the four question lists mentioned in the model representation section. The actual questions that can be activated depend upon the current model state, there being about 50 questions in the knowledge base, but only about half can be activated at any given time. In general RESAC only specifically asks questions the first time through the model. However, in the early clinical trials it was found that an anaesthetist would set a clinical sign such as 'patient is moving' to be true, but forget to inform RESAC that the patient had stopped moving later on. This would have the result that the suggested dose of anaesthetic would be higher than expected. To combat this problem the model was altered so that for some clinical signs, after a certain time, the anaesthetist would have to re-answer the

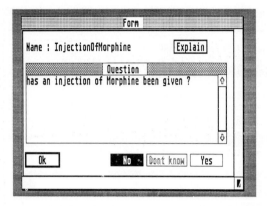

Figure 2.2 *Yes/no question form.*

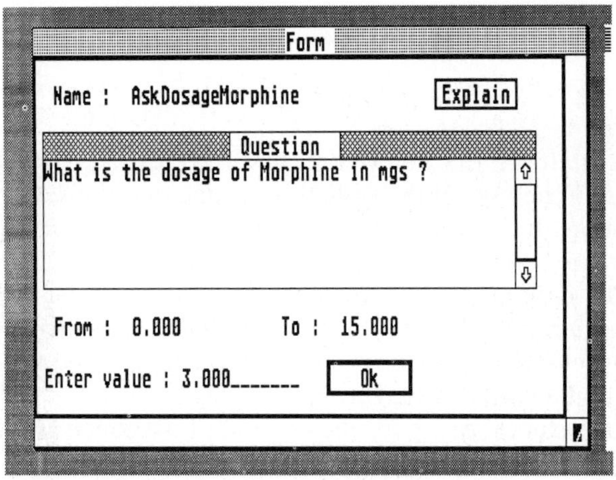

Figure 2.3 *Numeric question form.*

relevant question. Note that this forced re-answering would only occur if the clinical sign was in a state that was incompatible with a correctly anaesthetized patient.

All the question forms display the question text in a box with sliders to scroll through the text. However, long complicated questions were avoided, and as a result the sliders were only used when the 'explain' button on the form was activated. This button would place the associated explanation text beneath the question text. The multiple-choice question (figure 2.4) places the possible scenarios in a scrollable box. Questions with more than seven options were not used.

At the end of each model iteration the advice is displayed in a window, as

A real-time expert system for anaesthesia validated in clinical trials 29

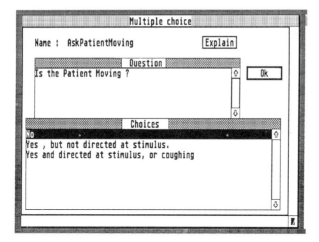

Figure 2.4 *Multiple choice question form.*

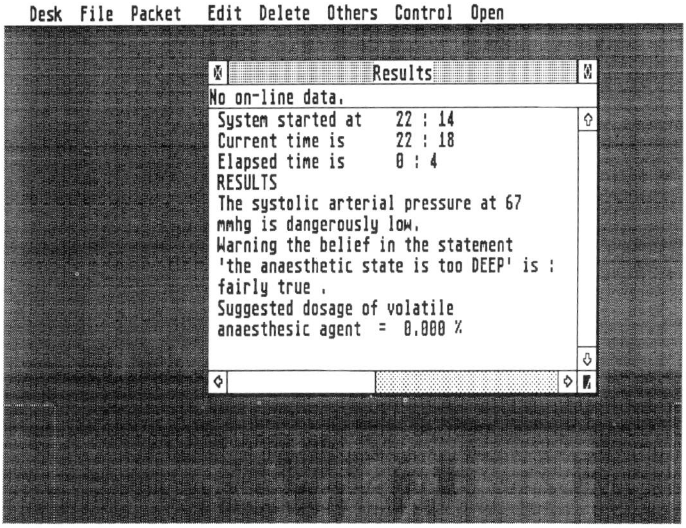

Figure 2.5 *Example of Results window.*

for example in Figure 2.5. As well as textual information, an optional graph could be displayed which would show trend information for the selected clinical sign.

For user-initiated questions, the forms can either be answered by clicking on the OK button, or ignored by clicking on the Cancel button. However, as questions asked by RESAC must be answered, the Cancel button is hidden under these circumstances, forcing the anaesthetist to supply an answer.

The use of canned speech to issue warning messages was investigated. However, this proved to be unsuccessful. Anaesthetists felt that such warning messages might adversely affect the surgeon. Care would also be required in the repetition rates of such messages. Possibly neutral messages such as 'please look at the results window', if not repeated too often, could be of value.

2.5 Clinical experiences

RESAC has been used in a series of clinical trials, where each trial consisted of several operations. For all operations the patients were given a pre-medication four hours before the start of the surgical procedure. During the procedure a mixture of nitrous oxide, oxygen and enflurane was supplied. Operations were performed both with patients breathing spontaneously, and patients being artificially ventilated. Patients were excluded from the clinical trial if some known condition would disturb the normal behaviour of the clinical signs to the procedure, examples being use of antihypertensive drugs, and patients who had had strokes.

The first two trials were aimed at validating the user-interface, together with knowledge acquisition. RESAC's model language was only fully implemented after clinical trial number two. From trial three to trial five the model was extensively altered, with additional clinical signs such as respiration rate being used. By trial five the following clinical signs were used:

Systolic arterial pressure (SAP) (from Dinamap)
Heart rate (from Dinamap)
Respiration rate
Sweating
Movement
Pupil size, movement, direction.

The last two trials were used to validate RESAC, with only minor changes being made to the model between trial six and seven. These changes included reducing the effect on the suggested dose due to high respiration and heart rates, and for high values of SAP. This section describes briefly the results obtained from these two trials, which are described fully by Greenhow (1991).

Information for validation was obtained from data logged by RESAC and from questionnaires filled in by anaesthetists during the operation. The latter allowed discrepancies between the suggested dose and the dose actually supplied to be recorded. The anaesthetist was also asked to write down the time the patient woke up versus the 'ideal' time for the operation.

A real-time expert system for anaesthesia validated in clinical trials 31

Table 2.1 *Results of clinical trial 6*

Operation	SAP RMSD	Heart rate RMSD	Respiration RMSD	Enflurane PerSt5	Quality
6	9.8	9.7	22.7	100	good
7	5.1	25.6	18.1	76	—
8	4.0	7.3	14.8	96	—
9	10.2	7.9	—	54	good
10	7.0	5.6	—	92	good
	7.2	11.2	18.5	83.6	

Table 2.2 *Results of clinical trial 7*

Operation	SAP RMSD	Heart rate RMSD	Respiration RMSD	Enflurane PerSt5	Quality
1	52.8	17.4	6	52	OK
2	25.8	1.3	—	44	OK
3	12.0	7.9	2.5	67	good
4	10.6	9.4	—	54	good
5	18.6	8.3	—	76	very good
6	64.9	12.4	13.8	34	good
7	14.7	21.6	—	70	very good
	28.5	11.2	33.3	56.7	

Finally the anaesthetist was asked to supply a subjective rating of the suggested anaesthetic on a range from 'very good' to 'very poor'.

From the logged data, calculations of the root mean standard deviation (RMSD) were calculated for *SAP*, heart rate and respiration rate (where appropriate). RMSD is given by:

$$\text{RMSD} = \sqrt{(\Sigma(x - \text{target})^2) \times 1/N}.$$

In order to establish the 'stability' of the suggested dose a calculation of the percentage of operation time that the suggested dose was stable for at least five minutes was made, the value being referred to as PerSt5.

Tables 2.1 and 2.2 show the RMSD values, PerSt5 and the subjective anaesthetic rating for operations in trials six and seven. Note that for trial six RESAC was unable to communicate with the Dinamap in operation one to five, and as a result these operations were ignored. Of the remaining operations in this trial the suggested dose was only supplied in the last two operations. For trial seven the suggested dose was supplied throughout for operations one, four, five and seven. Operations three and six had transitory

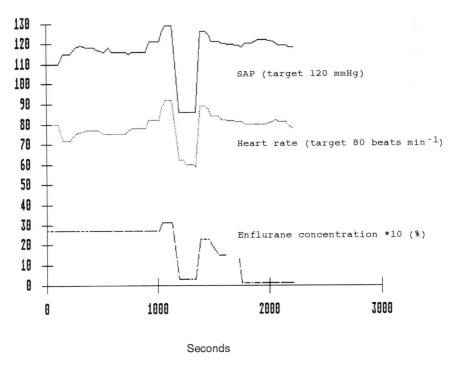

Figure 2.6 *On-line clinical signs and anaesthetic agent for patient 3 in trial 7.*

communication problems with the Dinamap, and hence the suggested dose was not supplied during these periods.

For both trials the difference between the ideal and actual waking up times was very minor, thus indicating that no major under- or over-anaesthetization occurred in the last 15 or 20 minutes of the operation.

The effect on *SAP* and heart rate due to problems with a Dinamap are shown in Figure 2.6, with both values decreasing dramatically. Figure 2.7 shows the effect on the output of RESAC due to this problem. Figures 2.8 and 2.9 show the progress of an operation that is rated as 'very good'.

2.6 Discussion and conclusions

RESAC has been successfully validated in a clinical situation, having been used with a variety of surgical procedures such as hydrocole repair, varicose veins, and laparotomy operations. In the later trials, anaesthetists felt able to use the advice of RESAC and supply the suggested dose, in effect becoming a closed-loop control system. This level of confidence was achieved after about forty operations. However, the reliability of the on-line information was a problem due to artefacts. As the Dinamap used a

A real-time expert system for anaesthesia validated in clinical trials

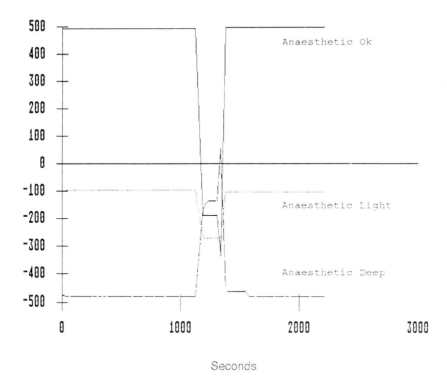

Figure 2.7 *Belief in the anaesthetic Goals for patient 3 in trial 7.*

pneumatic system any interference would have influenced the reading obtained from the Dinamap. Other activities such as flushing an arterial line would also cause problems.

The above problems could be partially solved by explicitly asking the anaesthetist if the on-line signs are reliable in cases where a clinical sign diverges by a large amount from the target value. In such cases the Relevance of the sign could be altered as appropriate.

The PerSt5 values shown in Tables 2.1 and 2.2 indicate that the suggested dose was stable for fairly long stretches of time during the operations, thus mimicking the behaviour of an anaesthetist. The subjective assessment for the advice was also highly encouraging with eight operations in the last two trials being rated as 'good' or 'very good'.

This series of trials highlighted clearly the different behaviour that patients can exhibit, whilst undergoing surgery, an example being the exceedingly high respiration rate encountered in operation six of trial six. In this operation RESAC suggested a high dose of anaesthetic which was ignored as the patient was considered to be correctly anaesthetized.

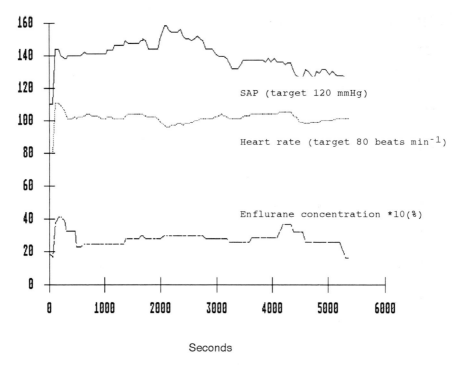

Figure 2.8 *On-line clinical signs and anaesthetic agent for patient 7 in trial 7.*

As a prototype RESAC worked very well, but it would be very difficult to extend the scope and size of the underlying knowledge base. For instance RESAC deals with drug dynamics but the model representation language is not really suitable for this task. As a result, increasing the number of drugs that RESAC knows about would greatly reduce the performance of the system. Another problem that would need to be addressed is the monolithic nature of the model language.

Work has started on a successor that would allow a large-scale expert system to be developed. This new system consists of a series of tightly coupled programs running concurrently, different aspects of the problem being dealt with by the various programs. Many of the programs are very simple, for instance one such program is concerned with extracting and validating information from a Dinamap monitor, whilst another deals with a drug dynamics database written in LISP.

Another program supports an enhanced version of the RESAC model language, the major change to the language being the creation of 'Packets'. A Packet consists of a group of model elements performing a defined task, for instance determining if *SAP* is relevant. The information entering and leaving a packet is closely controlled. An additional rule type has been created to control packet activation. This modification allows the knowledge

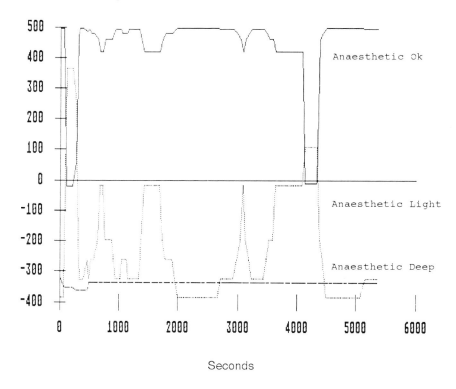

Figure 2.9 *Belief in the anaesthetic Goals for patient 7 in trial 7.*

base to be broken down into suitable chunks, which can be independently created and validated. In addition, only a few packets will be activated for any given operation, as many will deal with specific operation types and clinical conditions. This program does not have a user-interface, but relies on another program to provide one.

The user interacts with the system via an interface program. The user-interface is very similar to the one described for RESAC, with various question forms being displayed. This program coordinates the control of the other programs in the system, and can be considered to work like a telephone exchange, routing information between the separate sub-programs. For instance, the anaesthetic knowledge base will require information from the various monitoring programs and the drug database. In addition, the sub-programs can control aspects of the interface program. For instance, the inference engine can cause any of the question display forms to be shown. Adding more program modules is a relatively straightforward process.

This approach leads to the creation of reusable program modules, and supports a mixed language approach. Alternative inference strategies can be simply added to this system. These can be either to replace the current inference system or to work with it.

References

Alty, J.L. and Coombs, M.J., 1984, *Expert Systems: Concepts and Examples*, Manchester: NCC publications.

Chilcoat, R.T., 1980, A review of the control of depth of anaesthesia, *Transactions of the Institute of Measurement and Control*, **2**, 38–45.

Duda, R.O., Heart, P.E. and Nilsson, N.J., 1980, Subjective Bayesian methods for rule based inference systems, *National Computer Conference*, **45**, 1076–82.

Gaschnig, J., 1982, 'Prospector: An expert system for mineral exploration', in Michie, D. (Ed.) *Introductory Reading in Expert Systems*, pp. 47–64, New York: Gordon and Breach Science.

Greenhow, S.G., 1991, 'A knowledge based system for the control of depth of anaesthesia', PhD thesis, University of Sheffield.

Greenhow, S.G., Linkens, D.A. and Asbury, A.J., 1992, Development of an expert system advisor for the anaesthetic state, *Computer Methods and Programmes in Biomedicine*, **37**, 215–29.

Kraft, H.H. and Lees, D.E., 1984, Closing the loop: how near is automated anaesthesia? *Southern Medical Journal*, **77**, 7–12.

Schils, G.F., Sasse, F.J. and Rideout, V.C., 1987, Automatic control of anaesthesia using two feedback variables, *Annals of Biomedical Engineering*, **15**, 19–34.

Van Wyk, C.J., 1988, *Data Structures and C Programmes*, pp. 297–311, New York: Addison-Wesley.

Westenskow, D.R., 1987, Closed-loop control of blood pressure, ventilation, and anaesthetic delivery, *International Journal of Clinical Monitoring and Computing*, **4**, 69–74.

Chapter 3
Generalized predictive control (GPC) in the operating theatre

M. Mahfouf

3.1 Introduction

The major concerns of a clinical anaesthetist are drug-induced unconsciousness, muscle relaxation, and analgesia (i.e. pain relief). The first two of these are concentrated in the operating theatre, whereas the third is mainly related to post-operative conditions. Each of these areas has been researched in recent years for the possibility of using automated drug infusion via feedback strategies.

The question of measurement is a primary matter in each of the three areas of anaesthesia. The measurement of pain is the hardest of all, since it is heavily subjective, and liable to many levels of personal interpretation. However, some work has been done in this field with attempts to estimate wound healing and its associated pain level, using Kalman filtering (Jacobs et al., 1982). Analgesia, when not linked to unconsciousness, will not be considered further in this chapter. Depth of anaesthesia (i.e. unconsciousness) is hard to define, and hence to measure accurately. In practice, the anaesthetist has a number of clinical signs and on-line measurements which can be used selectively for the determination of the patient's state. Not surprisingly, therefore, a variety of methods have been used for feedback control of anaesthetic depth, based on different clinical measurements. One approach is that sensor data fusion is required together with an on-line expert system adviser which can reason with complex, uncertain data (see Chapter 2).

The measurement of muscle relaxation (or drug-induced paralysis) is considerably easier. A common approach is the monitoring of evoked electromyogram (EMG) signals produced at the hand via stimulation above the wrist. Supramaximal electrical pulse stimulation is applied, typically every 20 seconds. This stimulation ensures that all the nerve fibres are recruited, while suitable processing of the resultant EMG provides an analogue signal inversely proportional to the level of relaxation. The signal conditioning usually entails gating, rectifying and integrating. Commercial instruments are now available employing this principle, and this is the measurement basis for the work described in this chapter. An example of a typical EMG trace is shown in Figure 3.1 (the EMG level is represented in the form of bars, where bars of light intensity represent the relevant EMG values, while those of darker intensity represent the train-of-four (TOF) ratio), which also illustrates the difficulty of good regulation when using manual control. In this example an anaesthetist attempted to control relaxation by observing the EMG signal on-line and making manual adjustments to the infusion rate. This recording has also been used to elicit a human operator rule-base in fuzzy logic control of anaesthesia.

Early work on feedback control of drug infusion for muscle relaxation was performed on sheep (Cass et al., 1976). The feedback controller was based on a PID algorithm, as was the first set of human clinical trials performed by Brown et al. (1980). Similar simple control strategies have been used in more recent work using other drugs and in more extended clinical trials. Thus, Ebert et al. (1986) used a PD algorithm for vecuronium administration, and MacLeod et al. (1989) used a PI strategy for atracurium. Another emphasis has been on compact instruments for feedback control, examples being the work by Webster and Cohen (1987), and Jannett and De Falque (1990). Extreme simplification is provided by Wait et al. (1987) who merely added a relay to the output of a Datex Relaxograph alarm indicator. In this work there appears to be no attempt to smooth the measurements or add compensation to the relay control, and obviously oscillations are continuously induced via this technique. They claimed that the levels of oscillation were surgically acceptable. To achieve this, a 50 per cent higher drug consumption than in the classical PI approach used by MacLeod et al. (1989) was indicated. Similar reductions in drug consumption have been indicated in simulations undertaken to compare well-regulated control schemes with the multiple bolus[1] regime calculated via the manufacturers' recommendations[2]. One problem with feedback control in biomedicine is that there are enormous patient-to-patient variations in dynamic model

---

[1] This is a large dose of drug initially given by anaesthetists to patients to obtain a high level of relaxation in a relatively short time.
[2] Abbod, private communication.

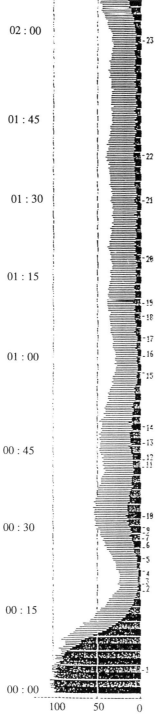

Stimulus artefact = 3%

Supramaximal stimulus 65 mA

Figure 3.1 *Typical relaxograph EMG tracing obtained via manual control of drug infusion. The light bars indicate the level of relaxation.*

parameters. This is compounded by large time-varying parameters for an individual patient during the course of an operation. This makes it difficult to design a fixed-parameter PID controller which will be suitable in all cases. This has already been noted in studies on hypertension control using sodium nitroprusside by Sheppard and co-workers (1979). Thus, in certain cases oscillations occurred, and this has been also observed in the muscle relaxation studies. This has led to the need to investigate self-adaptive control strategies, and later self-organizing controllers.

To facilitate the design of advanced controllers, it is necessary to have a good mathematical model of the process. Identification studies on animals have produced model structures and parameters which confirm the wide variability and also the non-linearity in the so-called pharmacodynamics for relaxant drug behaviour (Linkens et al., 1982 and Linkens and Asbury, 1985). This validated model has been used extensively in designing and simulating controllers based on either quantitative (e.g. self-tuning) or qualitative (e.g. self-organizing) techniques.

An early attempt at adaptive control used a pole-placement self-tuning algorithm in animal studies (Linkens et al., 1985). In this work two non-depolarizing drugs were used, together with the incorporation of a Smith Predictor to offset the time-delay inherent in the drug circulation which was also investigated. The simple and well-known nature of the PID controller suggests that self-tuning might be applied to that structure. Although this is now common-place in industry, the normal method of iterative adjustment of parameters via deliberately induced oscillations or large disturbances is not acceptable in an operating theatre. An alternative model-based self-tuning PID approach has been developed and evaluated clinically by Denai et al. (1990). This particular strategy is limited to systems with pure time delay and second-order dynamics, and is relevant for muscle relaxant control. Another model-based approach due to Olkkola and Schwilden (1991) uses an average population pharmacokinetic model, which is updated periodically on-line and then used for predictive control of drug administration. Earlier work by Rametti and co-workers had considered a dual-mode controller, with different strategies being adopted for initial and regulation phases for relaxation control. The initial phase controller used a sequence of small bolus doses, the amounts being adjusted to minimize the risk of excessive overshoot in the paralysis level (Rametti, 1985; Rametti et al., 1985). This protocol is not normally acceptable in theatre, and later work (Bradlow and O'Mahony, 1990) has emphasized the regulation phase controller comprising a state and parameter estimator which is used predictively to calculate the best current dosage.

Common to much of the above work is the theme of predictive control, and this is the background to this chapter which investigates generalized predictive control (GPC) (Clarke et al., 1987a; Clarke et al., 1987b) for on-line muscle relaxant drug administration. GPC has advantages over other forms of self-tuning control in that it is robust against variable and unknown time-delay, over-parameterization of system models, and has good disturbance rejection properties. It does, however, have a number of design 'knobs' which must be adjusted carefully to suit the particular application. In the following sections and in order to get to grips with the muscle relaxation concept in general, the mechanism of neuromuscular transmission together with that of the muscle relaxants' action are presented. A mathematical model for the drug pharmacology of atracurium is developed, together with off-line simulations of GPC based on this model. Design values were then transferred to an on-line simulation running 60 times faster than real-time. This validated software and hardware system was then transferred to the operating theatre, and the resulting clinical trials and their evaluation are described in later sections.

3.2 Physiological background pertaining to the muscle relaxation process

3.2.1 Neuromuscular transmission

In the chain of events that starts with the stimulation of a motor nerve and ends with the contraction of a muscle, the most vulnerable link is the synapse between the nerve and the muscle—the neuromuscular junction. The motor nerve is separated from the muscle by the synaptic cleft. This cleft is in fact a sub-division of the extracellular fluid (ECF) from which it is separated by the Schwann cell membrane. The neurotransmitter acetylcholine (Ach) is responsible for transmitting motor nerve activity across this junction. Early work by Birks *et al.* (1960) elucidated the fundamental anatomy of the neuromuscular junction, and modern techniques have allowed refinements of details relative to this structure. As shown in Figure 3.2, the motor nerve ends at that part of the muscle membrane known as the motor end plate. In this area, the membrane is folded into longitudinal gutters; the ridges of each gutter conceal orifices to secondary clefts. Around these orifices, a high concentration of a chemical substance known as cholinesterase (AchE) has been proved to be present. The end plate membrane potential is a reflection of the uneven distribution of ions across the surface membrane. In its resting state, this membrane is far more permeable to potassium ions (K^+) than those of sodium (Na^+) (ratio of 100). As a result, potassium ions pass out of the cell along their concentration gradient until the accumulation of positively charged ions on the outside of the membrane causes an opposing force to further migrations of potassium ions. The inside of the membrane has a negative potential, whereas the outside has a positive electrical charge. The membrane is said to be polarized. The transmembrane potential reaches a value of $-70\,mV$ to $-90\,mV$. The arrival of an impulse at the nerve terminals causes the release

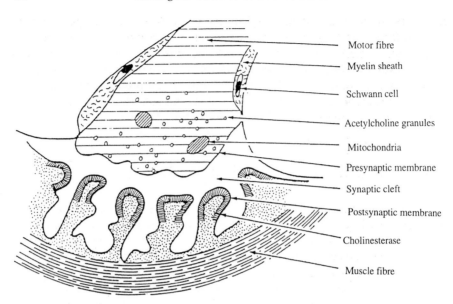

Figure 3.2 *A schematic representation of the neuromuscular junction (Birks et al., 1960).*

of Ach (Dale and Feldberg, 1934) which causes the opening of the sodium pores by reacting with specialized receptors on the post-synaptic membrane. This causes depolarization of the post-synaptic membrane by increasing its permeability to Na^+ relative to K^+. The end plate potential is reversed giving rise to an action potential propagation and subsequent muscle contraction. These events are quickly terminated as a result of interactions between Ach and AchE present in the orifices of the secondary clefts.

3.2.2 Muscle relaxant drugs and their mechanism of action

As seen in the previous section, the synaptic gap is the site which witnesses the unusual activity leading to a muscle contraction. Therefore, the process of neuromuscular transmission can only be blocked if relaxant drugs gain access to the synaptic cleft and break the previously described chain of events. Depending on their mechanism of action, muscle relaxant agents fall into two categories: depolarizing and non-depolarizing drugs; depolarizing drugs such as suxamethonium and decamethonium are believed to act by producing a continuous depolarization of the post-synaptic membrane, rendering it unresponsive to acetylcholine and at their first application a voluntary muscle contracts, but unlike acetylcholine, these agents are not destroyed by cholinesterase and the depolarization is maintained. Non-depolarizing agents, however, compete with acetylcholine for the cholinoreceptors. As a result, when acetylcholine reacts with these drugs, it fails to cause sufficient sodium pores to open to allow threshold depolarization to take place. These agents do not induce muscle pain following their administration and because of this they are preferred to the other category. Atracurium, a non-depolarizing fast-acting agent, which gained popularity over pancuronium and d-tubocurarine, is the subject of this research study and its associated mathematical model is presented next.

3.3 Atracurium mathematical model

In order to identify the muscle relaxation process associated with drugs, pharmacology is commonly used to describe the metabolism of such drugs. Pharmacology comprises two main categories known as pharmacokinetics and pharmacodynamics. Pharmacokinetics studies the relationship that exists between drug dose and drug concentration in the blood plasma as well as other parts of the body. Interpretation of this relationship can be given a mathematical meaning via the concept of compartmental models. Using this concept the body consists of several compartments each representing one part of the body that involves the drug metabolism. Pharmacodynamics, however, is concerned with the drug concentration and the effect produced. One key postulate of this is that there is a considerable delay separating the first administration of a muscle relaxant drug and the onset of relaxation; this non-linear effect is known as the 'margin of safety' (Paton and Waud, 1967; Waud and Waud, 1971), whereby no depression of twitch response can be detected until over 75 per cent of the receptors are occluded. Also, because of saturation effects, once initiated, paralysis cannot increase indefinitely as the drug dosage increases.

3.3.1. Pharmacokinetics

It has been shown that after a drug injection, the plasma concentration of atracurium declines rapidly in two exponential phases corresponding to distribution and elimination (Ward et al., 1983). Therefore, a conventional two-compartment model is used by adding an elimination path from the peripheral compartment obeying the so-called 'Hofmann elimination' (Ward et al., 1983; Weatherley et al., 1983). Figure 3.3 is a schematic diagram showing the different model components.

If x_i is the drug concentration at time t, $\dot{x}_i$ its rate of change, and u the drug input, then:

$$\begin{aligned} \dot{x}_1 &= -(k_{10} + k_{12})x_1 + k_{21}x_2 + u \\ \dot{x}_2 &= k_{12}x_1 - (k_{20} + k_{21})x_2. \end{aligned} \quad (3.1)$$

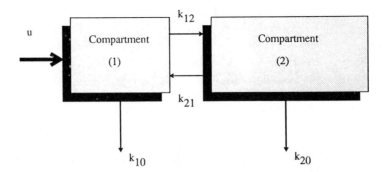

Figure 3.3 *A two-compartment model for atracurium with an additional elimination path (k_{20}).*

Using Laplace transforms, Equation (3.1) can be rewritten as:

$$sX_1 = -(k_{10} + k_{12})X_1 + k_{21}X_2 + U$$
$$sX_2 = k_{12}X_1 - (k_{20} + k_{21})X_2. \quad (3.2)$$

Hence

$$\frac{X_1(s)}{U(s)} = \frac{s + k_{20} + k_{21}}{(s + k_{10} + k_{12})(s + k_{20} + k_{21}) - k_{12}k_{21}}. \quad (3.3)$$

Experimental studies by Weatherley *et al.* (1983) gave the following mean values for the pharmacokinetics parameters:

$$k_{12} + k_{10} = 0.26 \text{ min}^{-1}$$
$$k_{21} + k_{20} = 0.094 \text{ min}^{-1}$$
$$k_{12} \times k_{21} = 0.015 \text{ min}^{-2}.$$

Substituting in Equation (3.3) leads to:

$$\frac{X_1(s)}{U(s)} = \frac{9.94(1 + 10.64s)}{(1 + 3.08s)(1 + 34.42s)} \quad (3.4)$$

which describes the pharmacokinetics of the muscle relaxation system relating to the drug atracurium in a transfer function form.

3.3.2. Pharmacodynamics

Simultaneous identification of pharmacokinetics and pharmacodynamics of d-tubocurarine (Sheiner *et al.*, 1979) led to the findings that the dynamics of

Generalized predictive control (GPC) in the operating theatre 45

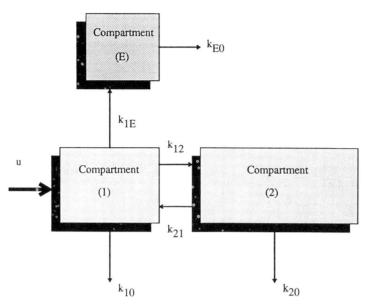

Figure 3.4 *Modification of the atracurium kinetics to include the 'effect' compartment E.*

the drug effect do not coincide with those of the plasma concentration. Similarly, in order to characterize temporal aspects of drug effect, a third compartment known as the 'effect compartment' is introduced. It is connected to the central compartment by a first-order rate constant k_{1E}, whereas the rate constant k_{E0} characterizes the drug dissipation from the effect compartment, as shown in Figure 3.4.

In this latter compartment, the drug concentration change is governed by the following equation:

$$\dot{x}_E = k_{1E} x_1 - k_{E0} x_E \tag{3.5}$$

which, using Laplace transforms, yields:

$$X_E = \frac{k_{1E} X_1}{s + k_{E0}}. \tag{3.6}$$

The Hill equation (Whiting and Kelman, 1980; Weatherley *et al.*, 1983) may be used to relate the effect to a specific concentration.

$$E_{\text{eff}} = \frac{E_{\text{max}}}{1 + \frac{X_E(50)^\alpha}{X_E^\alpha}} \tag{3.7}$$

where X_E is the drug concentration and $X_E(50)$ is the drug concentration at a 50 per cent effect.

Experimental work (Whiting and Kelman, 1980; Weatherley et al., 1983) has given the following parameters:

$$k_{E0} = 0.208 \text{ min}^{-1}$$
$$X_E(50) = 0.404 \text{ } \mu\text{g ml}^{-1}$$
$$\alpha = 2.98$$
$$k_{1E} = 10^{-4} \text{ min}^{-1}.$$

Combining Equations (3.6) and (3.4) and normalizing the overall open-loop gain at 1.0 leads to:

$$\frac{X_E}{U} = \frac{K(1+T_4 s)\,e^{-\tau s}}{(1+T_1 s)(1+T_2 s)(1+T_3 s)} \qquad (3.8)$$

where,

$$K = 1$$
$$\tau = 1 \text{ min}$$
$$T_1 = 4.81 \text{ min}$$
$$T_2 = 34.42 \text{ min}$$
$$T_3 = 3.08 \text{ min}$$
$$T_4 = 10.64 \text{ min}.$$

Finally, the overall non-linear model is obtained by combining Equation (3.8) together with the Hill equation (3.7), or alternatively a dead-space in series with a saturation element.

3.4 Development of an adaptive GPC controller

Long-range prediction algorithms enjoyed considerable popularity in the late 1970s especially with the development of a computer control algorithm called dynamic matrix control (DMC) (Cutler and Ramaker, 1980). Evolving from a technique that represents process dynamics with a set of numerical coefficients together with a least-squares formulation, it promised to solve complex control problems, especially those associated with systems exhibiting large dead-times. DMC's use of a non-parametric model was later challenged by another multi-step long-range predictive control algorithm: generalized predictive control (GPC) (Clarke et al., 1987a and Clarke et al., 1987b). It is a natural successor to the generalized minimum variance (GMV) design (Clarke and Gawthrop, 1975), and is considered to be very robust. Its development is reviewed in the next section.

3.4.1 Model description

The so-called CARMA (controlled autoregressive moving average) model (Wellstead, 1980; Clarke and Gawthrop, 1975) has found its place in many self-tuning designs, whereby an integrator is inserted in an *ad hoc* fashion to counteract any offset that may occur when regulating a process around a non-zero set-point. Another method suggested the use of a CARIMA (controlled autoregressive integrated moving average) model (Belanger, 1983; Tuffs and Clarke, 1985), in which the noise term is non-stationary. Good adaptive behaviour has been shown to be possible for this case.

Consider the following locally linearized discrete model in the backward shift operator z^{-1}:

$$A(z^{-1})y(t) = B(z^{-1})u(t-1) + x(t) \tag{3.9}$$

where,

$$A(z^{-1}) = 1 + a_1 z^{-1} + a_2 z^{-2} + \cdots + a_n z^{-n}$$
$$B(z^{-1}) = z^{-k}(b_1 + b_2 z^{-1} + b_3 z^{-2} + \cdots + b_m z^{-m+1})$$

and z^{-1} represents the backward shift operator, $u(t)$ the control input, $y(t)$ the measured variable, k the assumed value of time-delay, and $x(t)$ represents the disturbance upon which the model is based and is considered to be of moving average form, i.e.:

$$x(t) = C(z^{-1})\frac{\xi(t)}{\Delta} \tag{3.10}$$

where:

$$C(z^{-1}) = c_0 + c_1 z^{-1} + c_2 z^{-2} + \cdots + c_p z^{-p}$$
$$\xi(t) = \text{an uncorrelated random sequence}$$
$$\Delta = 1 - z^{-1}.$$

Thus, substituting Equation (3.10) into Equation (3.9) and appending the operator Δ gives:

$$A(z^{-1})\Delta y(t) = B(z^{-1})\Delta u(t-1) + C(z^{-1})\xi(t). \tag{3.11}$$

3.4.2 The control law

Before describing the mathematical background behind the algorithm, it is worthwhile outlining briefly the theory of long-range predictive control.

The strategy illustrated in Figure 3.5 can be summarized as follows (De Keyser and Van Cauwenberghe, 1983):

- At each present time t a forecast is made of the process output over a long-range time horizon by means of a mathematical model of the process dynamics.
- Several control actions will be proposed as a result of this forecast, but only the best strategy will be selected according to the predefined set-point.
- The chosen candidate is then applied as the control action at the same time t. The whole procedure is again repeated at the next sample. This procedure is also known as 'the receding horizon approach'.

The controller therefore computes the vector of controls using optimization of a function of the form:

$$\begin{cases} J = E[(Q1 + Q2)] \\ Q1 = \sum_{j=N_1}^{N_2} [(P(z^{-1})\hat{y}(t+j) - \omega(t+j))^2] \\ Q2 = \sum_{j=1}^{NU} [\lambda(j)(\Delta u(t+j-1))^2] \end{cases} \quad (3.12)$$

where, N_1 is the minimum costing horizon, N_2 is the maximum costing horizon, NU is the control horizon, ω is the future set-point usually presumed known, and $\lambda(j)$ is the control weighting sequence.

Omitting z^{-1} for the sake of brevity, one can then write:

$$P\hat{y}(t+j) = \bar{\bar{G}}_j \Delta u(t+j-1) + \Psi(t+j) \quad (3.13)$$

$$\Psi(t+j) = \bar{G}_j \Delta u^f(t-1) + \bar{F}_j y^f(t) \quad (3.14)$$

$$TP = E_j A \Delta + z^{-j} \bar{F}_j \quad (3.15)$$

$$P(z^{-1}) = \frac{P_n(z^{-1})}{P_d(z^{-1})} \quad (P(1) = 1) \quad (3.16)$$

$$T(z^{-1}) = 1 + t_1 z^{-1} + \ldots + t_{nt} z^{-nt} \quad (3.17)$$

$$\bar{F}_j = \frac{F_j}{P_d} \quad (3.18)$$

Generalized predictive control (GPC) in the operating theatre

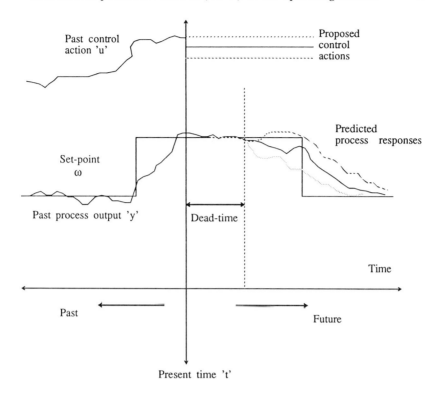

Figure 3.5 *Long-range predictive control (LRPC) principle.*

$$E_j B = \bar{\bar{G}}_j T + z^{-j} \bar{G}_j \tag{3.19}$$

$$\bar{\bar{G}}_j = \bar{\bar{g}}_0 + \bar{\bar{g}}_1 z^{-1} + \ldots + \bar{\bar{g}}_{j-1} z^{-j+1}$$

$$\bar{G}_j = \bar{g}_{j0} + \bar{g}_{j1} z^{-1} + \ldots + \bar{g}_{j(i-1)} z^{-i+1}$$

$$i = \text{from 1 to } \max(\delta B, \delta T)$$
$$1 \leq j \leq N_2$$

where superscript 'f' denotes signals filtered by $1/T(z^{-1})$ and P and T are user-chosen polynomials in z^{-1}. $1/T(z^{-1})$ is chosen as a low-pass filter, and is the so-called observer polynomial for the predictor of Equation (3.14) (Åström and Wittenmark, 1984). P is referred to as the model-following polynomial and the condition $P(1) = 1$ ensures an offset-free response (Clarke, 1985).

The minimization of the cost function described in Equation (3.12) leads to the following projected control increment:

$$\Delta u(t) = \bar{g}^T (\omega - \Psi) \tag{3.20}$$

where $\Psi = [\Psi(t+N_1), \ldots, \Psi(t+N_2)], \bar{g}^T$ is the first row of the matrix $(G_d^T G_d + \lambda I)^{-1} G_d^T$, and G_d is the dynamic (step-response) matrix of the form given by Clarke et al. (1987a).

3.5 Simulation studies

The simulation studies have been undertaken in two parts, the first being concerned with implementation of the GPC algorithm on a SUN workstation. The second consisted of evaluating the algorithm under real-time conditions using a VIDAC 336 analogue computer.

3.5.1 Implementation of the GPC algorithm on a SUN workstation

The overall non-linear muscle relaxant model describing atracurium dynamics has been simulated. For the continuous model being considered, a fourth-order Runge–Kutta method with fixed step length was used for the numerical integration, together with a sampling period of 1 minute. The pharmacokinetics of the drug are given by the three-time constant transfer function with a unit time-delay of Equation (3.8), whereas the pharmacodynamics are modelled by the Hill equation (3.7). Whenever the controller is operating in the non-linear region, parameter estimation is frozen and control is maintained with a fixed PI controller, and the self-tuner takes over as soon as the non-linear region is traversed. Figure 3.6 illustrates the structure of the overall control strategy.

As pointed out earlier, because the system exhibits a large dead-zone, a fixed PI controller, which includes gains obtained via optimization using a program called PSI (Van den Bosch, 1979), provides initial control for a 20-sample period after which the self-adaptive GPC took over. Parameter estimation, using incremental data, takes the form of a UD-factorization algorithm (Bierman, 1977) which is a modified robust version of the well-known Recursive Least-Squares (RLS) algorithm. A third-order discrete-time model was estimated with an assumed time-delay of 1 minute, i.e.

$$G_1(z^{-1}) = z^{-1} \frac{b_1 z^{-1} + b_2 z^{-2} + b_3 z^{-3}}{1 + a_1 z^{-1} + a_2 z^{-2} + a_3 z^{-3}}. \quad (3.21)$$

Parameter estimates were all set to 0.0 unless otherwise specified, the covariance matrix was made equal to $P = 10^4 I$, and a value of $\rho = 0.95$ was adopted for the forgetting factor. The control signal was clipped between maximum and minimum values of respectively 0.0 and 1.0. These limitations

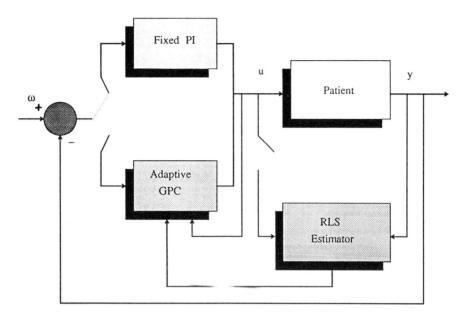

Figure 3.6 *Schematic diagram representing the overall structure of the muscle relaxation control system.*

were also reflected back to the estimator by recomputing the actual control sequence that was asserted (Clarke, 1985).

The experiments were conducted in two phases. Phase 1 utilized the basic GPC algorithm (Clarke *et al.*, 1987a), while phase 2 was concerned with the extended algorithm (Clarke *et al.*, 1987b) using the observer polynomial $T(z^{-1})$.

The performance of the self-adaptive GPC algorithm under the above initial and jacketting conditions together with a combination of (1, 10, 1, 0) for (N_1, N_2, NU, λ) is shown in Figure 3.7. The set-point command signal was 80 per cent then 70 per cent every 100 samples. The parameter estimates converged to the following final values:

$$\hat{a}_1 = -2.149 \quad \hat{a}_2 = 1.511 \quad \hat{a}_3 = -0.349$$
$$\hat{b}_1 = 0.010 \quad \hat{b}_2 = 0.002 \quad \hat{b}_3 = -0.005.$$

These are equivalent to the following positions in the z plane:

$$\text{zeros: } -0.85 \; ; \; 0.62$$
$$\text{poles: } 0.92 \; ; \; (0.61 \pm 0.04i).$$

These values could be considered as reflecting the compartmental idea since

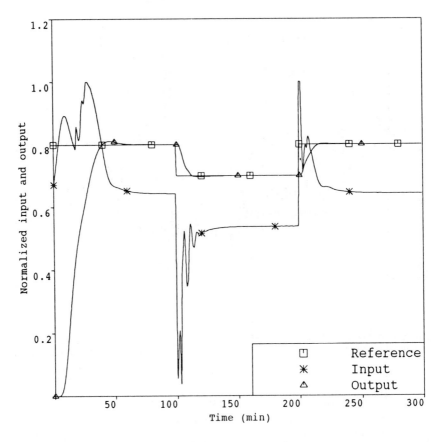

Figure 3.7 *Closed-loop response of atracurium model under self-adaptive GPC algorithm with* $N_1 = 1$; $N_2 = 10$; $NU = 1$.

the imaginary part of the conjugate poles is a negligible quantity compared to the real part.

In muscle relaxation, a pure time-delay has been shown to occur due to the transport of blood via the circulation system (Linkens *et al.*, 1982). Its value has been shown experimentally to vary from subject to subject with a ratio of approximately 4:1. To simulate such a situation, an experiment was conducted in which the dead-time value τ in Equation (3.8) was made to vary from 1 minute to 4 minutes every 100 samples. A noise sequence in the form of a pseudo-random binary sequence (PRBS) with 1 per cent amplitude was superimposed on the output. The same combination for the controller parameters was considered except that the observer polynomial $T(z^{-1})$ of the form $T(z^{-1}) = 1 - 0.97z^{-1}$, where 0.97 corresponds to the dominant time-constant of the process, was included this time, and any

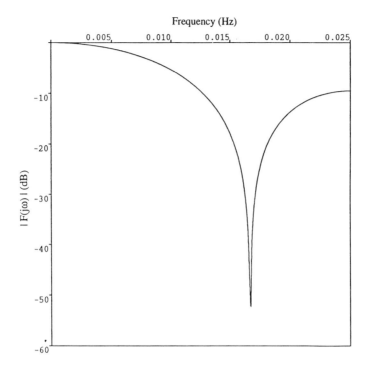

Figure 3.11 *Frequency response corresponding to the filter of Equation (3.24).*

results both in simulations and in real-time experiments. This was done by using a three-point non-recursive averaging filter of the form:

$$G_{AF}(z^{-1}) = \frac{1}{3} \sum_{i=0}^{i=2} z^{-i} \qquad (3.24)$$

where:

$$\begin{aligned} z^{-1} &= e^{-sh} \\ h &= 20 \text{ seconds}. \end{aligned} \qquad (3.25)$$

The log-magnitude plot response of the filter is shown in Figure 3.11, with the characteristic having a -3 dB point of 0.008 Hz. This provides low-pass filtering which reduces signal artefacts caused by fluctuations in the response due to inadequate positioning of the stimulating and recording electrodes and diathermy (severe electrical interference).

When closed-loop control is established, a PI controller is used to provide initial control allowing the parameter estimation routine to gather reasonable data. The PI parameters were obtained using Ziegler–Nichols techniques (1942) applied to open-loop step responses in an off-line study. The dose of atracurium is expressed in ml h^{-1} and is obtained using the following formula:

$$I \text{ (ml h}^{-1}) = K_p e + K_i(\Sigma e + P) \tag{3.26}$$

where, $K_p = k_p W_t$, $K_i = k_i W_t$, $k_p = 0.02$ kg^{-1}, $k_i = 0.0021$ kg^{-1}, I is the atracurium infusion rate, W_t represents the actual patient's weight, whereas e is the difference between the actual $T1\%$ and the target $T1\%$. These values were also used as a basis for an algorithm successfully applied in theatre (Denai et al., 1990).

At this stage it is worth noting that when a bolus dose is preloaded to induce muscle relaxation, the PI controller is initialized with some integral value P, so as to shorten the stabilization period when closed-loop control mode is entered. Nominal values between 150 and 333 were used throughout the trials for P.

3.6.2 Clinical preparation of patients before surgery

The patients were all selected knowing that they did not suffer from any known sensitivity to anaesthetic drugs or myoneural disorders, and had not been taking drugs known to affect neuromuscular transmission. They all underwent abdominal or orthopaedic surgery which normally requires muscle relaxation.

Approximately 60 minutes before surgery, they were all premedicated with temazepam by mouth. Anaesthesia was induced with methohexitane 1 mg kg^{-1}. The trachea was intubated when $T1$ rerached a value between 10 and 15 per cent. The lungs were inflated with 30 per cent oxygen, 70 per cent nitrous oxide and 1 per cent enflurane. During surgery, enflurane anaesthesia was supplemented with boluses of fentanyl at 1 μg kg^{-1}. While the patient was still in the anaesthetic room, the Relaxograph electrodes were carefully placed on the patient's arm, then the calibration proceeded. Once transferred to the theatre, the patient, already connected to the control system, was intravenously given an initial bolus dose of atracurium of 0.15 to 0.25 mg kg^{-1}.

The on-line controlled infusion was started when $T1$ (induced by the initial bolus) reached a level judged adequate by the anaesthetist (usually 10 to 15 per cent of the 100 per cent baseline[3] value). Muscle relaxation level was monitored until the surgeon requested cessation of paralysis. The

---

[3] A 100% EMG corresponds to 0% paralysis, whereas 0% EMG is equivalent to maximum paralysis.

Generalized predictive control (GPC) in the operating theatre 61

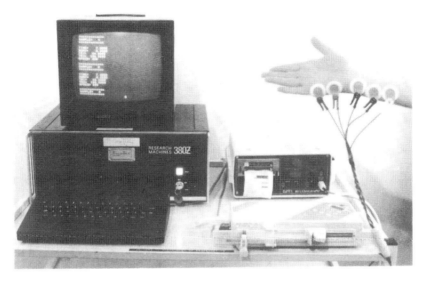

Figure 3.12 *Patient in the anaesthetic room while connected to the overall control system which includes (clockwise) the 380Z microcomputer system, the DATEX Relaxograph, and the CRITIKON syringe pump.*

control was then switched off immediately, and the residual blockade was reversed using antagonist agents such as neostigmine (2.5 mg) and atropine (0.8 mg). Figure 3.12 is a picture taken in hospital showing a patient connected to the overall muscle relaxation control system prior to undergoing surgery.

3.6.3 Results and discussions

After local Ethics Committee approval, ten patients (eight female, two male) were selected as being suitable for the experiments. Information relating to the patients is presented in Table 3.2. The atracurium concentrations used were all 1 mg ml^{-1} unless otherwise specified.

All ten trials were conducted using a sampling-time interval of 1 minute. Consequently, the three-point non-recursive averaging filter was included in all experiments. Control and estimation were performed every one minute, while EMG readings were obtained every 20 seconds. Parameter estimation was based on the UD-factorization algorithm and was triggered at the same time as the closed-loop control was established with a covariance matrix and forgetting factor values of $P = 10I$ and $\rho = 0.999$ respectively. A 20 per cent reference EMG level ($T1\%$) was required by the operating surgeon in all trials except for the last case corresponding to patient 10, where a 15 per

Table 3.2 *Summary of patients' personal details*

Personal details					
Patient	Sex	Age (years)	Weight (kg)	Duration of procedure (min)	Duration of control (min)
1	F	68	50	107	67
2	F	33	60	56	30
3	F	21	68	60	45
4	F	69	50	120	69
5	F	65	58	66	33
6	F	37	60	58	32
7	F	17	56	165	130
8	M	32	69	90	52
9	M	46	73	177	106
10	F	41	71	63	22

cent EMG reference level was targetted. Results corresponding to each patient are presented in two parts: the first part consists of two traces; the upper trace representing the recorded EMG level ($T1\%$), whereas the lower trace shows the variations of the infusion rate of atracurium in ml h^{-1}. The time axis is labelled in samples of 20 seconds, and it is worth noting that the infusion rate is constant over three samples of 20 seconds each. The second part of the results includes the parameter estimate variations plotted at one-minute intervals. Due to lack of space only some of the ten experiments will be described here, illustrating lessons learned from the trials.

3.6.3.1 Patient 3

For this experiment, whose results are shown in Figure 3.13(*a*), the atracurium drug concentration was halved to 500 μg ml^{-1}. The controller assumed a combination of $(1, 30, 1, 0)$ for (N_1, N_2, NU, λ) and a second-order observer polynomial $T(z^{-1}) = (1 - 0.7z^{-1})^2$. However, the estimator assumed a third-order model with a minimum time-delay of 1 minute. Mark 1 and Mark 2 on the upper trace of the same figure represent the times at which the anaesthetist administered bolus doses of 7.5 mg and 2.5 mg respectively in order to bring the EMG level down to approximately 15 per cent. At Mark 3, the closed-loop control mode was entered with the fixed PI allowed to run for 30 minutes, after which the self-adaptive GPC took over at Mark 4. Both control modes succeeded in keeping a remarkably steady level of paralysis with hardly any fluctuations at all, but looking at the infusion rate plot, the period corresponding to the GPC protocol was steader. Finally at Mark 5 the controller was switched off and the blockade reversed at Mark 6. Notice the return to a 100 per cent baseline suggesting that no unnecessary drug has been administered and that little drift in the relaxation calibration level has occurred. Figure 3.13(*b*) illustrates the variations of the parameter estimates which were steadier for this trial. They finally converged to the following values:

$$\hat{a}_1 = -1.1926 \quad \hat{a}_2 = 0.3059 \quad \hat{a}_3 = 0.0745$$
$$\hat{b}_1 = 0.8109 \quad \hat{b}_2 = -0.1358 \quad \hat{b}_3 = -0.0740.$$

These correspond to the following pole/zero positions in the z plane:

$$\text{zeros: } 0.3972 \; ; \; -0.2297$$
$$\text{poles: } (0.6702 \pm 0.2342i) \; ; \; -0.1478$$

with an estimated open-loop gain of 3.20. The presence of a pair of complex poles which does not reflect the compartmental idea is probably due to the lack of proper excitation necessary for the identification routine.

3.6.3.2 Patient 4

During this particular experiment, the subject, a young female, demonstrated very low sensitivity to the muscle relaxant drug. Indeed, as the EMG recording in Figure 3.14 shows, the patient was insensitive to the first bolus dose of 9 mg intravenously administered at Mark 2. Another 2 mg, then 3 mg were given at Mark 3 and Mark 4 respectively. At this stage, the anaesthetist decided to commence automatic control of the infusion at Mark 5 with the fixed PI allowed to run only for 5 minutes. The infusion rate of atracurium at 500 μg ml^{-1} began at approximately 60 ml h^{-1} then increased gradually to 80 ml h^{-1}, but even that did not cause the EMG to drop below the 50 per cent line. However, when the GPC took over at Mark 5, with a combination of $(1, 10, 1, 0)$ for (N_1, N_2, NU, λ) and $T(z^{-1}) = (1 - 0.95z^{-1})^2$, it was quick to drive the EMG level to the target in spite of the noise level estimated at ± 3 per cent persistently disturbing the output. The controller behaved rather well by rejecting these disturbances and produced a control signal, illustrated on the lower trace of the same figure, which was reasonably active. Undoubtedly, the use of a slower root in the $T(z^{-1})$ polynomial made the controller more robust. The parameter estimation routine, which in this case assumed a second-order model with a one-minute time delay, used filtered incremental data for the measurement vector. The parameter estimates converged to the following values:

$$\hat{a}_1 = -1.7674 \quad \hat{a}_2 = 0.7717$$
$$\hat{b}_1 = 0.0471 \quad \hat{b}_2 = -0.0386.$$

This is equivalent to a continuous second-order system of the following gain and time-constants:

$$\widehat{\text{Gain}} = 1.97 \quad \widehat{TC_1} = 4.19 \text{ min} \quad \widehat{TC_2} = 48.88 \text{ min}.$$

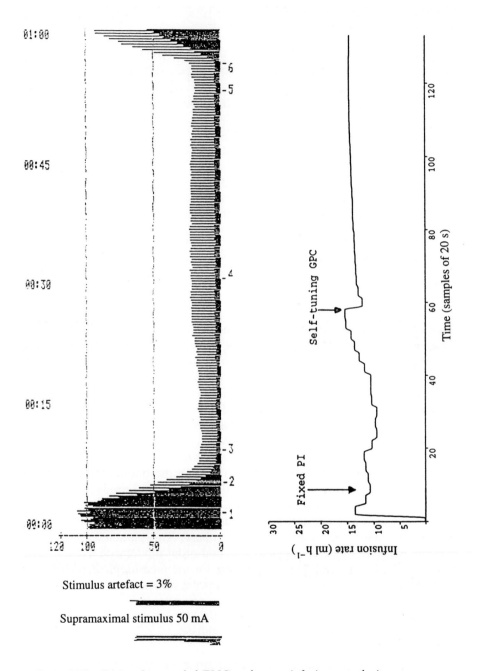

Figure 3.13a *Patient 3: recorded EMG and pump infusion rate during surgery.*

Generalized predictive control (GPC) in the operating theatre

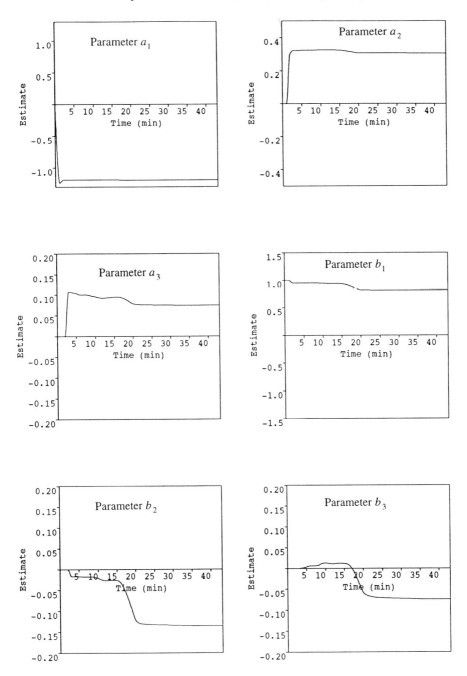

Figure 3.13b *System parameter estimates corresponding to Figure 3.13a.*

66

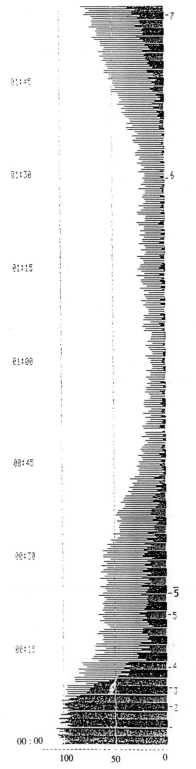
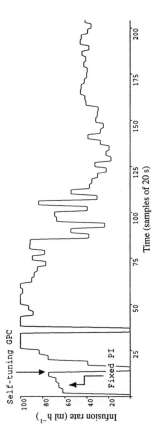

Figure 3.14 *Patient 4: recorded EMG and pump infusion rate during surgery.*

Before describing the remaining six clinical trials, it is worth noting that throughout the following, full-valued data (positional data) rather than incremental data were used in the measurement vector for estimation purposes. Although this would seem to contradict the idea of an integrative model, it was found to give satisfactory performances as the following results will demonstrate. Parameter estimation assumed a second-order model with a minimum time-delay of 1 minute unless otherwise specified, and initial conditions included a covariance matrix and a forgetting factor of $P = 10^2 I$, and $\rho = 0.995$, respectively. Parameter estimates were initialized so as to reflect a continuous second-order system with the following gain and time-constants:

$$\theta_i = [1.15, 0.34 \text{ min}, 16.13 \text{ min}].$$

3.6.3.3 Patient 8

After bolus doses of 8 mg then 3 mg administered at Mark 1 and Mark 2 respectively, shown on the upper trace of Figure 3.15 (again suggesting a low-sensitivity patient), the loop was closed at Mark 3 when the EMG level reached approximately 28 per cent. The PI was allowed to run for 5 minutes and produced an overshoot of 12 per cent. When the GPC took over at Mark $\overline{3}$ assuming a combination of $(1, 30, 1, 5)$ for (N_1, N_2, NU, λ) and no filter, it was quick to reduce the overshoot by making the EMG track efficiently the 20 per cent target. The control signal, whose variations are shown on the lower trace of the same figure, was good and reasonably active.

3.6.3.4 Patient 9

This experiment was the longest in the series of trials. The subject, a young male, underwent a three-hour surgery requiring muscle relaxation. Mark 1 on the trace of Figure 3.16 is the time at which suxamethonium was administered before the trachea was intubated. A return to a 100 per cent EMG level was achieved at Mark 4 when a large bolus dose of muscle relaxant drug of 24 mg was given intravenously, and this wiped out completely the EMG tracing, which only started to reappear again 12 minutes later. At Mark 5 the automatic control mode was entered with the PI providing initial control for 30 minutes until Mark 6. At this time the GPC took over with the same controller and estimation parameters as before, except that instead of assuming a minimum delay of 1 minute, the $B(z^{-1})$ polynomial structure was extended by one coefficient to absorb this value. Initial conditions for the estimates were taken to be:

$$\hat{a}_1 = -0.9927 \quad \hat{a}_2 = 0.0496$$
$$\hat{b}_1 = 0.0 \quad \hat{b}_2 = 0.0471 \quad \hat{b}_3 = 0.0183.$$

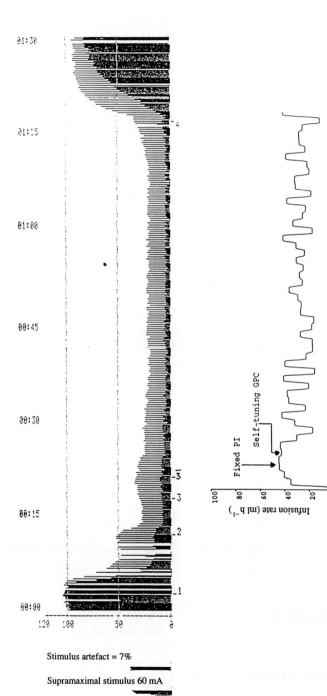

Figure 3.15 *Patient 8: recorded EMG and pump infusion rate during surgery.*

Generalized predictive control (GPC) in the operating theatre 69

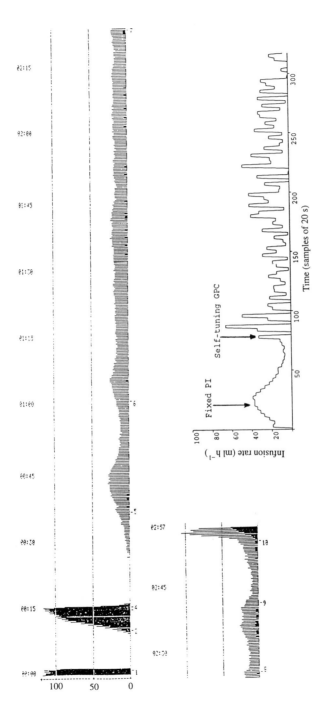

Figure 3.16 *Patient 9: recorded EMG and pump infusion rate during surgery.*

These were chosen to reflect the same gain, time-constants, and time-delay as in the previous case.

At Mark 7 the control had to be switched off due to a lack of computer disk-space. From then on, the anaesthetist had to resume manual control with bolus doses of 10 mg each at times indicated by Mark 8 and Mark 9. The large fluctuations in the EMG level during this phase indicate the difficulty of manual control via bolus injections. At Mark 10 the blockade was reversed with neostigmine. As shown in the same figure, the PI induced an 8 per cent overshoot followed by a 10 per cent undershoot of the EMG level, but this was quickly eliminated as soon as the GPC took over. The EMG level was quite steady, fluctuating between 17 per cent and 20 per cent leading to a highly activated control signal as the lower trace of the same figure illustrates, this occurring in spite of the relatively large value of the output horizon and the non-zero control weighting sequence. Parameter estimates suggest indeed a value of time-delay greater than or equal to 1 minute, since $\hat{b}_1$ was an insignificant value. These parameter estimates converged to the following final values:

$$\hat{a}_1 = -1.0149 \quad \hat{a}_2 = 0.0284$$
$$\hat{b}_1 = 0.0048 \quad \hat{b}_2 = 0.0228 \quad \hat{b}_3 = 0.0353.$$

This is equivalent to a continuous second-order system with the following gain and time-constants:

$$\widehat{\text{Gain}} = 4.66 \quad \widehat{TC_1} = 0.28 \text{ min} \quad \widehat{TC_2} = 71.44 \text{ min}.$$

These values suggest a high-sensitivity patient with a slow, dominant time-constant.

3.6.4 Analysis of the data

In order to analyse the data, three indices were used: the mean value, the standard deviation (SD), and the root mean square deviation (RMSD). These last two indices are commonly used to give an indication of the spread of a set of values around the mean value and the target value respectively. They are defined by the following two formulae:

$$\text{SD} = \sqrt{\frac{1}{N}\sum (X_i - \bar{X})^2} \tag{3.27}$$

where $X_i, \bar{X}$, and N are the current measurement, the mean value, and the total number of points considered respectively, and,

$$\text{RMSD} = \sqrt{\frac{1}{N}\sum (X_i - \text{TRGT})^2} \tag{3.28}$$

Table 3.3 *Summary of each patient's data*

Patient	Total number of points	Mean $T1$ (per cent)	SD (per cent)	RMSD (per cent)
1†	197	17.50	4.13	4.83
2†	58	19.92	1.36	1.37
3†	134	19.43	2.56	2.63
4†	123	18.49	3.51	3.82
5†	97	21.85	1.76	2.56
6†	94	21.59	3.57	3.91
7†	387	20.14	6.89	6.89
8†	99	20.29	1.02	1.07
9†	318	18.42	3.31	3.67
10‡	66	16.91	2.64	3.26

†A 20 per cent $T1$ target.
‡A 15 per cent $T1$ target.

here X_i is as defined previously and TRGT is the reference target. Table 3.3 summarizes these values for each of the ten patients in the trial.

The mean value of $T1\%$ for each patient was calculated for those trials where closed-loop infusion was started when $T1\%$ returned to 15 per cent after administration of the initial bolus dose of atracurium (patients 3, 6, 9 and 10). For those experiments where closed-loop control was initiated earlier, the mean was evaluated from the moment $T1\%$ crossed the target point for the first time. As shown in Table 3.3, the mean values of $T1\%$ suggest that the degree of neuromuscular blockade obtained with the ten patients was very satisfactory. Maximum overshoots were recorded with patients 7 (22 per cent), 9 (8 per cent), 1 (7 per cent), and 6 (7 per cent). This relates to the wrong time at which the closed-loop mode was entered. Indeed, with patient 7, automatic control was operational when $T1$ reached 19 per cent after recovery from the bolus, and the preloaded PI dose P was not large enough to shorten the stabilization period. This is probably the biggest problem facing such a controller because it is not always possible to switch to automatic control at $T1 = 15$ per cent as experiments with patients 1, 2, 4, 5 and 8 have demonstrated. These patients had very low sensitivity to the drug, so that even large bolus doses did not induce the expected drop in the EMG baseline. One solution to this problem of initial overshoot is of course to switch to the self-adaptive GPC a lot sooner as was the case for patients 8 and 10 who both produced a mean $T1\%$ level close to the target, i.e. 20.29 (SD 1.02) per cent and 16.91 (SD 2.64) per cent respectively. Perhaps more justice would have been done to the self-adaptive GPC, as far as Table 3.3 is concerned, if its corresponding values were evaluated only during the period GPC was operating, since all the bigger overshoots were induced by the PI controller. Obviously, the initiation of the self-tuning GPC at an earlier stage could be detrimental due to the fact that the estimator would not have gathered enough information about the patient to ensure adequate control. This may therefore produce a poor performance, especially if the wrong filter is used in the case of incremental data for the measurement vector. The use of positional data in this case would be advantageous. This has been demonstrated in the last six experiments, and particularly during the trial with patient 10 where in spite of the use of an operating point close to the non-linear region (15 per cent $T1$ target) (Mahfouf et al., 1992), the controller behaved sensibly by producing a good response and a reasonably active control. The same table also shows that the RMSD as well as the SD values were relatively low for all patients, except those of patient 7 which reached a value of $SD = RMSD = \pm 6.89$. However, these values include the case where the concentration was doubled halfway through the run, meaning that the pump should drive at approximately half speed but had to wait for the effect of the previous higher infusions to wear off. For patient 1, the RMSD and SD values were outside the 4 per cent range (4.83 per cent and 4.13 per cent respectively) due to the wrong choice of the filter $T(z^{-1})$ order, although otherwise the performance was good.

Regarding the infusion rate variations for the ten patients, an analysis of the mean atracurium drug consumption per minute and per kilogram body weight was performed, allowing for the corresponding muscle relaxant drug concentration. Table 3.4 summarizes this evaluation.

As shown in the table, the highest dose of muscle relaxant drug was recorded with patient 4 (6.81 $\mu g \, kg^{-1} \, min^{-1}$) who had a relatively low gain (1.97). The lowest drug dose was that for patients 3 and 2, where the GPC algorithm used the filter polynomial $T(z^{-1})$ which, as already seen, reduces the overall feedback gain, leading to smoother control actions. The mean dose consumed by patient 7 was surprisingly low at 5.38 $\mu g \, kg^{-1} \, min^{-1}$. Despite the severe concentration change made during this trial, the algorithm performed well. With this latter trial full-valued data were used for the estimator, and no filter was included to compensate for any unmodelled dynamics and to reduce high-frequency components. A summary of the results for the first nine patients is given in Table 3.5 where the mean and SD indices are displayed for the duration of automatic control, mean drug dose consumption, the mean, RMSD and the SD. The last experiment was excluded since the 15 per cent target was different from the other trials.

The value of 3.12 per cent for the mean of standard deviation of $T1$ indicates that, generally, a steady level of blockade was obtained. Moreover, the fact that this value was so close to the value of the mean of the root-mean square deviation of $T1$ (3.41 per cent) implies that the degree of neuromuscular blockade was close to the target. 19.74 per cent as the mean value of the mean of $T1\%$ reinforces the argument that the individual $T1\%$ values were also close to the target. At this stage it is too soon to draw conclusions about any clear correlation between the patient's reaction to the

Table 3.4 *Summary of each patient's drug consumption dose*

Patient	Total number of points	Mean dose (mg kg^{-1} per min)	SD (mg kg^{-1} per min)
1†	197	6.65	2.35
2†	58	2.65	0.007
3‡	134	1.57	0.28
4‡	123	6.81	2.78
5†	97	6.77	1.64
6†	94	5.27	2.39
7§	387	5.38	4.43
8†	99	6.34	1.75
9†	318	4.03	2.98
10†	66	5.30	1.81

†1 mg ml^{-1} concentration.
‡500 µg ml^{-1} concentration.
§Both concentrations used.

Table 3.5 *Summary of patients' data (n = 9)*

Parameter	Mean	SD	Range
Automatic control duration (min)	62.33	33.04	30–130
Dose (µg kg^{-1} per min)	5.05	1.80	1.57–6.81
Mean of $T1$ (per cent)	19.74	1.37	17.50–21.85
RMSD of $T1$ (per cent)	3.41	1.69	1.07–6.89
SD of $T1$ (per cent)	3.12	1.68	1.02–6.89

initial bolus and the overall control performance. Suffice it to say that from the three control modes used (manual, fixed controller, self-adaptive), the self-adaptive scheme proved more robust and efficient. Moreover, the mean dose of muscle relaxant drug (5.05 µg kg^{-1} min^{-1}) was far lower than that which would be obtained by the anaesthetist using bolus doses, and most of all was lower than the range recommended by the manufacturers of atracurium.

3.7 Conclusions

The application of self-adaptive GPC to on-line control of muscle relaxation has been successful in achieving two primary goals. These are the maintaining of a steady level of paralysis with minimum deviation from the set-point, and the reduction of total muscle relaxant dosage. The algorithm has proved to be robust with respect to external disturbances, such as the heavy electrical interference from surgical diathermy. This is particularly important since operating theatres are 'electrically dirty' environments. The overall computer control system proved to be easy to manage, with most of the clinical trials being performed without the presence of an engineer. The anaesthetist gained confidence in the controller as the trials proceeded and demonstrated good response, particularly in the case of low-sensitivity patients where the bolus doses were clearly inadequate at the beginning of the operation. They were conducive to implementing changes in the design parameters of the GPC algorithm, providing that these were explained to them clearly and rationally. Throughout the work it was emphasized that the closed-loop regulation was an assistance to the anaesthetist, relieving him of tedium during normal periods of operation and enabling him to concentrate on the higher-level supervisory control aspects for which no form of automation can be envisaged. The ability of adaptive GPC to cope with massively varying patient parameters, particularly relating to gain changes, has been demonstrated in the clinical trials.

From a design viewpoint, GPC offers considerable flexibility for goal-achievement via its 'tuning knobs'. This has been exploited extensively in this work via simulation studies. In addition to off-line selection of design parameters via a SUN workstation, the prior validation of the total systems software via on-line microcomputer-based simulations significantly reduced the initial time required to achieve successful clinical experiments. Several aspects of GPC were explored during the trials, one of which was the use of full-valued data for the estimation rather than incremental data. Although the effect of eliminating the offset from the data is absent, the estimates obtained were consistent and little biased, a problem which could certainly have occurred with incremental results and wrong filter choice.

Summarizing the best settings for the GPC design parameters obtained from the simulations and trials leads to the following conclusions. If full-valued data are being used for the measurement vector then values of $(1, 20, 1, 5)$ for (N_1, N_2, NU, λ) were found to be appropriate. Conversely, for incremental data, values of $(1, 10, 1, 0)$ for (N_1, N_2, NU, λ) together with a second-order filter having slow roots of the form $T(z^{-1}) = (1 - 0.95z^{-1})^2$ were found to be desirable.

For comparison, work concerning the extension of the GPC approach to simultaneous multivariable control of unconsciousness as well as muscle relaxation has also been considered (see Chapter 4). In addition, the use of a multivariable feedforward approach (GPCF) has been investigated, and shows considerable promise (Linkens and Mahfouf, 1992). Also, the possibility of an intelligent control approach has been investigated by superimposing fault detection isolation and accommodation (FDIA) on top of the multivariable GPC strategy (Linkens and Mahfouf, 1994). The performance of the overall supervisory control scheme has been evaluated in a series of simulations whose results are very encouraging.

References

Åström, K.J. and Wittenmark, B., 1984, *Computer-Controlled Systems—Theory and Design*, New Jersey: Prentice Hall.

Belanger, P.R., 1983, On type-1 systems and the Clarke-Gawthrop regulator, *Automatica*, **19**, 91–4.

Bierman, G.J., 1977, *Factorization Methods for Discrete Sequential Estimation*, New York: Academic Press.

Birks, R., Huxley, H.E. and Katz, B., 1960, The fine structure of neuromuscular junction, *Journal of Physiology (London)*, **150**, 134.

Bradlow, H.S. and O'Mahony, J.R., 1990, 'PC-based muscle relaxation controller and monitor', presentation at the Annual Conference of the IEEE Engineering in Medicine and Biology Society, pp. 947–48.

Brown, B.H., Asbury, A.J., Linkens, D.A., Perks, P. and Anthony, M., 1980, Closed-loop control of muscle relaxation during surgery, *Clinical Physics and Physiological Measurements*, **1**, 203–10.

Cass, N.M., Lampard, D.G., Brown, W.A. and Coles, J.R., 1976, Computer-controlled muscle relaxation: a comparison of four muscle relaxants in sheep, *Anaesthesia in Intensive Care*, **4**, 16–22.

Clarke, D.W., 1985, 'Implementation of self-tuning controllers', in Harris, C.J. and Billings, S.A. (Eds) *Self-tuning and Adaptive Control: Theory and Application* (IEE Control Engineering, **15**, 146–7).

Clarke, D.W. and Gawthrop, P.J., 1975, Self-tuning controller, *IEE Proceedings*, PtD, **122**, 929–34.

Clarke, D.W., Mohtadi, C. and Tuffs, P.S., 1987a, Generalised predictive control—Part I, the basic algorithm, *Automatica*, **23**, 137–48.

Clarke, D.W., Mohtadi, C. and Tuffs, P.S., 1987b, Generalised predictive control—Part II, extensions and interpretations, *Automatica*, **23**, 149–60.

Cutler, C.R. and Ramaker, B.L., 1980, 'Dynamic matrix control—a computer control algorithm', presentation at the Joint American Control Conference, San Francisco, USA, paper WP5-B.

Dale, H.H. and Feldberg, W., 1934, Chemical transmission at motor nerve endings in voluntary muscle, *Journal of Physiology (London)*, **81**, 39.

De Keyser, R.M.C. and Van Cauwenberghe, A.R., 1983, 'Microcomputer-controlled servo system based on self-tuning adaptive long-range prediction', in Tzafestas, S.G. and Hamza, M.H. (Eds) *Methods and Applications of Measurement and Control*, pp. 583–7, Canada: ACTA Press.

Denai, M., Linkens, D.A., Asbury, A.J., MacLeod, A.D. and Gray, W.M., 1990, Self-tuning PID control of atracurium induced muscle relaxation in surgical patients, *IEE Proceedings*, PtD, **137**, 261–72.

Ebert, J., Carrol, S.K. and Bradley, E.L., 1986, Closed-loop feedback control of muscle relaxation with vecuronium in surgical patients, *Anaesthesia and Anaesthesiology*, **65**, S44.

Jacobs, O.L.R., Bullingham, R.E.S., McQuay, H.J. and Reasbeck, M.P., 1982, 'On-line estimation in the control of post-operative pain', in Proceedings of the 6th IFAC Symposium on Identification of System Parameter Estimates, Washington, USA.

Jannett, T.C. and De Falque, R.J., 1990, 'Integrated instrumentation of closed-loop feedback control of muscle relaxation: initial clinical trials', presentation at the Annual Conference of the IEEE Engineering in Medicine and Biology Society, pp. 945–6.

Linkens, D.A. and Asbury, A.J., 1985, Non-invasive measurement of vecuronium pharmacokinetics and pharmocodynamics using systems identification techniques, *British Journal of Anaesthesia*, **57**, 829P.

Linkens, D.A. and Mahfouf, M., 1992, Generalized predictive control with feedforward (GPCF) for multivariable anaesthesia, *International Journal of Control*, **56**, 1039–57.

Linkens, D.A. and Mahfouf, M., 1994, Supervisory generalized predictive control (GPC) and fault detection for multivariable anaesthesia, *IEE Proceedings*, PtD, **141**, 70–82.

Linkens, D.A., Menad, M. and Asbury, A.J., 1985, Smith predictor and self-tuning control of muscle relaxant drug administration, *IEE Proceedings*, PtD, **132**, 212–8.

Linkens, D.A., Asbury, A.J., Rimmer, S.J. and Menad, M., 1982, Identification and control of muscle relaxant anaesthesia, *IEE Proceedings*, PtD, **129**, 136–41.

MacLeod, A.D., Asbury, A.J., Gray, W.M. and Linkens, D.A., 1989, Automatic control of neuromuscular block with atracurium, *British Journal of Anaesthesia*, **63**, 31–5.

Mahfouf, M., 1991, 'Adaptive control and identification for on-line drug infusion in anaesthesia', unpublished PhD thesis, Department of Automatic Control and Systems Engineering, University of Sheffield, UK.

Mahfouf, M., Linkens, D.A., Asbury, A.J., Gray, W.M. and Peacock, J.E., 1992, Generalized predictive control (GPC) in the operating theatre, *IEE Proceedings*, PtD, **139**, 404–20.

Menad, M., 1984, 'Feedback control of drug administration for muscle relaxation', unpublished PhD thesis, Department of Automatic Control and Systems Engineering, University of Sheffield, UK.

Olkkola, K.T. and Schwilden, H., 1991, Use of a pharmacokinetic-dynamic model for the automatic feedback control of atracurium, *European Journal of Pharmacology*, **49**, 293–6.

Paton, W.D.M. and Waud, D.R., 1967, The margin of safety of neuromuscular blockade transmission, *Journal of Physiology (London)*, **191**, 59.

Rametti, L.B., 1985, 'On-line control of d-tubocurarine-induced muscle relaxation', unpublished PhD thesis, University of Cape Town, South Africa.

Rametti, L.B., Bradlow, H.S. and Uys, P.C., 1985, On-line parameter estimation and control of d-tubocurarine-induced muscle relaxation, *Medical Biology and Engineering Computation*, **23**, 556–64.

Robinson, B.D. and Clarke, D.W., 1991, Robustness effects of a prefilter in generalized predictive control, *IEE Proceedings*, PtD, **138**, 2–8.

Sheiner, L.B., Stanski, D.R., Vozeh, S., Miller, R.D. and Ham, J., 1979, Simultaneous modelling of pharmocokinetics and pharmacodynamics: application to d-tubocurarine, *Clinical Pharmacology and Therapeutics*, **25**, 358.

Sheppard, L.C., Shotts, J.F., Robertson, N.F., Wallace, F.D. and Kouchoukos, N.T., 1979, 'Computer-controlled infusion of vasoactive drugs in post-cardiac surgical patients', IEEE Conference on Engineering Medicine and Biology, Denver, Colorado, pp. 280–4.

Tuffs, P.S. and Clarke, D.W., 1985, Self-tuning control of offset: a unified approach, *IEE Proceedings*, PtD, **132**, 100–10.

Van den Bosch, P.P.J., 1979, 'PSI: an extended interactive block oriented simulation program', presentation at the IFAC Symposium on CAD Control Systems, pp. 223–8.

Wait, C.M., Goat, V.A. and Blogg, C.E., 1987, Feedback control of neuromuscular blockade. A simple system for infusion of atracurium, *Anaesthesia*, **42**, 1212–7.

Ward, S., Neill, E.A.M., Weatherley, B.C., and Corall, I.M., 1983, Pharmacokinetics of atracurium besylate in healthy patients (after a single iv bolus dose), *British Journal of Anaesthesia*, **55**, 113.

Waud, D.R. and Waud, B.E., 1971, The relation between tetanic fade and receptor occlusion in the presence of competitive neuromuscular block, *Anaesthesiology*, **35**, 456.

Weatherley, B.C., Williams, S.G. and Neil, E.A.M., 1983, Pharmacokinetics, pharmacodynamics and dose response relationship of atracurium administered i.v., *British Journal of Anaesthesia*, **55**, 39S.

Webster, N.R. and Cohen, A.T., 1987, Closed-loop administration of atracurium. Steady-state neuromuscular blockade during surgery using a computer controlled closed-loop atracurium infusion, *Anaesthesia*, **42**, 1085–91.

Wellstead, P.E., 1980, 'Self-tuning control systems: the pole-zero assignment approach', presentation at the SERC Vacation School on Computer Control, University of Sheffield, UK, September, pp. 9.1–9.34.

Whiting, B. and Kelman, A.W., 1980, The modelling of drug response, *Clinical Science*, **59**, 311–4.

Ziegler, J.G. and Nichols, N.B., 1942, Optimum settings for automatic controllers, *Transactions of the American Society of Mechanical Engineers*, **64**, 759.

Chapter 4
A comparative study of generalized predictive control (GPC) and intelligent self-organizing fuzzy logic control (SOFLC) for multivariable anaesthesia

M. Mahfouf and M. F. Abbod

4.1 Introduction

In recent years, much attention has been given in control systems research and development to algorithms that have learning properties. Two common branches in a taxonomy of learning algorithms comprise self-adaptive systems (e.g. self-tuning control) and self-organizing systems. In both cases, one is concerned with the control of systems with unknown or time-varying structure or parameters. The purpose of this chapter is to explore these two forms of learning control in the area of biomedicine where structural uncertainty is the rule rather than the exception.

Much attention at both theoretical and applied levels has been given to self-tuning control based on quantitative models and algorithms. The approach was first proposed by Kalman (1958) who made an attempt to implement a self-tuner on an analogue computer. Figure 4.1 represents the structure of a self-tuner which immediately suggests that there is a constant but unknown parametric model which forms a fairly accurate description of the process response. The regulator of Figure 4.1 consists of three parts: the process to be regulated, a recursive estimator of the parameters emerging from the above model based on input–output data, and a control design

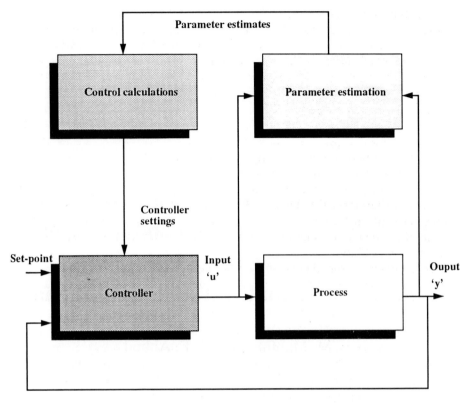

Figure 4.1 *Block diagram of a self-tuning regulator.*

procedure. However, despite the inclusion of all of these blocks in the structure, the algorithm can only pretend to the self-tuning property *if, as the number of samples approaches infinity, the controller parameters tend to those corresponding to an exactly known process model* (Clarke, 1988). Concomitant advantages in self-tuners, which constitute in effect their *raison d'être*, are their unchallenged robustness when applied to unknown or time-varying systems and their ability to track changes in process parameters, hence, they are known as adaptive controllers. However, the self-tuners' real power lies in the fact that when the process parameters are unknown or slowly time-varying, they can be replaced by their estimates (provided by the recursive estimator block of Figure 4.1) by evoking the principle of certainty equivalence (Åström and Wittenmark, 1984) which states that the self-tuning properties should still hold even if the *true* process parameters are represented by their estimates providing they are not totally biased. The principle represents, in fact, the cornerstone of the theory as it facilitates the solving of many practical problems, especially those of a non-linear nature.

Self-tuners can, however, be based on several techniques which although different in structure use the same philosophy, i.e. regulating around a particular operating point, be it a single input–single output (SISO) or a multi-input–multi-output (MIMO) situation. Space prohibits mentioning all of them, but for high-performance objectives pole-placement (Wellstead et al., 1979), general minimum variance (GMV) (Clarke and Gawthrop, 1975) and recently generalized predictive control (GPC) (Clarke et al., 1987a; Clarke et al., 1987b) are among the best known algorithms. They fall into two categories: explicit and implicit algorithms. The first category implies that the regulator parameters are updated indirectly via estimation of the process parameters, whereas in the second category, and by a proper choice of the model structure, the regulator parameters are updated directly avoiding, therefore, the design calculations. GPC, as used in this chapter, falls into the first category, and represents a currently popular algorithm which has shown considerable success in both theoretical extensibility and practical feasibility.

In contrast to the theory of self-tuning adaptive control, another area which has seen growing interest among control engineers is that of intelligent control. It, like the former technique, had to wait until significant development had occurred in computer technology before its associated algorithms could be implemented. Indeed, for many years it has been the scientists' dream to be able to duplicate as faithfully as possible a human's behaviour simply by using computers. One consequence of this, as far as feedback control systems are concerned, is that if the designed control strategy bears similarities to that of a human brain, the control could in some sense be optimal. Fuzzy control is one qualitative strategy that endeavours to do that, and originates in the theory of fuzzy logic, first introduced by Zadeh (1965, 1973). The theory has proved to be partly successful in representing fuzziness in human decision-making behaviour. From a structural point of view the controller is represented by a set of rules built via guidelines normally provided by an experienced operator well aware of the process under investigation. Consequently, the controller looks at the process as a black box and does not need an accurate model description. Following some successful applications of fuzzy control in automation by pioneers such as Assilian and Mamdani (1974), the so-called self-organizing fuzzy logic controller (SOFLC) was later introduced by Procyk (1977). The algorithm is able to realize adaptation by building its fuzzy rules on-line as it controls the process, altering and adding as many rules as it judges necessary from off-line criteria. This approach has seen several successful applications (Daley and Gill, 1986; Harris and Moore, 1989; Linkens and Hasnain, 1991) and it is suggested that it represents a serious contender to quantitative approaches for control.

Hitherto, little work has been reported apart from that by Al-Assaf (1988) in which the two approaches, different perhaps in their concept but having the same aim, are experimentally compared, and in which disadvantages as well as advantages of both strategies are discussed. The experimental area is that of control of anaesthetic drug administration in the operating theatre.

Automated on-line drug infusion schemes for patient care have been investigated in recent years for a number of medical applications (Linkens and Hacisalihzade, 1990). While fixed control structures, such as a three-term PID, may be satisfactory in certain situations, it has been found that instability can occur in hypertensive blood pressure control for post-operative patients (Sheppard et al., 1979) and in muscle relaxant anaesthesia (Linkens et al., 1982). This is due to very large patient-to-patient variability in pharmacological parameters, and also due to parameter drift during operations. Thus, adaptive control offers the possibility of improved on-line performance for drug infusion as already seen in Chapter 3. The development of multivariable GPC and some initial simulation results are described in Linkens et al. (1991). The use of intelligent control strategies has also been considered for SISO muscle relaxant drug administration (Linkens and Hasnain, 1991).

To investigate the performance associated with the two approaches of multivariable self-tuning adaptive GPC and multivariable SOFLC, we have considered the possibility of simultaneous control of relaxation and unconsciousness during anaesthesia. To do this, it was necessary to identify an adequate two-input, two-output mathematical model, which is described in Section 4.2. Although the model presented here is well defined structurally, it should be noted that in reality there is considerable uncertainty attached to it. The model does, however, offer a realistic multivariable challenge to the two approaches, particularly because of the severe non-linearity in the relaxant pharmacodynamics. Following a brief review of the multivariable GPC method in Section 4.3 and the multivariable SOFLC in Section 4.4, a series of comparative simulation results follow in Section 4.5, with concluding remarks from the study in Section 4.6.

4.2. Identification of the multivariable anaesthetic model

Chapter 3 outlined a number of on-line drug infusion strategies in medicine that have been developed in recent years. On-line control of neuromuscular blockade (muscle relaxation) and depth of anaesthesia (unconsciousness) have been investigated by several researchers (e.g. Robb et al., 1988; Schwilden et al., 1987 and Schwilden et al., 1989). Both of these areas are prime responsibilities for anaesthetists in the operating theatre. It has already been mentioned in the previous chapter that, for muscle relaxation, continuous monitoring can be done via evoked EMG responses using commercial instruments such as a Datex Relaxograph. The drug used throughout this study is similar to the one previously considered (see

Chapter 3), i.e. atracurium, which is a modern fast-acting agent suitable for infusion via a motor-driven syringe pump. In contrast, depth of anaesthesia is more difficult to quantify accurately. Thus one approach has been to merge a number of clinical signs and on-line data to produce an expert system advisor for the anaesthetist similar to the one described in Chapter 2 and called RESAC. In spite of the multi-sensor nature of the above approach, it appears that during the majority of operating periods when no unusual emergency conditions occur, a good indication of depth of anaesthesia can be obtained from a single on-line monitored variable. Thus, the use of arterial blood pressure, monitored via an inflatable cuff using a Dinamap instrument, has been investigated for feedback control with simple PI strategies by Robb *et al.* (1988, 1991). In this case the control actuation is via a stepper motor driving the dial on a gas vaporizer. This concept forms the basis for the modelling and control aspects of unconsciousness in the following study. In particular, the drug isoflurane has been considered throughout, it being commonly used in modern surgery.

The necessary transfer function components for the model used in this study have been elicited via a combination of literature surveys and clinical experiments conducted by our research group. The individual pathways are described in the following sections.

4.2.1 The atracurium mathematical model

4.2.1.1 Pharmacokinetics

The study described in Chapter 3 allowed us to obtain the following equation:

$$G_1(s) = \frac{9.94(1 + 10.64s)}{(1 + 3.08s)(1 + 34.42s)}. \tag{4.1}$$

Equation (4.1) describes the pharmacokinetics of the muscle relaxation system relating to the drug atracurium.

4.2.1.2 Pharmacodynamics

Similarly, to characterize different aspects of drug effect a hypothetical 'effect' compartment is introduced in the above structure leading to the following transfer function:

$$G_{11}(s) = \frac{K_1(1 + T_4 s) e^{-\tau_1 s}}{(1 + T_1 s)(1 + T_2 s)(1 + T_3 s)} \tag{4.2}$$

where $\tau_1 = 1$ min, $K_1 = 1$, $T_1 = 4.81$ min, $T_2 = 34.42$ min, $T_3 = 3.08$ min, $T_4 = 10.64$ min. Moreover, the following non-linearity represented by a Hill equation is used to relate the effect to a specific drug concentration:

$$E_{\text{eff}} = E_{\max} \frac{X_E^\alpha}{X_E^\alpha + (X_E(50))^\alpha} \quad (4.3)$$

where X_E is the drug concentration, α the power and $X_E(50)$ the drug concentration at 50% effect with the following values:

$E_{\max} = 100\%$, $X_E(50) = 0.404\ \mu\text{g ml}^{-1}$, $\alpha = 2.98$.

4.2.2 The isoflurane unconsciousness model

There is no doubt that anything that is related to the human brain represents a very complex entity, and anaesthesia or unconsciousness which affects the brain has indeed been the subject of many conflicting views even about its definition! However, agreement about its objective has been reached and this can also be regarded as its general definition: *it is to produce a reversible pharmacological state in which the patient, while being subject to surgical stimulation, has no memory of events and whose physiological variables lie in the zone appropriate to natural sleep, and who makes no reflex response.* Halothane, enflurane and isoflurane are common inhalational agents known to produce adequate anaesthesia. There is no direct method of measuring depth of anaesthesia. Previous research work, namely by Schwilden *et al.* (1987, 1989) and Savege *et al.* (1978), used quantitative EEG (electroencephalogram) analysis in humans to give an indication of the anaesthetic state. However, the interpretation of the tracings is a difficult and subjective task. The information proved unreliable even when interpreted by experienced staff, since the characteristic patterns are often disturbed by factors such as anoxia, surgical stimulations, and anaesthetic agents used (Breckenridge and Aitkenhead, 1983). Consequently, anaesthetists have to resort to the merger of several clinical signs such as blood pressure, respiration, heart rate, etc, to obtain the closest possible indication of how lightly anaesthetized the patient is. Indeed, in a study conducted by Asbury (1990), anaesthetists were asked to give a personal rank for the relative importance of ten clinical signs. These signs were ranked on a scale of 1 to 10 based on the mean of these personal ranks assigned to each one of them. Table 4.1 illustrates the results of such a survey. From these ten clinical signs investigated, blood pressure has been used as one variable to give indication of depth of anaesthesia. Robb and coworkers (1991) describe a system that controls systolic arterial pressure (*SAP*) using enflurane and morphine. The algorithm, a simple PI controller, achieved a quality of control judged to be satisfactory, and in most operations the patient

Table 4.1 *Anaesthetists' classification of the ten clinical signs indicating unconsciousness by order of importance*

Clinical Sign	Mean of Raw Ranks	Order of Mean Rank
Movement and response to surgery	7.40	1
Respiration rate	5.80	2
Heart rate	5.30	3
Low muscle tone	5.00	4
Lacrimation	4.90	5
Arterial pressure	4.84	6
Sweating	4.77	7
Pupil position	4.60	8
Pupil diameter	3.40	9
Capillary refill	2.50	10

recovered fairly quickly. It was concluded from this study that when no emergency conditions occur, blood pressure could be used to provide good indication of the patient's anaesthetic state. In fact, recent published work by Schils and coworkers (1987) used mean arterial pressure and a measure of EEG frequency to control halothane anaesthesia via an on–off control strategy which was found to be less sensitive to parameter mismatches. It has also been argued that the lowest blood pressure that occurs normally during sleep is 15 to 20 per cent less than the average pressure whilst awake. Elderly and hypotensive persons have a margin at about 10 per cent. Consequently, mean arterial pressure (MAP) is used as the second variable for the multivariable model considered throughout this study. Isoflurane, a relatively new agent which has gained popularity over halothane, is used as the anaesthetic agent throughout.

Hence, in a study conducted by Millard and coworkers (1988), step responses to changes in inspired concentration of isoflurane from a vaporizer were performed. The patients' blood pressure responses showed a transport delay which was subject to slight variations due primarily to breathing cycles of about 6 seconds. In fact in the five patients studied, plus twelve in other similar conducted experiments (Millard *et al.*, 1986), dead-times in the range 16 to 30 seconds have been observed. Moreover, if the changes in inhaled isoflurane concentration are small (≤ 5 per cent), the responses could be approximated by linear characteristics. However, if the changes do not fall within this range, the responses are in general non-linear and time-varying.

Thus, a first-order linear model with dead-time has been adopted, having a time-constant of 1–2 minutes. The magnitude of the time-constant is long enough to absorb some inaccuracy of dead-time estimate due to breathing variation. On the other hand, in order to estimate the steady-state gain, it is assumed that a relatively sensitive patient needs 2 per cent isoflurane for a 30 mmHg reduction in MAP. Therefore, the model describing variations of blood pressure to small changes in inhaled isoflurane concentration can be written as:

$$G_2(s) = \frac{\Delta MAP(s)}{U_2(s)} = \frac{K_2 e^{-\tau_2 s}}{(1 + T_5 s)} \qquad (4.4)$$

where, $\tau_2 = 25$ s, $T_5 = 2$ min, $K_2 = -15$ mmHg/per cent.

4.2.3 Interactive component model

4.2.3.1 'Atracurium to arterial pressure' interaction

This interaction has been investigated in human beings and there seems to be a small increase in heart rate when the above drug is administered. This is said to be due to the release of local cathecolamines from the nerve terminals around the heart. It is a transient effect lasting no more than a few minutes and does not appear in every patient (Asbury, 1990). As an initial approximation, therefore, this pathway has been ignored in the dynamic model. It should be noted, however, that this may not be appropriate for other drugs used for unconsciousness, such as other inhalational agents like enflurane.

4.2.3.2 'Isoflurane to muscle relaxation' interaction

To identify this type of interaction which is small but significant, an experiment was performed by Asbury (1990), in which a patient, a man of 47 without a kidney but having a renal transplant, was anaesthetized. Step changes of 0–1 per cent isoflurane infusions were superimposed on steady relaxation levels achieved 50 minutes into the operation via atracurium infusion. Transient responses for both *on* and *off* conditions were obtained, and dynamics estimated for each case.

Because there was not a large difference between the phases, an averaged transfer function was obtained as follows:

$$G_4(s) = \frac{K_4 e^{-\tau_4 s}}{(1 + T_6 s)(1 + T_7 s)} \qquad (4.5)$$

where, $\tau_4 = 1$ min, $T_6 = 2.83$ min, $T_7 = 1.25$ min, $K_4 = 0.27$.

4.2.4 The overall multivariable anaesthetic model

In light of the above identification studies, the overall linear multivariable system combining muscle relaxation together with unconsciousness (in terms

A comparative study of generalized predictive control (GPC)

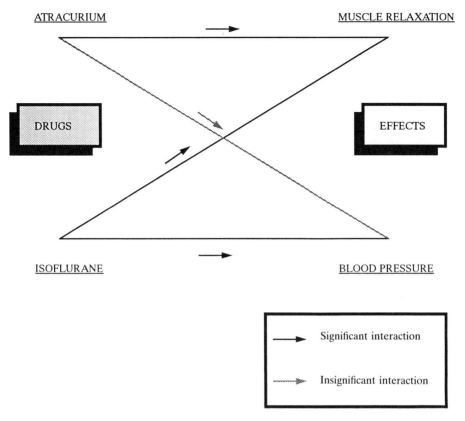

Figure 4.2 *Diagram representing the different pathways forming the multivariable anaesthetic model structure.*

of blood pressure measurements), whose components are also illustrated in Figure 4.2, can be summarized by the following system:

$$\begin{bmatrix} \text{Paralysis} \\ \Delta MAP \end{bmatrix} = \begin{bmatrix} G_{11}(s) & G_{12}(s) \\ 0 & G_{22}(s) \end{bmatrix} \begin{bmatrix} U_1 \\ U_2 \end{bmatrix} \quad (4.6)$$

where,

$$G_{11}(s) = \frac{1.0\,e^{-s}(1+10.64s)}{(1+3.08s)(1+4.81s)(1+34.42s)}$$

$$G_{12}(s) = \frac{0.27\,e^{-s}}{(1+2.83s)(1+1.25s)}$$

$$G_{22}(s) = \frac{-15.0\,e^{-0.42s}}{(1+2s)}.$$

Finally, the overall *non-linear* multivariable system combining all the effects is obtained by including the non-linearity described in Section 4.2.1, which involves the atracurium drug only, since the other drug-effects are considered to reflect linear characteristics within a range already specified in the preceding sections.

4.3 Review of multivariable GPC controller

As already mentioned in the previous chapter, the theme of predictive control and that of GPC has dealt successfully with many problems currently encountered in modern control theory, i.e. non-linearities, time-delay, offsets, etc. Its multivariable version, which no longer requires prior information with respect to the interactor matrix (Mohtadi, 1986), has already been used in many successful applications which include cement mills (Al-Assaf, 1988), and an industrial soap spray drying tower (Lambert, 1987). Its popularity has also been enhanced recently by the development of the frequency response characteristics for the whole multivariable structure (Mohtadi *et al.*, 1991). Its basic and extended forms were used in this study, and the necessary design parameters are referred to in the following.

Consider the following m input and n output, linear, discrete time-system where the interactions are represented in a feedforward manner (Kam *et al.*, 1985)

$$\mathbf{A}(z^{-1})Y(t) = \mathbf{B}(z^{-1})U(t-1) + \mathbf{C}(z^{-1})\frac{\zeta(t)}{\Delta} \tag{4.7}$$

where

$$\mathbf{A}(z^{-1}) = \mathbf{I} + A_1 z^{-1} + A_2 z^{-2} + \ldots + A_{na} z^{-na}$$

I is the indentity matrix and the individual $\mathbf{A}_i$ are diagonal matrices

$$\mathbf{B}(z^{-1}) = B_0 + B_1 z^{-1} + B_2 z^{-2} + \ldots + B_{nb} z^{-nb}$$
$$\mathbf{C}(z^{-1}) = C_0 + C_1 z^{-1} + C_2 z^{-2} + \ldots + C_p z^{-p}$$

and,

$$Y(t) = [y_1(t), y_2(t), \ldots, y_n(t)]$$
$$U(t) = [u_1(t), u_2(t), \ldots, u_m(t)]$$
$$\Delta = 1 - z^{-1}$$

$Y(t)$, $U(t)$ are vectors of 'n' measurable outputs $y(t)$ and 'm' measurable inputs $u(t)$ respectively. $\zeta(t)$ denotes a vector of uncorrelated sequences of

A comparative study of generalized predictive control (GPC)

random variables with zero mean and covariance σ. Any extra time-delay can be absorbed in the structure of the $\mathbf{B}(z^{-1})$ polynomial.

GPC considers a cost function of the form

$$\begin{cases} J = E[(Q_1 + Q_2)] \\ Q1 = \sum_{j=N_1}^{N_2} [P\hat{Y}(t+j) - \omega(t+j)]^T [P\hat{Y}(t+j) - \omega(t+j)] \\ Q2 = \sum_{j=1}^{N_2} [\Delta U(t+j-1)^T \Lambda(j) \Delta U(t+j-1)] \end{cases} \quad (4.8)$$

where N_1 is the minimum costing horizon, N_2 is the maximum costing horizon, NU is the control horizon, ω is the future set-point, usually presumed known, $\Lambda(j)$ is the control weighting sequence. Omitting z^{-1} one can write:

$$P\hat{Y}(t+j) = \bar{\bar{G}}_j \Delta U(t+j-1) + \Psi(t+j) \quad (4.9)$$

$$\Psi(t+j) = \bar{G}_j \Delta U^f(t-1) + \bar{F}_j Y^f(t) \quad (4.10)$$

$$TP = E_j A \Delta + z^{-j} \bar{F}_j \quad (4.11)$$

$$P(z^{-1}) = P_N(z^{-1})(P_D(z^{-1}))^{-1} \quad (P(1) = \mathbf{I}) \quad (4.12)$$

$$T(z^{-1}) = T_1(z^{-1}) \mathbf{I} \quad (4.13)$$

$$T_1(z^{-1}) = 1 + t_1 z^{-1} + \ldots + t_{nt} z^{-nt} \quad (4.14)$$

$$\bar{F}_j = F_j(P_D)^{-1} \quad (4.15)$$

where superscript f denotes signals filtered by $1/T_1(z^{-1})$

$$E_j B = \bar{\bar{G}}_j T + z^{-j} \bar{G}_j. \quad (4.16)$$

where

$$\bar{\bar{G}}_j = \bar{\bar{G}}_0 + \bar{\bar{G}}_1 z^{-1} + \ldots + \bar{\bar{G}}_{j-1} z^{-j+1}$$

$$\bar{G}_j = \bar{G}_{j0} + \bar{G}_{j1} z^{-1} + \ldots + \bar{G}_{j(i-1)} z^{-i+1}$$

$i = $ from 1 to max(degree of B, degree of T)

$1 \leq j \leq N_2$

P and T are user-chosen polynomials in z^{-1}. $1/T_1(z^{-1})$ is chosen as a low-pass filter, and is the so-called observer polynomial for the predictor of

Equation (4.10) (Åström and Wittenmark, 1984; Robinson and Clarke, 1991; Shook et al., 1991 and McIntosh et al., 1989). P is referred to as the model-following polynomial, and the condition $P(1) = \mathbf{I}$ ensures an offset-free response (Clarke, 1985).

The minimization of the cost function described in Equation (4.8) leads to the following projected control increment:

$$\Delta U(t) = \bar{g}^{\mathrm{T}}(\omega - \Psi) \tag{4.17}$$

where,

$$\Psi = [\Psi(t + N_1), \ldots, \Psi(t + N_2)]$$

$\bar{g}^T$ is the first m rows of the matrix $(G_\mathrm{d}^\mathrm{T} G_\mathrm{d} + \Lambda \mathbf{I})^{-1} G_\mathrm{d}^\mathrm{T}$

and G_d is the dynamic step-response matrix of the form given in Clarke et al. (1987a).

It is worth noting that the choice of a P canonical form for Equation (4.7) (implying a diagonal structure for the $\mathbf{A}(z^{-1})$ matrices) and identical elements for the matrix polynomial $\mathbf{T}(z^{-1})$ reduces considerably the computational burden, and this structure was the one adopted throughout this study.

4.4 Review of multivariable SOC using fuzzy logic

As illustrated in Figure 4.3, the self-organizing fuzzy logic controller (SOFLC) comprises two main levels. The first level consists of a simple fuzzy controller, whereas the second acts as a monitor and a performance evaluator of the previous level and is usually called the self-organizing mechanism. It includes four blocks: the performance index, the process reference model, the rules modifier, and the state buffer.

In the first level, the input signal to the controller is taken at each sampling instant in the form of error and change-in-error. Each signal is mapped to its correspondent discrete level by using the error and change-in-error scaling factors respectively, and sent to the SOFLC. According to the control rules issued by the second level the SOFLC calculates the outputs with respect to the inputs. The output signals are scaled to actual values using the output scaling factors and afterwards sent to the process being controlled.

The first level is a simple fuzzy logic controller, containing a set of control rules. The latter are derived from linguistic expressions and interpreted by fuzzy logic (King and Mamdani, 1977). Many parameters affect the design of this crucial part such as: the fuzzification procedure, the choice of the input and output variables, the type of fuzzy control rules, the implication

A comparative study of generalized predictive control (GPC)

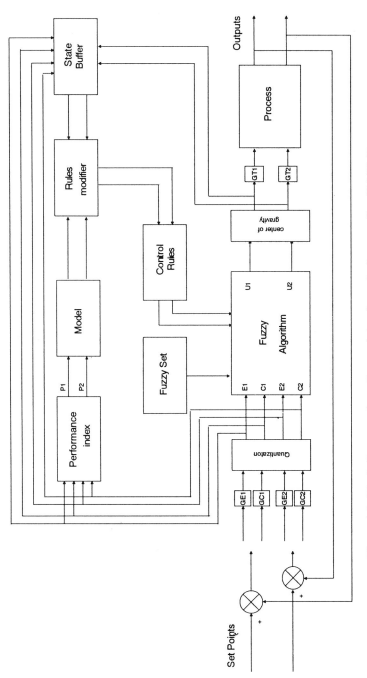

Figure 4.3 Block diagram of a self-organizing fuzzy logic controller (SOFLC).

and inference procedure, as well as the defuzzification operation. In this work, the fuzzy sets associated with the input and the output variables were formed upon discrete universes of discourse of 14, 13, and 15 elements for error, change-in-error, and output, respectively. The choice of the membership function forming a particular fuzzy set is based on Mizumoto's findings (Mizumoto, 1988) that the fuzzy sets are best selected when the fuzzy labels are not isolated and not too much overlapped. Therefore, the linguistic labels are the same as those reported previously in other studies, where the terms PO and NO respectively define values slightly below zero. They were mainly introduced to obtain finer control around the equilibrium state. The control rules are linguistic conditional statements, symbolized in the form of a relational matrix **R**, with the fuzzy output being obtained using Zadeh's compositional rule of inference (Zadeh, 1973; Harris and Moore, 1989). Several procedures allow one to reduce this fuzzy set to a single value, via 'defuzzification'. Among these methods are the mean of maxima (MOM) procedure (Assilian and Mamdani, 1974), and the centroid of area method (COA) (Harris and Moore, 1989). Because the latter allows for smoother variations in the control signal, it was adopted in these studies.

The second level is basically the part that realizes the adaptation referred to above. Based on observations of the trajectory of the process being controlled, any deviation from the desired path is corrected by modifying the rules responsible for that particular undesirable deviation.

The performance index function is an evaluation criterion of the controller performance, and is derived from linguistic conditional statements using standard fuzzy operations as shown in Table 4.2. The entries in this table have the usual fuzzy linguistic connotation of N = negative, P = positive, O = zero, B = big, S = small, and M = medium. The rule modification procedure can be explained as follows. Assuming that the process has a time-delay of m samples, then the control action at sample $(nT - mT)$ has most contributed to the process performance at the sampling instant nT,

Table 4.2 *The performance index table*

	Change in Error						
Error	NB	NM	NS	ZO	PS	PM	PB
NB	NB	NB	NB	NM	NM	NS	ZO
NM	NB	NB	NM	NM	NS	ZO	PS
NS	NB	NB	NS	NS	ZO	PS	PM
NO	NB	NM	NS	ZO	ZO	PM	PM
PO	NB	NM	ZO	ZO	PS	PM	PB
PS	NM	NS	ZO	PS	PS	PB	PB
PM	NS	ZO	PS	PM	PM	PB	PB
PB	ZO	PS	PM	PM	PB	PB	PB

A comparative study of generalized predictive control (GPC) 93

thus the modification is made to the controller output mT samples earlier, and therefore the rule to be included will be

$$E(nT - mT) \to CE(nT - mT) \to U(nT - mT) + P_i(nT) \quad (4.18)$$

where $P_i(nT)$ is issued by the performance index. To avoid contradictory rules, only rules with similar antecedents to the new rule must be removed. An algorithm for rules removal has been presented (Daley and Gill, 1986) which can be expressed linguistically as:

Delete all the rules that are the same ones as to be added.

The process reference model relates the input changes to the output changes, and can be derived simply by considering a two-input two-output process characterizing a general state-space equation (Procyk and Mamdani, 1979). For small changes in the inputs, one can write:

$$\begin{bmatrix} \Delta X \\ \Delta Y \end{bmatrix} = \begin{bmatrix} T \partial \dot{X} \\ T \partial \dot{Y} \end{bmatrix} = M \begin{bmatrix} \Delta U \\ \Delta V \end{bmatrix} \quad (4.19)$$

where M is regarded as an incremental model of the process. Therefore, if the performance index outputs are $P_{i1}(nT)$ and $P_{i2}(nT)$, then the necessary input corrections $P_{o1}(nT)$ and $P_{o2}(nT)$ are given by:

$$\begin{bmatrix} P_{i1}(nT) \\ P_{i2}(nT) \end{bmatrix} = M^{-1} \begin{bmatrix} P_{o1}(nT) \\ P_{o2}(nT) \end{bmatrix} \quad (4.20)$$

where

$$M = \begin{bmatrix} m_{11} & m_{12} \\ m_{21} & m_{22} \end{bmatrix}.$$

The model M should be scaled from real values to normalized values using scaling factors for each variable, details of which follow. Thus,

$$P_i(nT) = (GT)^{-1}(M)^{-1}(GY)^{-1}P_o(nT) \quad (4.21)$$

P_o should not exceed the maximum or the minimum range defined initially. The condition is therefore satisfied if:

$$\begin{aligned} (S_1)^{-1} &= \frac{m_{11}}{GY_1 GT_1} + \frac{m_{12}}{GY_1 GT_2} \leq 1 \\ (S_2)^{-1} &= \frac{m_{21}}{GY_2 GT_1} + \frac{m_{22}}{GY_2 GT_2} \leq 1. \end{aligned} \quad (4.22)$$

This yields:

$$M = \text{scale}\,(GT)^{-1}(M)^{-1}(GY)^{-1} \quad (4.23)$$

where

$$\text{scale} = \min[S_1, S_2].$$

The state buffer is a FIFO (first-in/first-out) register which records the values of the error and change-in-error, as well as the output. The output from the register will be recorded after a time equal to the delay-in-reward (DLS). This latter parameter plays a vital role in modifying the rules, since it specifies which input in the past contributed to the present performance. It is suggested that a value equal to the dead-time of the process is appropriate (Procyk, 1977).

4.4.1 Selection of the controller parameters

As mentioned before, the different variables used are scaled before entering the algorithm, and the selection of the respective scaling factors is not entirely subjective since their magnitude is a compromise between the sensitivity during the rise time and the required steady-state accuracy. Useful guidelines leading to the choice of these parameters are given below, and these were used in initial tuning of the simulation results which follow.

The error scaling factor was chosen according to the percentage value and is given by the following:

$$GE = \frac{6.0}{\text{full error}}$$

$$\text{full error} = \text{error percentage} \times \text{set-point} \quad (4.24)$$

The value of the error percentage (EP) decides the sensitivity of the previous scaling factor. Associated high values mean small scaling factors, while low values imply large ones.

The change-in-error scaling factor (GC) was chosen according to the maximum real change-in-error for each variable giving:

$$GC = \frac{6.0}{\text{max real error change}}. \quad (4.25)$$

In contrast to the previous ones, the output scaling factor was chosen to accommodate the controller output to the process input according to the following relation:

$$GT = \frac{\text{max process input}}{\text{max controller output}}. \quad (4.26)$$

Further details about recommendations for the selection of these scaling factors can be found in Linkens and Abbod (1992).

4.5 Simulation studies

The simulation studies were undertaken in two parts, the first being concerned with evaluation of both algorithms via nominal process parameters. In each case, the design parameters were refined by extensive simulation studies carried out by one of the authors. The second consisted of selecting the process parameters using a randomized Monte Carlo approach. For all the continuous models being considered, a fourth-order Runge–Kutta method with fixed step length was used for the numerical integration.

4.5.1 Simulation studies using nominal parameter values

The non-linear multivariable model described in Section 4.2 was simulated in continuous form. A series of simulations was considered for both algorithms on different machines, the GPC being implemented on a SUN workstation, whereas the SOFLC was run on a single T800 transputer with a host PC.

The study used a step length of 0.1 and a sampling interval of 1 minute. Initial conditions were 0 per cent relaxation and 140 mmHg arterial pressure. For both algorithms, the set-point command signal was 80 per cent for relaxation, and 110 mmHg for blood pressure.

As well as discussing the performances of both designs, a comparison of the respective execution times is also given.

4.5.1.1 Performance of the adaptive GPC algorithm

In this case, during the first 25 samples, initial control was provided by the self-tuner but with fixed parameter estimates obtained from the nominal linear model. The input signal was clipped between 0 and 1.0 for the atracurium drug input, and between 0 per cent and 5 per cent for the isoflurane input. A further maximum limit of 0.5 was placed on the atracurium input during the initial 25 samples (where the parameter estimates were fixed) to prevent wild fluctuations in drug demand. For parameter estimation, a UD-factorization method (Bierman, 1977) was used on incremental data, with an initial covariance matrix and forgetting factor given by:

$$P = 10^2 I \quad \rho = 0.995.$$

A discrete multivariable model with five diagonal $\mathbf{A}(z^{-1})$ and six $\mathbf{B}(z^{-1})$

parameters was estimated with an assumed time-delay of one sample. The experiments were conducted in three phases to determine suitable tuning parameter settings.

Phase 1 investigated the base algorithm, in contrast to phases 2 and 3 which were concerned with the extended algorithm using respectively the model-following polynomial $\mathbf{P}(z^{-1})$ and the observer polynomial $T(z^{-1})$. Figure 4.4 shows one result from phase 1 where the controller parameter settings were different between the two channels: $N_1 = 1$, $N_2(\text{chan}\,1) = 10$, $N_2(\text{chan}\,2) = 20$, $NU(\text{chan}\,1) = 1$, $NU(\text{chan}\,2) = 2$. This result gave fast responses particularly for arterial pressure.

Phase 2 was concerned with the model-following polynomial $\mathbf{P}(z^{-1})$. Based on the particular dynamics as well as the sampling period, a value of time constant of approximately 10 minutes (identical for both channels) was selected for assignment of the $\mathbf{P}$ matrix. Figure 4.5 shows how this could be used to produce a smooth response in the relaxation channel as well as minimizing the interaction, at the cost of overdamping in the arterial pressure channel.

Finally, phase 3 considered the inclusion of the important observer polynomial $T(z^{-1})$. Figure 4.6 shows how the effect of disturbances could be reduced without affecting the closed-loop responses. In this result, output changes were made during the run, being 5 per cent at time 90 minutes in the relaxation dynamics, and 10 per cent at time 150 minutes in the arterial pressure model. From these figures, it can be seen that the control action for atracurium is severe during the initial transient, but this is reduced significantly by inclusion of the observer polynomial.

4.5.1.2 Performance of the fuzzy SOC algorithm

Under the same conditions as those described in Section 4.5.1, the study considered two versions of the algorithm. The simple version consists of a fixed set of scaling factors, while the extended one includes switching from one set of scaling factors to another. Multi-run tests with a maximum of three runs for each case were conducted starting with an initially empty controller (i.e. no rules). The rules were then stored at the end of each run and used as a starting point for the following one.

Figure 4.7 shows a result where the simple controller with the following small scaling factors was used:

$$GE_1 = 11.36 \quad GC_1 = 30.0 \quad GT_1 = 0.166 \quad \text{for channel 1}$$
$$GE_2 = 0.333 \quad GC_2 = 0.30 \quad GT_2 = 0.45 \quad \text{for channel 2.}$$

With these settings the controller gave a fair control policy for the two channels. In the first run, the output for channel 1 exhibited an undershoot due to the fact that the controller started with no rules at all, whereas the output for channel 2 was fast and adequately damped. During the second

A comparative study of generalized predictive control (GPC)

Table 4.3 *Parameters of the simple controller*

Figure number	Run	EP (per cent)	Number of rules	
			Paralysis	ΔMAP
4.7	1st	66.66	15	10
	2nd	66.66	22	12
	3rd	66.66	22	13
4.8	1st	16.66	18	15
	2nd	16.66	21	20
	3rd	16.66	27	22

and third runs, the previous undershoot was removed. The presence of a steady-state error for the first channel (muscle relaxation) could be explained by the choice of low scaling factors which scale the error to positive or negative fuzzy labels which suggest that there is no process output error at all. Table 4.3 also summarizes the number of rules generated at the end of each run which was on average 22 and 12 respectively for the first and second channels.

Using the same controller, another experiment was conducted but this time using high scaling factors. The following values were adopted:

$GE_1 = 45.18 \quad GC_1 = 35.0 \quad GT_1 = 0.166$ for channel 1
$GE_2 = 1.205 \quad GC_2 = 0.45 \quad GT_2 = 0.45$ for channel 2.

As shown in Figure 4.8, the controller removed the undershoot in the first channel produced during the first run, as well as reducing the steady-state error making the controller therefore highly accurate. It did, however, produce a highly active control signal in the relaxation channel. Also, Table 4.3 shows that the number of rules generated increased to 27 and 22 respectively for the first and second channels due to the higher sensitivity with the chosen scaling factors.

Taking into account the fact that low scaling factors lead to a relatively good transient response on one hand and a large steady-state error on the other, and that high scaling factors give generally good accuracy in the steady-state period but with a larger rule-base size and active control signals, the idea of merging the two techniques seems attractive. This was the object of the third experiment within the framework of an extended controller. To reduce the number of generated rules and also to obtain a good control strategy during the transient response, the controller started with small scaling factors then switched to higher ones. The switch of the scaling factors from one mode to another was programmed in such a way as to occur when the output reached 83 per cent of its final value ($Y_s = 83$ per cent). Depending on four adopted regimes, the switch could occur on none of the

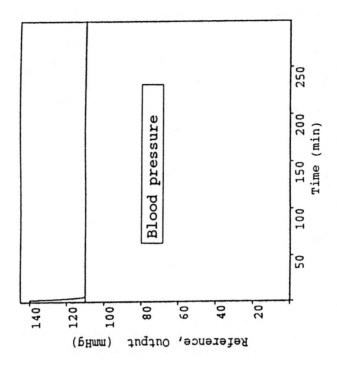
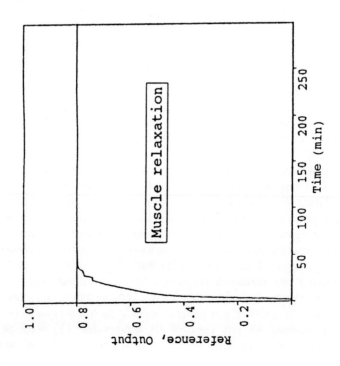

A comparative study of generalized predictive control (GPC)   99

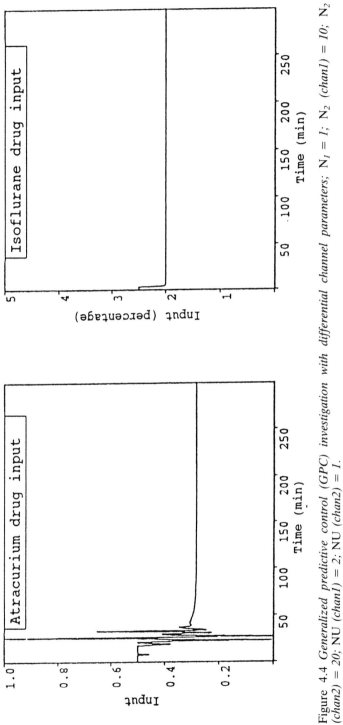

Figure 4.4 *Generalized predictive control (GPC) investigation with differential channel parameters;* $N_1 = 1$; N_2 *(chan1)* $= 10$; N_2 *(chan2)* $= 20$; *NU (chan1)* $= 2$; *NU (chan2)* $= 1$.

100 *Intelligent Control in Biomedicine*

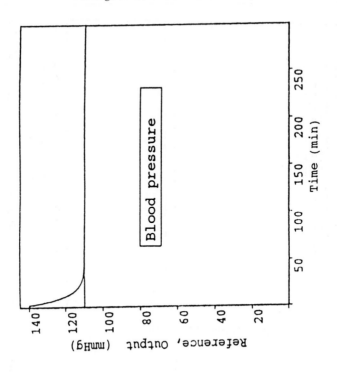

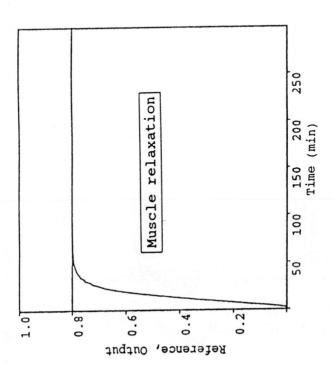

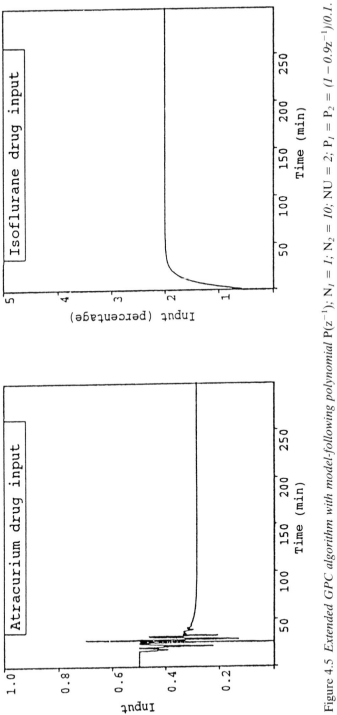

Figure 4.5 *Extended GPC algorithm with model-following polynomial* $P(z^{-1})$; $N_1 = 1$; $N_2 = 10$; $NU = 2$; $P_1 = P_2 = (1 - 0.9z^{-1})/0.1$.

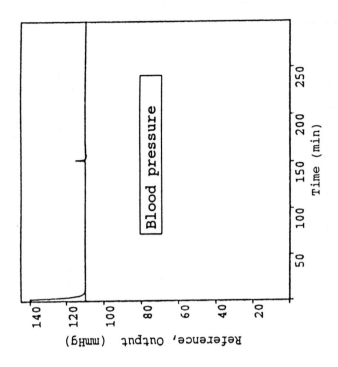
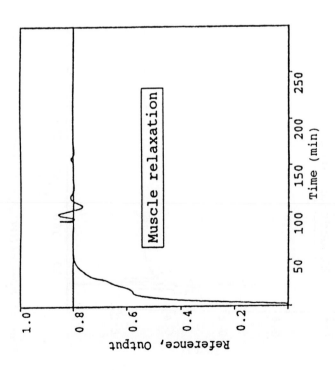

A comparative study of generalized predictive control (GPC) 103

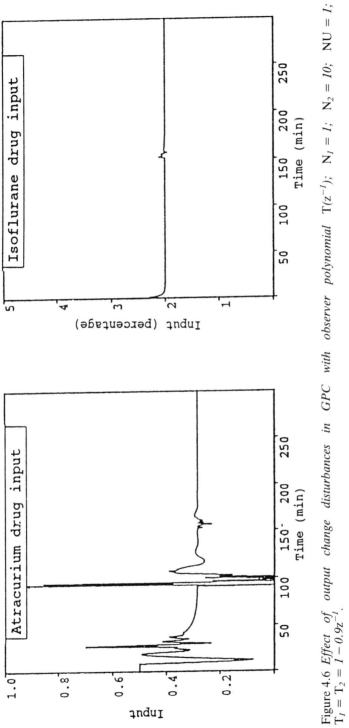

Figure 4.6 *Effect of output change disturbances in GPC with observer polynomial* $T(z^{-1})$; $N_1 = 1$; $N_2 = 10$; $NU = 1$; $T_1 = T_2 = 1 - 0.9z^{-1}$.

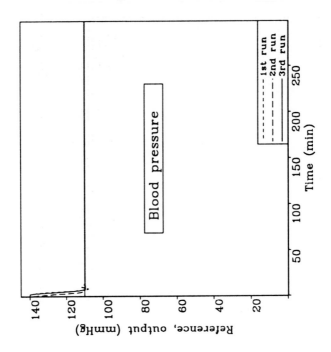
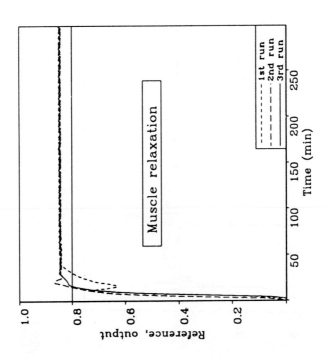

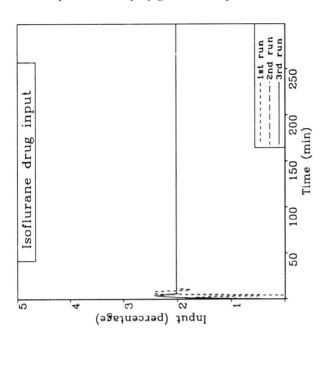
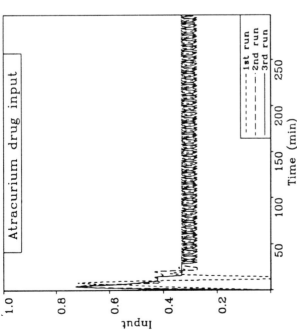

Figure 4.7 Response of a simple SOFLC using low scaling factors, with three successive runs commencing with the rule-base from the previous run.

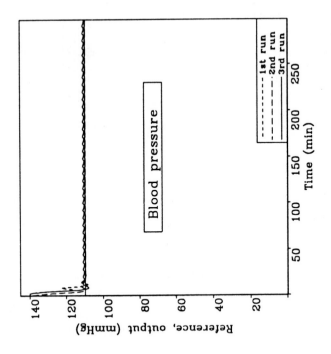
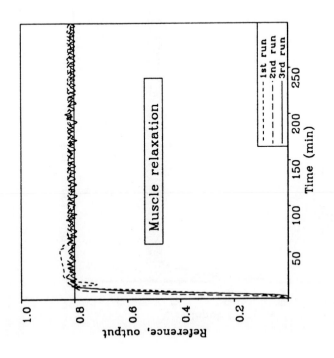

A comparative study of generalized predictive control (GPC) 107

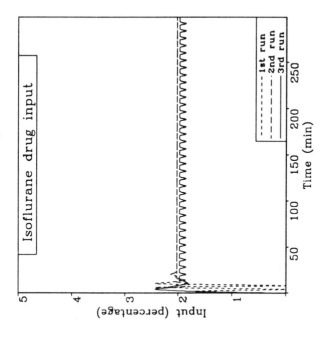
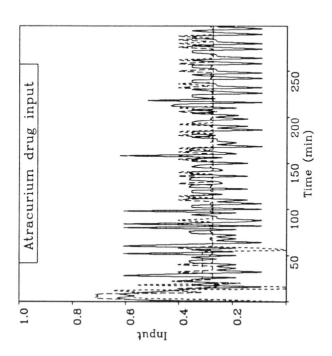

Figure 4.8 *Response of a simple SOFLC using high scaling factors.*

Table 4.4 *The different regimes for the extended fuzzy controller*

Regimes	Switch dependent
0	No switch
1	Paralysis channel
2	ΔMAP channel
3	Independent

Table 4.5 *Parameters of the extended fuzzy controller*

Figure number	Run	Y_s (per cent)	Regime	EP (per cent) Before	EP (per cent) After	Number of rules Paralysis	Number of rules ΔMAP
4.9	1st	83	3	66.66	16.66	20	12
	2nd	83	3	66.66	16.66	23	16
	3rd	83	3	66.66	16.66	23	18

channels, the first channel only, the second channel only, or both channels. Table 4.4 summarizes the four regimes.

Extensive simulation studies, beyond the scope of this chapter, showed that regime 3 gave the best performance as far as size of the rule-base and control signal activity were concerned. Therefore, an experiment was conducted along these lines and gave responses as shown in Figure 4.9 which demonstrate a good control even during the first run for both channels. These tended to improve even more during the second and third runs without an increase in the rule-base size as Table 4.5 illustrates.

Through simulation studies performed on the nominal process model, examples of which have been presented in Section 4.5.1, experience was gained on the selection of the crucial design parameters for GPC and SOFLC. Like many biomedical systems, however, anaesthetic models have very large inter-patient variability for which there is no information prior to an operation. The next section describes the use of the experience gained from the nominal model in the case of randomized model investigations.

4.5.2 Simulation studies via Monte Carlo parameter selection method

Clearly, the application of these algorithms to this particular multivariable non-linear anaesthetic model requires many design parameters to be selected, and this selection is very important in a safety-critical situation such as an operating theatre. Therefore, in order to validate further the robustness of these control strategies, Monte Carlo simulations were chosen

Table 4.6 *Selected model parameters using the Monte Carlo method*

Monte Carlo simulation method

Case number	Anaesthetic model parameters									
	T_1	T_2	T_3	T_4	K_1	T_5	K_2	T_6	T_7	K_4
1	2.54	4.17	27.88	14.89	2.01	1.57	−17.26	2.79	1.19	0.24
2	2.45	4.28	16.44	7.30	1.69	1.54	−17.70	3.01	1.33	0.27
3	2.35	5.95	27.88	10.88	2.16	1.15	−14.61	3.06	1.26	0.24
4	1.18	5.10	31.26	10.31	1.34	1.14	−15.94	2.99	1.26	0.24
5	1.36	3.84	32.00	7.31	2.46	1.20	−10.48	2.42	1.25	0.27
6	1.55	2.58	32.74	13.31	2.08	1.26	−15.02	2.85	1.24	0.25
7	1.73	5.32	33.48	10.31	1.71	1.31	−19.55	3.28	1.22	0.27
8	1.91	4.06	34.22	7.31	1.33	1.37	−14.09	2.71	1.21	0.25
9	2.09	2.80	34.96	13.30	2.45	1.43	−18.63	3.14	1.20	0.27
10	2.27	5.54	15.70	10.30	2.07	1.49	−13.61	2.57	1.18	0.25

to undergo such tests. Equation (4.27) describes the model with parameters which are known to vary from patient to patient:

$$\begin{bmatrix} \text{Paralysis} \\ \Delta \text{MAP} \end{bmatrix} = \begin{bmatrix} \dfrac{K_1(1+T_4s)e^{-\tau_1 s}}{(1+T_1s)(1+T_2s)(1+T_3s)} & \dfrac{K_4 e^{-\tau_4 s}}{(1+T_6s)(1+T_7s)} \\ 0 & \dfrac{K_2 e^{-\tau_2 s}}{(1+T_5s)} \end{bmatrix} \begin{bmatrix} U_1 \\ U_2 \end{bmatrix}.$$

(4.27)

The non-linearity is still represented by the Hill equation (4.3) described in Section 4.2.1 using the same parameters, although these could have been randomized.

The Monte Carlo simulations consisted of choosing the model parameters in a random manner using the following formula:

$$\text{Monte Carlo parameter} = \min + \text{random} \times (\max - \min)$$

where $0 < \text{Random} < 1$, and Random is obtained from a random number generator. The *Min* and *Max* values for each parameter were chosen to reflect probable pharmacological ranges known to exist. In this way many combinations could be produced. Table 4.6 shows a sample of ten cases that were studied, but due to lack of space only three of these will be presented for discussion. Cases 4, 5 and 7 were selected for a comparison of the multivariable GPC and SOC algorithms. These cases were chosen to indicate the best, worst and medium performance conditions for each algorithm. The conditions as described in Section 4.5.1 remained unchanged

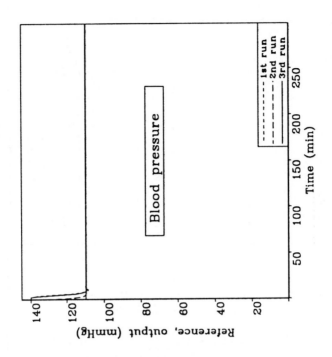

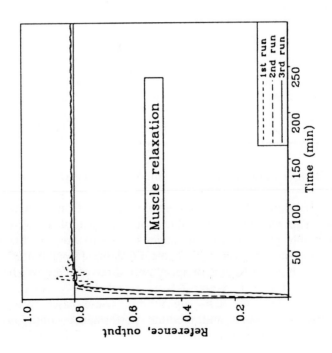

A comparative study of generalized predictive control (GPC) 111

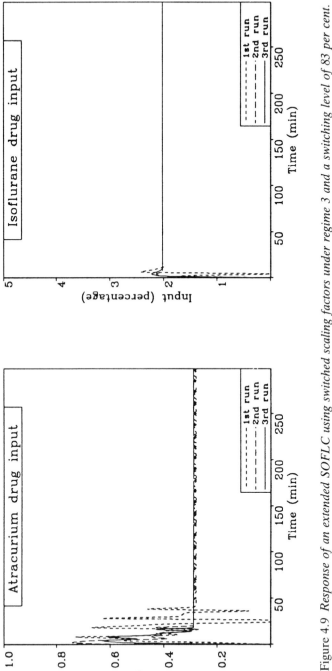

Figure 4.9 *Response of an extended SOFLC using switched scaling factors under regime 3 and a switching level of 83 per cent.*

except that the fixed GPC mode was operational only for the first ten samples, during which the control signal was clipped between 0 and 0.50. For the multivariable SOC algorithm, the extended version of regime 3 was adopted using the same scaling as before with the exception of the change-in-error scaling factors where a compromise set of values suiting most cases had to be found. The adopted values were:

$$GC_1 = 1.0 \quad GCE_2 = 0.10.$$

Figure 4.10 shows the performance of the extended version of GPC using case 4 with the model following polynomial $\mathbf{P}(z^{-1})$ having a relatively fast time-constant of 1.44 minutes. The responses in both channels were fast and well damped with the overshoot reduced to a low level in channel 1 which exhibits severe non-linearities.

Case 5 represented a severe test for the chosen GPC configuration, as was also the case for the SOC. It corresponds to a high-gain muscle relaxation model, and a low-gain blood pressure model. Figure 4.11 shows a good performance for blood pressure, but a heavy initial overshoot in the relaxation channel and subsequent saturation of drug signals. Finally, case 7 represented a medium condition with inferior blood pressure response to that of Figure 4.10, but similar paralysis behaviour, as shown in Figure 4.12.

The next series of experiments considered the fuzzy SOC algorithm. Figure 4.13 illustrates how the controller behaved on the model with the parameters of case 4. The responses in both channels were quite good although the control signals were active. The worst performance was recorded when using the model parameters of case 5. The responses shown in Figure 4.14 demonstrated large steady-state errors in both channels, mainly because the switch from a set of low scaling factors to a set of high scaling factors did not take place. For case 7 shown in Figure 4.15, the control signals were active and led to a limit cycle in channel 1. Table 4.7 summarizes the controller parameters and the number of generated rules during the three experiments.

To complement the visual indications of control performance, an objective measure of error performance over the simulation runs was made using ISE (integral of squared errors) and ITAE (integral of time and absolute error) criteria. Table 4.8 gives the ISE and ITAE values for GPC and SOC respectively for Figures 4.4–4.15. The unit of time for the ITAE criterion was minutes in each case. The criteria were evaluated over the whole 300-minute run in each case. This length of run is much longer than the transient settling time, and hence accentuates any steady-state error in the ITAE evaluation. This is particularly evident in the SOFLC values.

In general, all the ITAE values were greater than the ISE values, because of the time-scale involved. Similarly, all the blood pressure ITAE and ISE values were greater than for paralysis, simply because of the non-normalized values for blood pressure. Approximate normalization of blood pressure

Table 4.7 The fuzzy controller parameters

Figure number	Case	Run	Y_s (per cent)	EP (per cent) Before	EP (per cent) After	Number of rules Paralysis	Number of rules ΔMAP
4.13	4	1st	83	66.66	16.66	10	8
		2nd	83	66.66	16.66	13	8
		3rd	83	66.66	16.66	13	8
4.14	5	1st	83	66.66	16.66	5	2
		2nd	83	66.66	16.66	7	2
		3rd	83	66.66	16.66	7	2
4.15	7	1st	83	66.66	16.66	11	8
		2nd	83	66.66	16.66	12	10
		3rd	83	66.66	16.66	12	11

ISE could be obtained via division by 10 000 and ITAE via division by 100. This would give lower figures for blood pressure than paralysis in both GPC and SOC. This reflects clearly the better dynamic performance for the simpler and linear dynamic of that channel. In Figures 4.4–4.9 the GPC and SOFLC parameters were experimentally tuned to obtain a good control performance for the particular design selection and scaling factor choice. This is reflected in the ISE and ITAE entries for these figures, where it is seen that there is little difference between the values for Figures 4.4–4.6 and Figures 4.7–4.9. The well-known sensitivity of ITAE to errors at large time is shown clearly in the case of Figure 4.9. Whereas the ISE for paralysis shows little differential indication between the runs, the ITAE measure for the third run shows a definite degradation in performance. This is also indicated in the blood pressure response, where the large increase in ITAE is hardly evidenced visually in Figure 4.9.

Turning now to the Monte Carlo results, we can discuss differences in performance between GPC and SOC. For case 4, which both algorithms found easy to control, SOFLC gave better ISE for paralysis (indicating a faster initial response), but worse ITAE and ISE for blood pressure. Both GPC and SOFLC found case 5 difficult to manage, which is not surprising because of the extreme nature of the parameters. SOC gave large ISE and ITAE because of its inability to reduce steady-state errors for either paralysis or blood pressure, this being true for each of the runs. In contrast, GPC provided reasonable control. The third case, selected visually as giving moderate performance, indicated a better performance by SOFLC in terms of ISE for paralysis, but better blood pressure performance for GPC.

4.5.3 Execution time considerations

An execution time evaluation for both algorithms was conducted for all the previous experiments. For implementation reasons, the algorithms were run

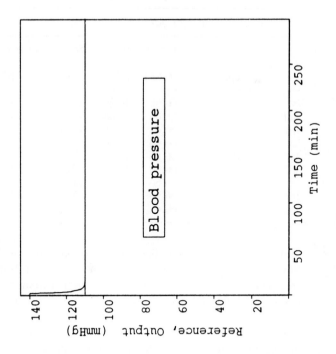
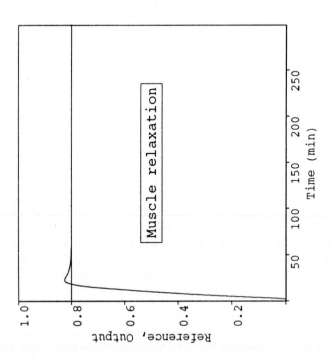

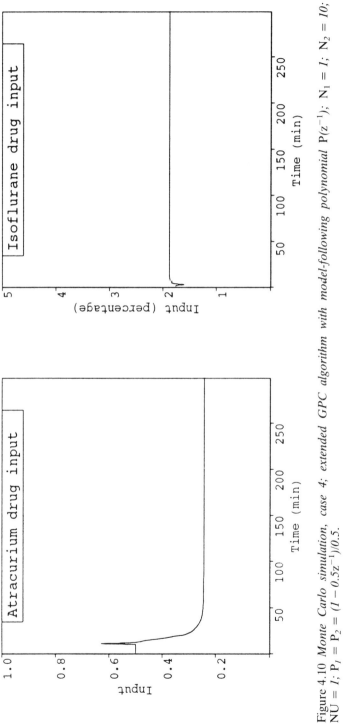

Figure 4.10 *Monte Carlo simulation, case 4; extended GPC algorithm with model-following polynomial* $P(z^{-1})$; $N_1 = 1$; $N_2 = 10$; $NU = 1$; $P_1 = P_2 = (1 - 0.5z^{-1})/0.5$.

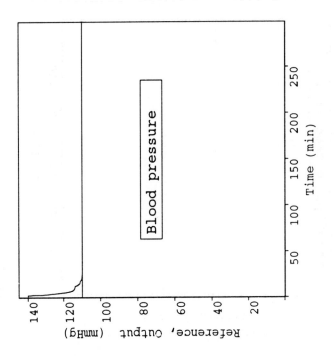
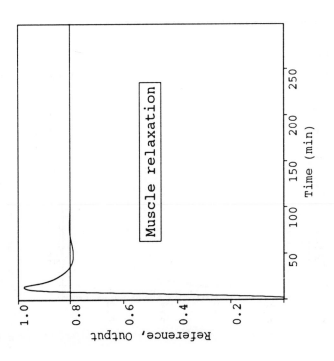

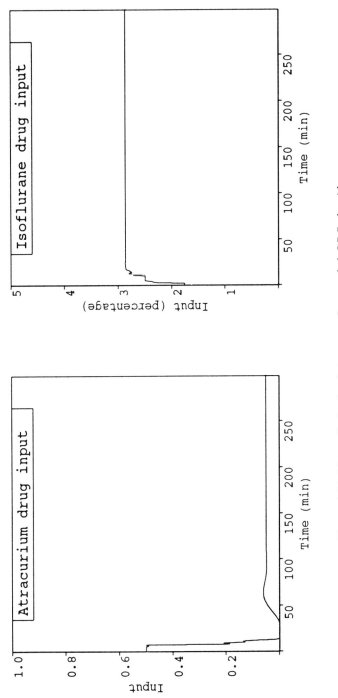

Figure 4.11 *Monte Carlo simulation, case 5; extended GPC algorithm.*

118   *Intelligent Control in Biomedicine*

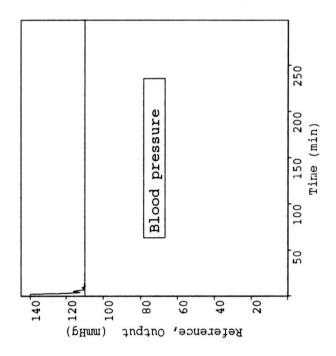

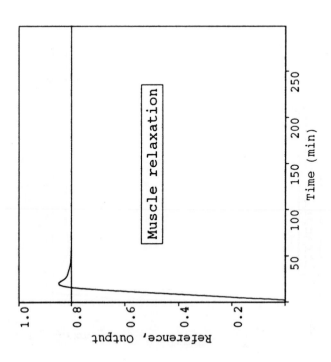

A comparative study of generalized predictive control (GPC)

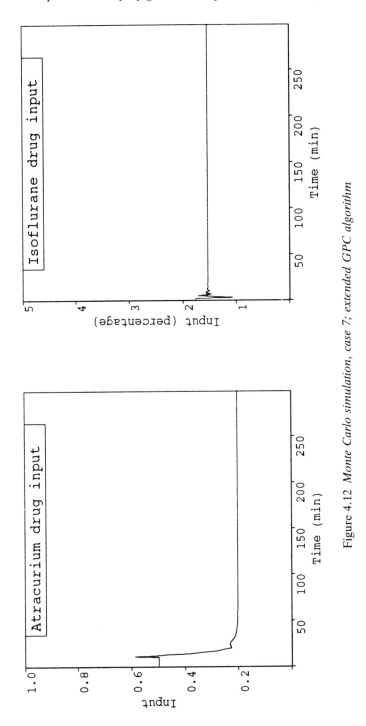

Figure 4.12 *Monte Carlo simulation, case 7; extended GPC algorithm*

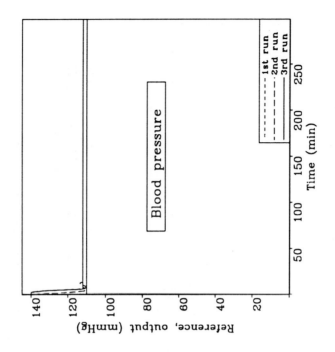
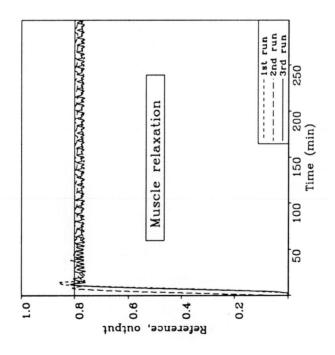

A comparative study of generalized predictive control (GPC) 121

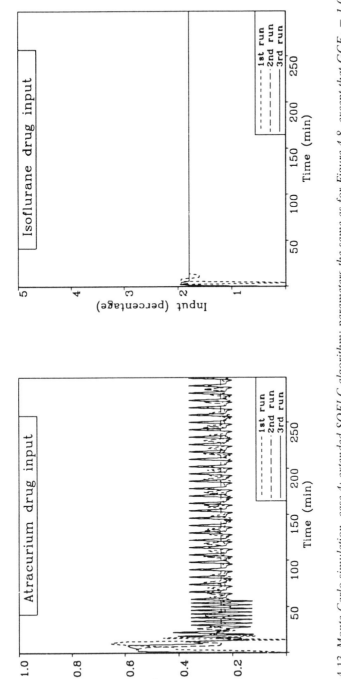

Figure 4.13 *Monte Carlo simulation, case 4; extended SOFLC algorithm; parameters the same as for Figure 4.8, except that $GCE_1 = 1.0$; $GCE_2 = 0.10$.*

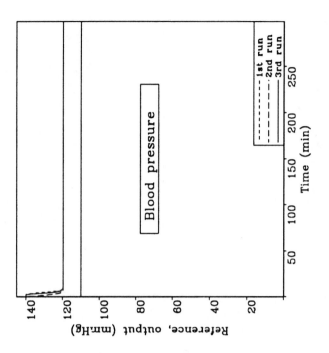
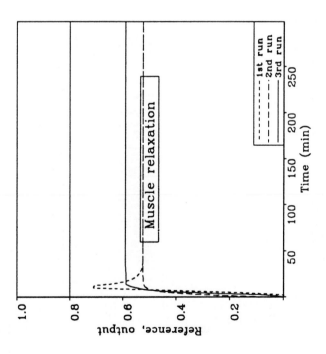

A comparative study of generalized predictive control (GPC)

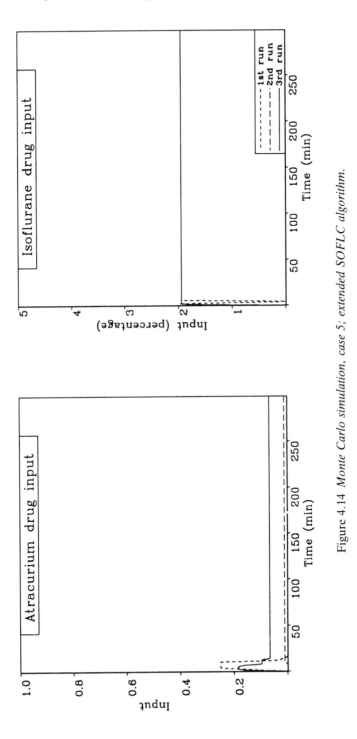

Figure 4.14 *Monte Carlo simulation, case 5; extended SOFLC algorithm.*

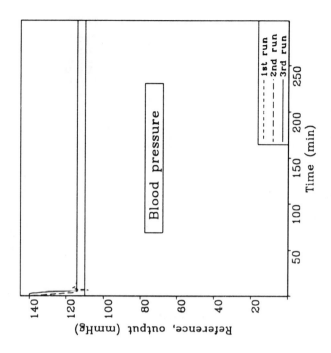
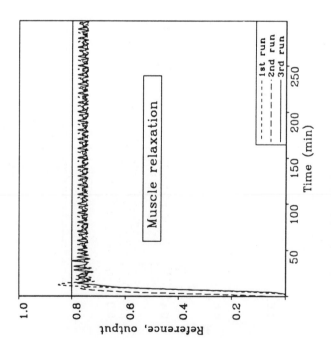

A comparative study of generalized predictive control (GPC) 125

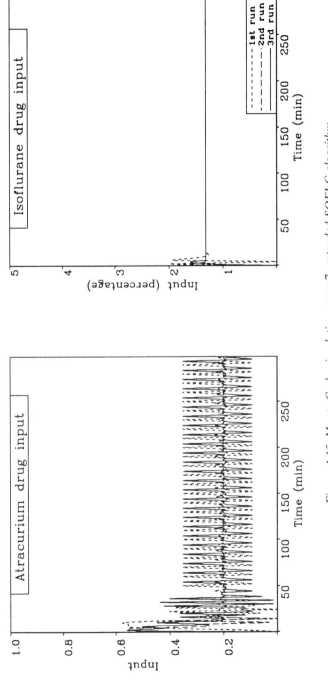

Figure 4.15 *Monte Carlo simulation, case 7; extended SOFLC algorithm.*

Table 4.8 *Table representing the ISE and ITAE criteria for equivalent GPC and SOFLC runs*

GPC					SOFLC					
	Paralysis		ΔMAP				Paralysis		ΔMAP	
Figure number	ISE	ITAE	ISE	ITAE	Figure number	Run number	ISE	ITAE	ISE	ITAE
4.4	3.34	60	2073	84	4.7	1st	3.52	307	2435	4151
						2nd	3.34	297	2411	4140
						3rd	3.33	297	2410	4140
4.5	5.93	112	5096	2316	4.8	1st	4.65	242	4058	15172
						2nd	3.96	227	3289	15011
						3rd	3.95	227	3285	15008
4.6	3.91	189	2215	2081	4.9	1st	3.22	56	2565	7254
						2nd	3.03	94	2427	4631
						3rd	3.95	227	3285	15008
4.10	3.75	42	2126	63	4.13	1st	3.16	226	2943	12699
						2nd	2.89	113	2530	12946
						3rd	3.13	250	2584	11954
4.11	2.98	60	2707	584	4.14	1st	10.5	1488	13510	53503
						2nd	11.7	1561	13510	53503
						3rd	10.1	1442	13510	53503
4.12	3.84	43	1979	139	4.15	1st	3.13	207	2750	11603
						2nd	2.99	205	2935	15862
						3rd	2.91	151	2981	15865

on different machines. The multivariable GPC was run on a SUN computer, whereas the multivariable SOC used a single T800 transputer. The study produced Tables 4.9 and 4.10 where the corresponding execution times in seconds for each type of algorithm are shown for a standard simulation run of 5 hours. The study suggests that both algorithms would perform adequately here, considering a real-time sampling of 1 minute in this anaesthetic application! It took on average 0.35 second for the GPC to finish one iteration for calculations, whereas 0.033 second was needed for the fuzzy SOC execution. The fuzzy SOC formulation was considerably faster than the GPC algorithm, but the use of a transputer constitutes a big advantage over a normal processor. A previous study using SOFLC has, in fact, shown a tenfold increase in speed by using a transputer-based system against a SUN 3 workstation (Linkens and Hasnain, 1991). In this case, a single T800 transputer was also used, albeit in a slightly different hardware configuration. It is, however, worth noting that the choice of controller parameters is crucial not only for the final performance but also for the computer burden. For instance, in the case of GPC, larger N_2, NU, etc., give bigger matrix calculations. In the case of SOFLC, the size of the rule-base produced by modifying, deleting and adding rules is directly

Table 4.9 *Table representing the speed of execution for different settings of the multivariable GPC algorithm*

Speed performances relating to GPC; 5-hour simulation run

Figure number	Type of algorithm	Execution time (s)
4.4	Basic multivariable algorithm; $N_1 = 1$, $N_2(\text{chan1}) = 10$; $N_2(\text{chan2}) = 20$; $NU(\text{chan1}) = 1$; $NU(\text{chan2}) = 2$	124.8
4.5	Extended multivariable algorithm with model following polynomial $P(z^{-1})$; $N_1 = 1$; $N_2 = 10$; $NU = 2$; $P_1 = P_2 = (1 - 0.9z^{-1})/0.1$	116.3
4.6	Extended multivariable algorithm with observer polynomial $T(z^{-1})$; $N_1 = 1$; $N_2 = 10$; $NU = 1$; $T_1 = T_2 = 1 - 0.9z^{-1}$	94.4
4.10, 4.11 and 4.12	Extended multivariable algorithm with model following polynomial $P(z^{-1})$; $N_1 = 1$; $N_2 = 10$; $NU = 1$; $P_1 = P_2 = (1 - 0.5z^{-1})/0.5$	99.4

Table 4.10 *Table representing the speed of execution for different versions of SOFLC*

Speed performance relating to SOC; 5-hour simulation run

Figure number	Type of algorithm	1st Run	2nd Run	3rd Run
4.7	Simple controller; low scaling factors	2.8	3.1	3.1
4.8	Simple controller; high scaling factors	2.8	3.1	3.2
4.9	Extended controller; Regime 3	3.6	3.8	4.0
4.13	SOC with switch mode	3.2	3.6	3.7
4.14	SOC with switch mode	2.2	2.4	2.3
4.15	SOC with switch mode	3.2	3.6	3.7

influenced by the choice of the performance model as well as the scaling factors for the error, change-in-error and the output.

4.6 Discussions and conclusions

The multivariable anaesthetic model represents a challenging and realistic basis on which to compare control strategies. The system dynamics are of moderate complexity, but more importantly they contain significant and pharmacologically valid non-linearities. Of particular relevance, however, is the large patient-to-patient variability in model parameters. This is a well-known phenomenon in the life sciences, where parameter variations of 4:1 are endemic, known examples being in muscle relaxation (Linkens *et al.*, 1982) and blood pressure (Slate, 1980). It was because of oscillations observed in some operations performed using parameter PID control strategies that advanced adaptive methods have been introduced. Thus, pole-placement self-tuning was applied to muscle relaxation (Linkens *et al.*, 1985), while a mixed switching controller with Smith prediction for delay compensation, together with gain adaptation, was introduced for blood pressure control (Slate, 1980).

The examples cited above for self-adaptive control refer to SISO systems. Similarly, self-organizing approaches have been studied for biomedicine. Fuzzy logic control for biomedicine is attractive, since it offers the possibility of good control without the knowledge of a detailed mathematical model of the process. The problem of rule elicitation is obviated using SOFLC. For muscle relaxation it has been shown that SOFLC can perform well, even with large model mismatches and with an initially empty knowledge base (Linkens and Hasnain, 1991). Similarly, the GPC algorithm used in the current studies has been evaluated in the muscle relaxation SISO case, both via simulation and clinical trials (Mahfouf, 1991).

For the multivariable anaesthesia problem the GPC algorithm has been refined via extensive simulations reported elsewhere (Linkens *et al.*, 1991). Suitable settings of the many design parameters for the application of GPC were obtained via these studies and previous SISO experience, and have been used in this comparative study. They represent a serious attempt by one of the authors to obtain the best performance via this control strategy. The major design feature of SOFLC is the settings of the scaling factors. Considerable experience has been gained in heuristic methods for selecting these scaling factors via a number of SISO and MIMO laboratory-based engineering rigs (Linkens and Abbod, 1991). Again, this knowledge has been used by another of the authors to obtain the best performance of the same pharmacological process via SOFLC. It remains then to discuss the relative performance between serious best attempts at control using the two different approaches.

In general, the GPC results show a smoother performance both in the individually adjusted examples of Figures 4.4–4.6 and in the Monte Carlo runs of Figures 4.10–4.12. The control of paralysis is considerably harder than for control of unconsciousness. This is partly due to differences in linear pharmacokinetics, but is mainly caused by the severely non-linear pharmacodynamics. To obtain smooth control action, however, it was necessary to perform many trials using the model-following and observer polynomials of the extended form of GPC (see Figures 4.4–4.6). Using this approach it was possible to trade stability and rise-time between the two channels (see Figure 4.5). This was not easily possible, however, for the Monte Carlo runs where the design parameters were 'frozen'.

The SOFLC, in general, gave more active control signals, and in several cases approached limit cycle conditions. This is a well-known feature of fuzzy logic control. Although the scaling factors (three for each channel) had to be selected heuristically, this was greatly helped via previous experiments on engineering rigs. In particular, the switching regime of Figure 4.9, giving effectively coarse/fine control, produced a fast initial response together with good steady-state accuracy. This regime also performed well on laboratory rigs. In nearly all the results, it can be seen that the SOFLC needed a second run to obtain a set of rules which would give good performance. This is not surprising, since the controller had an empty rule-base at the commencement of the first run in each case. The second run also seemed necessary to obtain an adequate number of rules in the knowledge-base. Further runs beyond the third seemed to extend the rule-base excessively and increase the computer burden. This has the implication that it would be desirable in a clinical setting to choose initial design values for the scaling factors and a tentative rule-base via prior simulation studies based on an average population model. Although the initial transient response was impressive, the steady-state performance was inferior to that of GPC, as evidenced by the generally larger ITAE measures. A fast initial transient response is, however, an important issue in many operations since the surgeon wishes to commence procedures as soon as possible after patient entry into the operating theatre. In contrast, some deviation from set-point is tolerable particularly for the muscle relaxation channel.

It is difficult to make computational speed comparisons between the methods, since the studies were performed on different computing platforms. However, the SOFLC execution on a single T800 transputer was impressive. In fact, it was implemented in this way on a PC-hosted transputer system to enable multivariable SOFLC to be studied on a laboratory scale coupled electric drive rig, where a sampling period of 20 milliseconds was necessary (Linkens and Abbod, 1991). It performed adequately in this case.

The model utilized in this study was not truly multivariable, since it has only one-way interaction. It belongs to a category of systems known as triangular systems which does not necessarily render it easy to control. Although the structure of the model used considered the interactions in a feedforward manner by adopting a *P*-canonical form structure, other forms of control, such as feedforward compensation, could have been employed, instead of feedback GPC and SOFLC. However, other drugs, especially inhalational anaesthetic agents, have different dynamic effects and hence the general feedback structure was retained for experimental comparisons. Also, other instances of multivariable control in biomedicine are being explored. One example is that of blood pressure management in intensive care, providing simultaneous control of blood pressure and cardiac output via simultaneous infusion of two drugs. Cases such as this give strongly cross-interactive systems for which GPC and SOFLC in full feedback configuration are necessary.

In conclusion it can be stated that self-adaptive strategies such as GPC give a superior control performance to a self-organizing approach. It achieves this, however, from a detailed knowledge of the process dynamics. It has been assumed that the multivariable model used here is an accurate description of process structure, albeit with massive parameter uncertainty. In reality, such a model structure is at best an over-determined abstraction, and therefore simplification, of life science systems. In the event of large structural uncertainties in process dynamics, the concept of self-organizing control is attractive. This comparative study has shown it to be a tolerable runner-up in a situation which clearly favours the self-adaptive methodology. These conclusions are similar to those obtained by Al-Assaf (1988) who compared GPC and SOFLC applied to a cement grinding mill. He noted the need to apply a start-up signal to the process for obtaining suitable GPC paramount settings, and also the need for experimentation to fill the empty rule-base for SOFLC. His findings of inferior speed and steady-state performance for SOFLC were based on single scale factor settings. This contrasts with the present study which used switched scaling factors to improve performance via a 'coarse/fine' control strategy. Of course, we expect to see improvements in algorithms for both approaches. It is, however, in the area of self-organizing control that we may expect to see more rapid advances in the near future. The principle of SOFLC has been around for many years, but it still needs more detailed attention and comparison with its neural network equivalents which are currently fashionable. Recent work (Harris and Moore, 1990; Moore, 1991) has introduced the concept of indirect SOFLC whereby a fuzzy model of the process is first identified, followed by inversion to provide a control algorithm. This is analogous to explicit self-tuning control, of which GPC is one example. It does, however, require *a priori* knowledge about the process in terms of its dynamical order, but provides self-organization in terms of rules which allow for non-linear situations.

References

Al-Assaf, Y., 1988, 'Self-tuning control: theory and applications', unpublished DPhil thesis, Oxford University.
Asbury, A.J., 1990, unpublished correspondence.
Assilian, S. and Mamdani, E.H., 1975, An experiment in linguistic synthesis with a fuzzy logic controller, *International Journal of Man-Machine Studies*, **7**, 1–13.
Åström, K.J. and Wittenmark, B., 1984, *Computer-Controlled Systems—Theory and Design*, New Jersey: Prentice Hall.
Bierman, G.J., 1977, *Factorization Methods for Discrete Sequential Estimation*, New York: Academic Press.
Breckenridge, J.L. and Aitkenhead, A.R., 1983, Awareness during anaesthesia: a review, *Annals of the Royal College of Surgeons of England*, **6**, 93–6.

Clarke, D.W., 1985, 'Implementation of self-tuning controllers', in Harris, C.J. and Billings, S.A. (Eds) *Self-tuning and Adaptive Control: Theory and Application*, (*IEE Control Engineering*, **15**, 146–7).

Clarke, D.W., 1988, Introduction to self-tuning control, in Warwick, K. (Ed.) *Implementation of Self-Tuning Control*, vol. 35, pp. 3–22, London: Peter Peregrinus.

Clarke, D.W. and Gawthrop, P.J., 1975, Self-tuning controller, *IEE Proceedings*, PtD, **122**, 929–34.

Clarke, D.W., Mohtadi, C. and Tuffs, P.S., 1987a, Generalised predictive control—Part I. the basic algorithm, *Automatica*, **23**, 137–48.

Clarke, D.W., Mohtadi, C. and Tuffs, P.S., 1987b, Generalised predictive control—Part II. extensions and interpretations, *Automatica*, **23**, 149–60.

Daley, S. and Gill, K.F., 1986, A design study of a self-organising fuzzy logic controller, *Proceedings of the Institution of Mechanical Engineers*, **200**, 59–69.

Harris, C.J. and Moore, C.G., 1989, 'Intelligent identification and control for autonomous guided vehicles using adaptive fuzzy based algorithms', Internal Report, Southampton University, October.

Harris, C.J. and Moore, C.G., 1990, 'Real-time fuzzy-based self-learning predictors and controllers', in Proceedings of the 11th IFAC World Congress, Tallinn, USSR, vol. 7, pp. 180–186.

Kalman, R.E., 1958, Design of a self-optimizing control system, *ASME Transactions Journal of Basic Engineering*, **80**, 468–78.

Kam, W.Y., Tham, M.T., Morris, A.J. and Warwick, K., 1985, 'Multivariable self-tuning: structure identification and control', in Proceedings of the IFAC Conference on Identification and Parameter Estimation. York, UK, pp. 385–90.

King, P.J. and Mamdani, E.H., 1977, Application of fuzzy control systems to industrial processes, *Automatica*, **13**, 235–42.

Lambert, E.P., 1987, 'Process control applications of long-range prediction', unpublished DPhil thesis, Oxford University.

Linkens, D.A. and Abbod, M., 1991, 'Self-organising fuzzy logic control for real-time processes', in Proceedings of IEE International Conference 'Control 91', Edinburgh, Vol. 2, pp. 971–76, March.

Linkens, D.A. and Abbod, M., 1992, Self-organising fuzzy logic control and the selection of its scaling factors, *Transactions of the Institute of Measurement and Control*, **14**, 114–25.

Linkens, D.A. and Hacisalihzade, S.S., 1990, Computer control systems and pharmacological drug administration: a survey, *Journal of Medical Engineering and Technology*, **14**, 41–54.

Linkens, D.A. and Hasnain, S.B., 1991, Self-organising fuzzy logic control and its application to muscle relaxant anaesthesia, *IEE Proceedings*, PtD, **138**, 274–84.

Linkens, D.A., Mahfouf, M. and Asbury, A.J., 1991, 'Multivariable generalised predictive control for anaesthesia', in Proceedings of the First European Control Conference 'ECC1', Vol. 2, pp. 1630–5.

Linkens, D.A., Menad, M. and Asbury, A.J., 1985, Smith predictor and self-tuning control of muscle relaxant drug administration, *IEE Proceedings*, PtD, **132**, 212–8.

Linkens, D.A., Asbury, A.J., Rimmer, S.J. and Menad, M., 1982, Identification and control of muscle relaxant anaesthesia, *IEE Proceedings*, PtD, **129**, 136–41.

Mahfouf, M., 1991, 'Adaptive control and identification for on-line drug infusion in anaesthesia', unpublished PhD thesis, Department of Automatic Control and Systems Engineering, University of Sheffield, UK.

McIntosh, A.R., Shah, S.L. and Fisher, D.G., 1989, 'Selection of tuning parameters for adaptive generalized predictive control', in Proceedings of the American Control Conference, Pittsburgh, pp. 1828–33.

Millard, R.K., Hutton, P., Pereira, E. and Roberts, C.P., 1986, 'On using a self-tuning controller for blood pressure regulation during surgery', presentation at the IMEKO Conference on Measurement in Clinical Medicine, Edinburgh, pp. 173–8.

Millard, R.K., Monk, C.R., Woodcock, T.E. and Roberts, C.P., 1988, Controlled hypotension during ENT surgery using self-tuners, *Computational Biology and Medicine*, **17**, 1–18.

Mizumoto, M., 1988, Fuzzy controls under various fuzzy reasoning methods, *International Journal of Man-Machine Studies*, **7**, 129–51.

Mohtadi, C., 1986, 'Studies in advanced self-tuning algorithms', unpublished DPhil thesis, Oxford University.

Mohtadi, C., Shah, S.L. and Fisher, D.G., 1991, 'Frequency response characteristics of MIMO GPC', in Proceedings of the First European Control Conference 'ECC1', Vol. **2**, pp. 1845–50.

Moore, C.G., 1991, 'Indirect adaptive fuzzy controllers', unpublished DPhil thesis, Southampton University.

Procyk, T.J., 1977, 'Self-organising control for dynamic processes', unpublished DPhil thesis, Queen Mary College, London.

Procyk, T.J. and Mamdani, E.H., 1979, Linguistic self-organising process controller, *Automatica*, **15**, 15–30.

Robb, H.M., Asbury, A.J., Gray, W.M. and Linkens, D.A., 1988, 'Towards automatic control of general anaesthesia', presentation at the Conference 'Medical informatics' 88, Nottingham, pp. 121–6.

Robb, H.M., Asbury, A.J., Gray, W.M. and Linkens, D.A., 1991, Towards a standardized anaesthetic state using enflurane and morphine, *British Journal of Anaesthesia*, **66**, 358–64.

Robinson, B.D. and Clarke, D.W., 1991, Robustness effects of a prefilter in generalized predictive control, *IEE Proceedings*, PtD, **138**, 2–8.

Savege, T.M., Dubois, M., Frank, M. and Holly, J.M.P., 1978, Preliminary investigation into a new method of assessing the quality of anaesthesia: the cardiovascular response to a measured noxious stimulus, *British Journal of Anaesthesia*, **50**, 481–7.

Schils, G.F., Sasse, F.J. and Rideout, V., 1987, Automatic control of anaesthesia using two feedback variables, *Annals of Biomedical Engineering*, **15**, 19–34.

Schwilden, H., Schuttler, J. and Stoeckel, H., 1987, Closed-loop feedback control of methohexital anaesthesia by quantitative EEG analysis in humans, *Anesthesiology*, **67**, 341–7.

Schwilden, H., Stoeckel, H. and Schuttler, J., 1989, Closed-loop control of propofol anaesthesia by quantitative EEG analysis in humans, *British Journal of Anaesthesia*, **62**, 290–6.

Sheppard, L.C., Shotts, J.F., Robertson, N.F., Wallace, F.D. and Kouchoukos, N.T., 1979, 'Computer-controlled infusion of vasoactive drugs in post-cardiac surgical patients', IEEE Conference on Engineering Medicine and Biology, Denver, Colorado, pp. 280–4.

Shook, D.S., Mohtadi, C. and Shah, S.L., 1991, Identification for long-range predictive control, *IEE Proceedings*, PtD, **138**, 75–84.

Slate, S.L., 1980, 'Model-based design of a controller for infusing sodium nitroprusside during post surgical hypertension', unpublished DPhil thesis, University of Wisconsin, USA.

Wellstead, P.E., Edmunds, J.M., Prager, D. and Zanker, P., 1979, Self-tuning pole/zero assignment regulators, *International Journal of Control*, **30**, 1–26.

Zadeh, L.A., 1965, Fuzzy sets, *Information and Control*, **12**, 94–102.

Zadeh, L.A., 1973, An outline of a new approach to the analysis of complex systems and decision processes, *IEEE Transactions*, **SMC-3**, 28–44.

Chapter 5
Hierarchical supervisory self-organizing fuzzy control for muscle relaxation anaesthesia

M. F. Abbod

5.1 Introduction

Supervisory expert control concentrates on general information about the process and the controller. The decision-making in the supervisory control system is related to situations involving major disturbances, technical faults, inappropriate human actions, and a combination of such events (Rasmussen, 1985). In such events the established control algorithm does not apply, and the planning for proper actions by the controller depends on knowledge about the functional properties of the system. The planning for a new control strategy will depend on information about the process characteristics in a specific situation. Such a system should be capable of performing the following tasks: monitoring the performance of the controller and the process, detecting possible system component failure or malfunctioning and replacing the control algorithm to maintain stability, and selecting the appropriate control algorithm best suited for a particular situation. Such a system can be formed in a closed loop to provide a conceptualized hierarchical system which consists of a supervision level as the highest hierarchical level, and the basic control level as the lowest. In general, more tasks can be handled by the supervisory control algorithm (deSilva and MacFarlane, 1988) e.g. start up and shut down procedures, process optimization, fault diagnosis, response to malfunctioning behaviour, pattern recognition, start and stop parameters estimation procedure, and alarm handling procedure.

5.2 Muscle relaxation in surgical patients

The medical system considered in this chapter represents the control of muscle relaxation of human beings during surgical operations. For certain operations such as eye surgery it is required to block the muscle movement, this being done by infusing the patient with muscle relaxant drugs such as atracurium or pancuronium. Such a process is usually done by anaesthetists who, based on their experience, infuse the patient in order to obtain a predefined degree of paralysis. Sometimes such tasks may not be done properly due to the patient-to-patient sensitivity to drugs which results in increased consumption of drug by the patient. A better method is to use a closed-loop control system by measuring the muscle relaxation using a monitor such as 'Relaxograph' and infusing the drug into the patient with a digitally driven syringe.

For a more complete description of the muscle relaxation process and the mathematical modelling of the system and the non-linearities involved, refer to Chapter 3, section 3.3.

5.2.1 Fault conditions in muscle relaxant control

The major sources of potential error in the drug delivery system, as described by Miller (1990) can be classified into three classes: the host computer, the infusion device, and the patient. The types of fault occurring in the host computer could be split into hardware faults and software faults. Hardware faults, such as power failure, are to be considered as uncontrollable faults since the control algorithm will no longer be running. Software faults could be represented by an error in the control algorithm which may divert the system, where a manual control recommendation will be issued to the anaesthetist. Other faults in the host computer could be a communication error with the Relaxograph or the syringe drive, which will be reported as a communication fault signal. The last source of error in the host computer is the drug mathematical model, in which case such a fault will not be reported since the self-organizing feature of the controller will adapt the rule-base to suit the new environment.

Faults in the infusion section can be considered as follows: incorrect infusion, incorrect delivery, and communication error. The two former cases are corrected with the self-organizing feature as stated in the last paragraph, while the communication error is reported as a software fault. The last source of fault is the patient, who is considered to be the major source of faults in the system. Faults in the patient are represented by the following:

drug infusion line disconnected, pharmacokinetics variability, acute pharmacokinetics change, pharmacodynamic variability, and sampling error. The first type of error is recognized as a fault in the syringe drive where an alarm signal is given to the anaesthetist to check the syringe drive. The pharmacokinetic and pharmacodynamic variability are not considered to be faults, rather these are considered to be on-line dynamic changes where the control algorithm is modified via the self-organizing and the parameter-tuning features. An acute change in the pharmacokinetics is considered to be due to a change in the patient sensitivity, and the modification procedure will involve a change in the rule-modification factor.

A change in the pharmacodynamics is considered to occur due to movements of the relaxograph electrodes which are due to movement of the patient's hand. In this case the relaxograph will not indicate the actual relaxation, and this is considered as a change in the non-linear parameters. A correction procedure is a change in the set-point to account for the new faulty relaxation measurement since the measure represents the same muscle relaxation but with shifted values. The last source of error is the patient sampling error. Sampling error could be of two kinds: the first is an impulsive reading, and the second is a relaxograph failure to supply the measured data. The former type of error is not considered to be a fault since the impulsive noise is removed using the filtering technique provided. The latter error is considered to be a fault in the Relaxograph since it is supposed to supply data every 20 seconds. In this case if the Relaxograph fails to supply data for two successive periods, then a fault in the Relaxograph is reported. However, if it happens once only then it is considered to be an impulsive noise and is filtered out.

5.2.2 Muscle relaxant simulator

For robustness tests on the control algorithm, it was necessary to test the algorithm under real-time conditions. Previous studies by Menad (1984), Denai *et al.* (1990), and Linkens *et al.* (1991) adopted a similar approach using different control algorithms and this proved to be a very useful robustness study. The real-time simulation study presented in the next section is concerned with applying the supervisory control algorithm to control the muscle relaxant model running on an Atari machine. The host PC and the Atari machine communicate with each other via analogue-to-digital/digital-to-analogue (ADC/DAC) converters mounted on both machines.

The digital simulator has been constructed using PASCAL on an Atari machine equipped with ADC/DAC facilities. A set of initial information has to be fed to the simulator via the keyboard. Such information includes the patient sensitivity, the drug concentration, the initial bolus amount, the sampling time, and the noise contamination. Also, fault conditions can be set to simulate a specific fault at a specified time. Such features give the simulator great flexibility in terms of choosing the required parameters to simulate the patient response. As well as having such facilities, the simulator is supported by a graphics facility which gives a graphical representation of the muscle relaxation and the amount of the infused drug. This approach is much more flexible than using an analogue computer, and therefore this simulator was considered for the studies reported in this chapter.

5.3 Supervisory hierarchical control

Supervisory control concentrates on general information about the process and the controller. Such a system must monitor the system and the controller performance, detect any malfunctioning of the controlled system and modify the control algorithm to maintain basic requirements such as stability, and select the right control algorithm best suited to the particular situation. Such a system may have a hierarchical structure described by three levels as shown in Figure 5.1.

The highest supervision level does all the decision-making like choosing the control algorithm, searching for system faults and diagnosing them. The dialogue level provides an interface between different levels of the controller as well as to the outside world, i.e. the human–machine interface. The lower level acts as a simple control loop using any type of controller with the parameters being adapted at the supervisory level.

In every system there are some types of behaviour that are acceptable and others that are not. Acceptable behaviour would be the normal operating conditions, which may include distorted signals due to noise contamination. In contrast, unacceptable behaviour occurs due to changes in the physical structure of the system. Some types of unacceptable behaviour may be simple, resulting from process parameter changes, others are not, being in the form of faults in the system due to the actuators, sensors, or in the internal system structure. Although it is possible to identify types of behaviour resulting from changing parameters in the system, they are not observable explicitly. Instead, they are observed indirectly through a set of performance characteristics abstracted from measurements, such as bandwidth, rise time, overshoot. Other behaviour which results from faulty instrumentation may be detected by comparing the actual system output with the system reference.

It is now possible to define two unacceptable types of behaviour, malfunctioning and faulty behaviour. Malfunctioning behaviour is caused by changes in the process parameters and is corrected by adapting the controller, i.e. by modifying the controller parameters in order to overcome the malfunctioning. In contrast, faulty behaviour should be diagnosed to find the faulty part, and then rectified via primary or adaptive control action

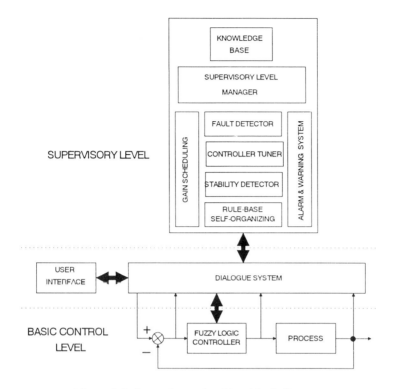

Figure 5.1 *Supervisory algorithm block diagram.*

being applied to ensure acceptable behaviour. The supervisory level must also have an alarm-handling facility, so that when a fault occurs and is detected an alarm signal is issued.

5.4 Fuzzy logic control

The concept of fuzzy set theory was introduced by Zadeh (1965) to represent the method of human reasoning involving imprecise information. For example, many of the strategies employed in the control and scheduling of industrial plant cannot be described by standard mathematical equations. However, they can be written down in linguistic form such as 'IF . . . THEN . . . ELSE . . .' rules. Fuzzy set theory provides a tool for representing the operator's linguistic rules in a manner suitable for implementation on digital computers. The early work of Assilian and Mamdani (1975) applied fuzzy set theory to the control of a steam engine by replicating the human operator's behaviour in the form of heuristic 'IF . . . THEN . . .' control rules. A survey of the early work is given by Tong (1977), and an extended self-organizing fuzzy logic controller was proposed by Procyk and Mamdani (1979).

Most of the fuzzy logic controllers work on the concept of classifying the behaviour of the controller process by a set of fuzzy control rules describing the error and change-in-error as an antecedent of the control rules and the controller output as the consequent of the rules. The control cycle starts by calculating the error and change-in-error, and fuzzifying them into fuzzy sets, then a fuzzy control output set is calculated given the fuzzy control rules and the fuzzy input sets using a rule inference procedure. Lastly, the fuzzy control output is defuzzified into a quantitative value to be used as the control signal. The rule-base is generated using the self-organizing method.

5.4.1 Rule-based fuzzy logic controller

A fuzzy logic controller is designed to use linguistic variables to express the control rules and manipulate incoming data from the process. Since the linguistic variables are formulated in a fuzzy number form, the incoming data from the process should be converted to fuzzy numbers after being scaled.

For a fuzzy controller a fixed number of linguistic labels are defined, so that the numerical inputs need to be quantized into different quantization levels in order to convert them into fuzzy linguistic variables.

The design procedure for the fuzzy logic controller is that first of all the fuzzy sets are formed upon a discrete support universe of discourse of 14 elements for the error (± 6), 13 elements for the change-in-error (± 6), and 15 elements for the output (± 7). The choice of the membership function that forms a particular fuzzy set is based on the Mizumoto (1988) study which found that the best fuzzy set is when the fuzzy sets of the fuzzy control rules are not isolated and not too much overlapped. The linguistic labels were chosen to be the same as in most of the reported studies, the terms being represented as:

PB: positive big   NB: negative big
PM: positive medium   NM: negative medium
PS: positive small   NS: negative small
PO: positive zero   NO: negative zero

The terms PO and NO are introduced to obtain finer control about the equilibrium state, where NO defines values slightly below zero and PO defines values slightly above zero. Such a procedure requires changing the real input values to integer numbers that suit the quantization level. Having done that, the input variables would change their real values into integer values. That leads to the fuzzy controller being less sensitive to small changes in the output of the process.

The control rules should be viewed as linguistic conditional statements and symbolized in the form of a relation matrix **R** given by the Cartesian product.

$$\mathbf{R} = \mathbf{E}_k \times \mathbf{CE}_k \times \mathbf{U}_k \tag{5.1}$$

The overall relation matrix **R** obtained from the control rules is calculated as the union of n individual relation matrices. The output from the fuzzy controller can be obtained from its inputs **E** and **CE** using Zadeh's compositional rules of inference:

$$\mathbf{U} = (\mathbf{E} \times \mathbf{CE}) \circ \mathbf{R}. \tag{5.2}$$

The output fuzzy set is defuzzified to obtain a crisp control action using the centre of area method.

5.4.2 Three-term controller

The rule-based fuzzy logic controller presented in the last section is linguistically classified as a PD controller which has the disadvantage of giving steady-state error. Kwok *et al.* (1990) presents different types of linguistic PID fuzzy logic control algorithms. The best performance was achieved by combining PD and I control rules are shown in Figure 5.2.

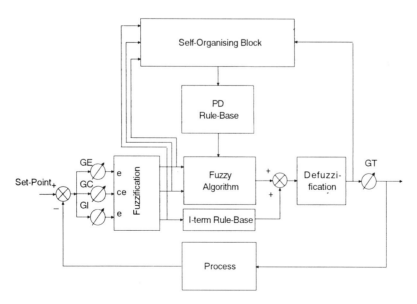

Figure 5.2 *Three-term (PID) fuzzy logic controller.*

The calculation of the output for the three-term controller will be as follows:

$$\text{Output(PID)} = \text{Output(PD)} + \text{Output(I)}$$

5.4.3 Pseudo-continuous fuzzification

A method has been proposed here to ignore the quantization procedure and fuzzify the real numbers to linguistic labels with adjustable membership function according to the input value. This method is represented in Figure 5.3 which involves two representations of a number after being fuzzified. For example, suppose the input number to be fuzzified is 2.6. In order to fuzzify this number, it should be quantized first. Its value after quantization is 3 which represents a positive medium linguistic label. In this case the membership function distribution will be as follows:

Universe of discourse	−6 . . . −1 0 +1 +2 +3 +4 +5 +6
Membership function	0.0 . . . 0.0 0.0 0.3 0.7 1.0 0.7 0.3 0.0

In reality, however, the number should not have a maximum membership value at 3 if it were not quantized. The new method involves keeping the same linguistic value where the membership function is defined but giving the real membership value of the input without quantization. This method would guarantee keeping the real value of the input variables.

The calculation of the membership function uses the following algorithm. Let y be the input, then the new membership function will be defined as follows:

$$\text{IF } y > Q(y) \text{ THEN } \mu(y) = \mu(Q(y)) - \mu(d)$$
$$\text{IF } y < Q(y) \text{ THEN } \mu(y) = \mu(Q(y)) + \mu(d)$$

and the membership function adjustment is calculated as follows:

$$\mu(d) = (Q(y) - y) \times \text{slope}(Q(y))$$

where $Q(y)$ is the quantized value.

The new universe of discourse for the same value (2.6) using the new method will be as follows:

Universe of discourse	−6 . . . −1 0 +1 +2 +3 +4 +5 +6
Membership function	0.0 . . . 0.0 0.12 0.42 0.86 0.88 0.54 0.18 0.0

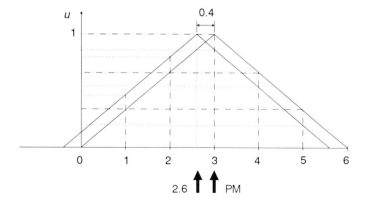

Figure 5.3 *Quantized and continuous fuzzy sets.*

5.5 Supervisory expert control

The development of the supervisory level was based on applying the control algorithm to the medical system where most of the system specifications were derived from the specifications of the medical system. The first thing encountered is the filtering of the incoming data from the controlled environment, as medical systems tend to be noisy and the sensors are affected by many types of disturbance. The second feature of the medical system is the use of a big initial bolus of drug for a fast reaction which leads to the concept of gain scheduling, since the drug bolus can be considered as an auxiliary input to the system. Other features of the supervisory control algorithms are the performance monitoring and controller tuning, and the self-organizing procedure which generates and modifies the rule-base. The last feature in the supervisory level is fault detection and diagnosis. All these features are supervised by a top-level supervisory level manager that has an embedded rule-base describing the system specifications and operation modes. In the following sections a brief explanation of each procedure is presented.

5.5.1 Rule-base self-organizing

The self-organizing level is considered to be a second hierarchical layer which provides on-line rule generation and modifications. It incorporates performance feedback where the performance index operates locally by assigning a credit or reward value to individual control actions that contribute to the present performance. It consists of the following functional blocks: the performance reference index, the process model, the rules modifier and the state buffer.

5.5.1.1 The performance index

The performance index measures the deviation from the path of the desired trajectory and issues the appropriate changes that are required at the output of the controller. It can be written in the form of a 'look-up' table. If the antecedents of the performance rules are the process output error $e(nt)$ and the change in the process output error $ce(nt)$, then the credit value of a particular process output U at a sample instance (nT) is given by:

$$P_o(nT) = f(e(nT), ce(nT)). \qquad (5.3)$$

This credit represents the required change in the system output and consequently it determines the rule modifications. The dimension of the performance index must be chosen to be the same dimension as the fuzzy set which is chosen for its error, change in error, and output. The linguistic performance rules are written to achieve the following objectives (Procyk, 1977): to achieve good speed of recovery form disturbance, good damping as the set-point is approached, and the output is confined within a certain tolerance band around the set-point. The linguistic performance-index table is shown in table 5.1.

The ZO elements represent states where the performance is acceptable, but note that there are few of these in the performance rules. This occurs because the rules are written to generate control rules from an empty controller and therefore it makes the controller more active. It is seen that the ZO elements form a diagonal band in the performance-index table. It is better to make this band have a certain width instead of making it a line in order to allow the process to take more than one trajectory. Making the band have the form of a line yields only one trajectory. Therefore, it is preferred to choose a medium-width zero-band in order to make the convergence of learning better.

Table 5.1 *The performance index*

Error	Change-in-error						
	NB	NM	NS	ZO	PS	PM	PB
NB	NB	NB	NB	NM	NM	NS	ZO
NM	NB	NB	NM	NM	NS	ZO	PS
NS	NB	NB	NS	NS	ZO	PS	PM
NO	NB	NM	NS	ZO	ZO	PM	PB
PO	NB	NM	ZO	ZO	PS	PM	PB
PS	NM	NS	ZO	PS	PS	PB	PB
PM	NS	ZO	PS	PM	PM	PB	PB
PB	ZO	PS	PM	PM	PB	PB	PB

For a continuous performance-index output, rather than a quantized one, Sutton and Jess (1991) incorporated the concept of weightings to give pseudo-continuous variables. This is achieved by applying a suitable weighting to the two nearest integer values for a given measured value. For example, if the error is 2.4 then the calculation will be performed as follows:

$$\text{Error}(2.4) = \text{Error}(2) \times 0.6 + \text{Error}(3) \times 0.4.$$

Accordingly the weighted output will be the product of the weighted error and change-in-error using the following relationship:

$$W(i,j) = W_e(i) \times W_{ce}(j)$$

where:

$W(i,j)$ is the weighting for $e = i$ and $ce = j$
$W_e(i)$ is the weighting for $e = i$
$W_{ce}(j)$ is the weighting for $ce = j$.

Therefore, the rule inference mechanism needs to be performed four times for each combination of the error and the change-in-error. To ensure that the compilation of the weightings do not consume extensive computation time, threshold values were applied. This method was applied for the performance-index calculations.

5.5.1.2 The process reference model

The design of the SOFLC involves the selection of a real-world process model which reflects the degree of the input/output coupling. For a single-input–single-output process, the control rule modifications are given by the following:

$$P_i(nT) = K^{-1} P_o(nT) \qquad (5.4)$$

where P_o is the correction issued by the performance index, P_i the manipulated input variable to the process, K is the process gain.

5.5.1.3 Rule modification

The rule modification procedure is based on reformulating the set of rules in the rule-base and can be explained by the following example. Assume the process has a time-lag of m samples. This means that the control action at sampling instant $(nT - mT)$ has most contributed to the process performance at sampling instant nT. Therefore the original implication:

$$E(nT - mT) \to CE(nT - mT) \to U(nT - mT) \qquad (5.5)$$

should be changed to:

$$E(nT - mT) \rightarrow CE(nT - mT) \rightarrow V(nT - mT) \quad (5.6)$$

where

$$E(nT - mT) = F\{e(nT - mT)\} \quad (5.7)$$

$$CE(nT - mT) = F\{ce(nT - mT)\} \quad (5.8)$$

$$U(nT - mT) = F\{u(nT - mT)\} \quad (5.9)$$

$$V(nT - mT) = F\{u(nT - mT) + P_i(nT)\} \quad (5.10)$$

and $P_i(nT)$ is the correction issued by the performance index. For a three-term (PID) controller the learning mechanism (performance-index modification) would be as follows:

Performance-index correction (PID) = Performance-index correction (PD) + Integral correction term (I).

Linguistically this operation can be expressed as: *if the rule exists then modify it, else add it to the rule base*. The inference procedure adopted here improves the computational efficiency of the algorithm that generates and controls the output as follows.

The control rule IF E THEN IF CE THEN U is a fuzzy relation

$$R = E \times CE \times U \quad (5.11)$$

where E = error, CE = change-in-error, and U = output.

$$\mu_R(E, CE, U) = \min\{\mu_E(E), \mu_{CE}(CE), \mu_U(U)\}. \quad (5.12)$$

If the inputs to the controller at some instance are the fuzzy set e and ce, then an implied output set is u which can be obtained from the above rule using the process of fuzzy composition.

$$u = (e \circ (ce \circ (E \times CE \times U))) \quad (5.13)$$

which has a membership function given by

$$\mu_u(u) = \max_e \min\{[\max_{ce} \min\{\mu_R(E, CE, U), \mu_{ce}(ce)\}], \mu_e(e)\}. \quad (5.14)$$

For several control rules, the output set U is characterized by the membership function:

$$\mu_u = \max_{\text{rules}}\{\mu_u(u)\}. \tag{5.15}$$

The rule modification method involves a modification procedure for both the rule antecedents and consequents, depending on the recommended modification assigned by the state buffer and the performance index. The rule consequents modification is a conditional procedure. It involves either modifying the rule membership function, or the rule linguistic label depending on the modification amount. This procedure is required in order to avoid contradictory rules. If the recommended modification to the rule consequent exceeds the linguistic value width then a linguistic value modification is performed, otherwise if the recommended modification does not exceed the rule linguistic width then only a membership function modification will be performed. Such a procedure may be represented as follows:

Let y be the rule consequent

IF $Q(y + \delta M) \geqslant Q(y)$ THEN linguistic modification
IF $Q(y + \delta M) < Q(y)$ THEN membership modification

where $Q(y)$ is the linguistic value of the variable y and δM is the recommended modification.

5.5.1.4 The state buffer

For a process with a large dead-time or delay, the control action should be rewarded an adequare amount of time earlier. The state buffer is a first-in/first-out register (FIFO) which records the values of the scaled error, scaled change-in-error, and the defuzzified controller output before scaling, and produces the registered values in the buffer output after a time equal to the delay-in-Reward parameter.

5.5.2 Rule-base manipulation

The rule-base manipulation involves the control of the rule-base modification, growth and optimization. The rule modification selects either to start or to stop the rule-base modification and generation procedure, depending on the recommendation of the supervisory level. In normal operation mode, the rule-base modification is kept on-line for obtaining an adaptive rule-base that satisfies the on-line changes in the controlled process dynamics. But if a fault occurs in the system, the supervisory level will recommend rule-base freezing which stops the rule-base modification procedure. This is performed in order to keep a normal-operating-conditions rule-base, so avoiding spoiling the rule-base by the modification procedure assigning a faulty-behaviour-rule modification. As the system recovers from the fault, the rule-base modification procedure will be put on-line again.

The rule-base growth and optimization procedure involves classifying the rules into long-term and short-term memory rules. Minimizing the number of rules is essential since big rule-bases give uncertain control actions. This procedure is accomplished by assigning a decay factor for each rule. The decay factor represents the survival of the rule; the more the rule participates in calculating the control signal, the lower the decay factor assigned to it thus becoming a long-term memory rule, and vice versa where the rules become short-term memory rules. As a new rule is generated, modified, or selected as an initial rule, a minimum decay factor is assigned to it. The decay factor for each rule is updated each sample time. Once the decay factor of the rule becomes maximum, then the rule is disabled and not deleted so it is not used in the rule inference to reduce the calculation time.

When special events occur, the decay factor of each rule is reset to give them a full survival strength. Such events include a change in the set-point, or a fault in the system. This is for controlling the new environment or the new task using the initial rule-base, since new states or behaviour are expected where the optimized rule-base does not include rules relating to the new conditions.

5.5.3 Filtering library

The filtering library includes a number of low-pass filter types which are selected for the appropriate application, depending on the controlled system and the noise contamination. There are five types of filter in the library as follows:

1. Three-point non-recursive average filter.
2. Six-point non-recursive average filter.
3. Median filter.
4. Non-recursive hybrid median filter (NRHMF).
5. Recursive hybrid median filter (RHMF).

The moving average filter is represented by:

$$G_F(z^{-1}) = \frac{1}{n} \sum_{i=1}^{n} z^{-1} \qquad (5.16)$$

where n is the number of points.

The other types of filter are of the median type. A median filter incorporates a non-linear filtering technique known for preserving sharp changes in signal and for being particularly effective in removing impulsive noise. The median filter algorithm is a simple operation of choosing the median value of the sample inside a moving average window of fixed length.

Let S_N be a set of N samples $\{x_1, x_2, \ldots, x_i, \ldots, x_N\}$, where $N = 2k + 1$. The median is defined by:

$$Y(N) = \text{MED}\{x_i | x_i \in S_N\} \tag{5.17}$$

By definition, the median Y is both the $(k+1)$st largest and the $(k+1)$st smallest element in S_N (Tuckey, 1974). The connection between the moving average and the moving median filters is that the output of the former is an unbiased estimate of the mean distribution while the latter is an unbiased estimate of the centre of the distribution. Several modifications of the standard median filter have been represented by other authors. Two general types of median filters were represented by Astola *et al.* (1989). The class called linear median hybrid (LMH) filters contains the standard median filter, recursive and non-recursive median hybrid filters.

LMH filters utilize subfilters and a median operation typically over three samples. LMH filters consider the following structure:

$$Y(N) = \text{MED}\{\phi_L(x(N)), \phi_C(x(N)), \phi_R(x(N))\} \tag{5.18}$$

The filters ϕ_L and ϕ_R are low pass filters following slower trends in the input signals. The ϕ_L filter is designed to react quickly to signal level changes allowing the whole filter to move swiftly from one level to another. Subscripts R, L and C denote right, left and centre, indicating the corresponding filter's position with respect to the current output value being calculated.

The use of median filters for medical applications was represented by Makivirta *et al.* (1989) for data filtering of systolic blood pressure which has the properties of impulsive noise, physiological fluctuation and sampling error. A median filter was compared to a moving average filter where better data interpolation was achieved using the median filter. In a comparative study for the different types of filter included in the library acting on a sinusoidal noisy signal, the moving average filters do not reject the impulsive-type noise. Better rejection could be achieved by increasing the order of the filter. The median filter type gives better rejection for the impulsive noise. The non-recursive LMH filter gives the smoothest signal. The selection of the filter type is performed by the supervisory level depending on the noise contamination percentage during the controller initialization.

5.5.4 Gain scheduling

The gain scheduling procedure is based on the amount of the initial bolus of drug which is considered as an auxiliary input signal, and the time response due to the effect of the drug bolus. More precisely, the gain is estimated by calculating the time point where the paralysis reaches the maximum point and starts to drop. At this point, the time difference between this point and the time when the bolus was injected is calculated and considered as a parameter for the model response to an impulse and is used for calculating the gain as follows.

The linear part of the model is described by the following:

$$\frac{X_E}{U} = \frac{K(s+t_4)}{(s+t_1)(s+t_2)(s+t_3)} \quad (5.19)$$

where K is the model gain, X_E is the drug concentration and U is the drug input.

Equation (5.19) can be written as follows:

$$X_E = \frac{\acute{K}(1+m_4 s)}{(1+m_1 s)(1+m_2 s)(1+m_3 s)} \quad (5.20)$$

where

$$\acute{K} = \frac{UKt_4}{(t_1 t_2 t_3)} \quad (5.21)$$

$$m_1 = \frac{1}{t_1}, \; m_2 = \frac{1}{t_2}, \; m_3 = \frac{1}{t_3}, \; m_4 = \frac{1}{t_4}.$$

Using the partial fractions method, the roots of the equation are as follows:

$$a = \frac{(m_4 - m_1)}{(m_2 - m_1)(m_3 - m_1)} \qquad b = \frac{(m_4 - m_2)}{(m_2 - m_1)(m_2 - m_3)}$$

$$c = \frac{(m_4 - m_3)}{(m_3 - m_1)(m_3 - m_2)}. \quad (5.22)$$

Solving the equation in terms of time:

$$X_E = (a e^{-m_1 t} + b e^{-m_2 t} + c e^{-m_3 t}) \acute{K}. \quad (5.23)$$

Solving equation (5.19) for the gain

$$\acute{K} = \frac{X_E}{(a e^{-m_1 t} + b e^{-m_2 t} + c e^{-m_3 t})}. \quad (5.24)$$

The non-linear part is represented by a Hill equation as follows:

$$E_{\text{eff}} = \frac{E_{\max}}{1 + X_E(50)^\alpha / X_E^\alpha}. \quad (5.25)$$

Solving for the value of X_E:

$$X_E = \left\{ \frac{E_{\text{eff}} X_E(50)^\alpha}{1 - E_{\text{eff}}} \right\}^{1/\alpha}. \quad (5.26)$$

Combining equations (5.21), (5.24) and (5.26) results in the following:

$$\text{Gain} = \frac{(t_1 t_2 t_3) \left(\dfrac{E_{\text{eff}} X_E(50)^\alpha}{1 - E_{\text{eff}}} \right)^{1/\alpha}}{(Ut_4)(a e^{-t/t_1} + b e^{-t/t_2} + c e^{-t/t_3})}. \quad (5.27)$$

The time constants used for the equation are the nominal values since deviating values do not have a large effect on the estimation.

5.5.5 Controller setting

The controller initialization includes setting the delay-in-reward, the scaling factors, and the selection of an initial rule-base. According to the patient gain estimated by the gain scheduler, the patient is classified into one of the three defined categories (low sensitivity, medium sensitivity and high sensitivity) as follows:

$0.5 < K \leqslant 1.0$ (low sensitivity)
$1.0 < K \leqslant 3.0$ (medium sensitivity)
$3.0 < K \leqslant 10.0$ (high sensitivity).

The delay-in-reward is selected to be 1 minute which is kept fixed for all the cases where an estimation for the delay is not possible in the initial response because of the non-linear characteristics.

The scaling factors are defined as the error scaling factor (GE), the change-in-error scaling factor (GC), the integral term scaling factor (GI), and the output scaling factor (GT). The values specified below are the scaling factors default settings. The change-in-error scaling factor is set according to the maximum change-in-error detected within the period between the gain scheduling and setting the control algorithm on-line.

The scaling factor selection is set as follows for the three cases:

case 1: low sensitivity
$GE = 0.33 \quad GC = 6.0/\text{max}CE \quad GI = 1.0 \quad GT = 16.66$

case 2: medium sensitivity
$GE = 0.33 \quad GC = 6.0/\text{max}CE \quad GI = 0.75 \quad GT = 16.66$

case 3: high sensitivity
$GE = 0.33 \quad GC = 6.0/\text{max}CE \quad GI = 0.5 \quad GT = 16.66.$

Three rule-bases of 15 rules each were developed, starting the controller with an empty rule-base and modifying it with a multi-run procedure in order to develop a rule-base for each operating category.

5.5.6 Performance monitor and controller tuning

The objective of the performance monitor block is to observe the response pattern of the system and detect if the system is within the acceptable operation limits. The pattern to be recognized is the error versus time. The absence or presence of peak heights, the time between peaks and steady-state error are the features which are monitored in the process response. This concept was first implemented in the Foxboro self-tuning PID commercial controller using the EXACT control algorithm (Kraus and Myron, 1984).

The performance monitor in this application uses three parameters to evaluate the process response: the error tolerance, oscillation amplitude tolerance and acceptable range of error convergence. Accordingly, the performance is evaluated with respect to the accuracy, oscillation, speed of response, divergence and steady-state error. Figure 5.4 shows the five distinguished behaviours; steady-state behaviour, oscillation behaviour, convergence behaviour, divergence behaviour, and steady-state behaviour with noise. The accuracy measure defines a noise tolerance band such that fluctuation within this band is considered to be the noise effect. The oscillation measure checks for the oscillatory behaviour by detecting the peaks in the response. The speed-of-convergence measure checks for the system response whether it is within the desired response speed limit or exceeds it. The divergence measure checks whether the system is stable or starts to diverge to unstable behaviour. The last measure checks for the steady-state error in the response.

The extracted observations from the response are then converted into a set of linguistic statements that describe the system response. Then the

Hierarchical supervisory self-organizing fuzzy control 151

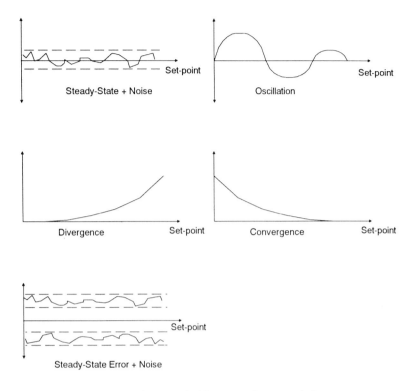

Figure 5.4 *Five distinguishable types of process behaviour.*

controller is re-tuned according to the inferred tuning recommendation from a rule-base that describes the expert knowledge of tuning the fuzzy logic controller. The rules are expressed in an 'IF . . . THEN' form that has the observed behaviours as antecedents and the tuning action as consequents of the rules. The recommended tuning will be either an increment or decrement to the specified term.

The development of the tuning fuzzy rule-base starts by defining linguistic labels for the process behaviours as follows: oscillation (OSC), convergence (CON), divergence (DIV) and steady-state error (SSE). The linguistic variables defined for this case are as follows: acceptable behaviour (ACP), not-acceptable behaviour (NOA), high-speed response (HI), and low-speed response (LO). Another conditional statement to be considered as the rules antecedent is the classification of the process category as follows: low gain, medium gain, and high gain (LO, MED, HI). The consequences of the rules would be either no-change, increment, or decrement to the appropriate parameter. Seven linguistic labels have been established for this purpose: negative big (NB), negative medium (NM), negative small (NS), zero or no-change (NC), positive small (PS), positive medium (PM), and positive big (PB).

However in the present situation, the linguistic rules can be expressed in the following example:

IF the error response has steady-state error AND the process class is MED THEN change in the error integral scaling factor is PM

In order to define the rules, Figure 5.5 shows the notations used for the fuzzy quantities. In order to define the universe of discourse for the linguistic variables, the noise contamination percentage allowed should be defined, as well as defining a time-limit period in which the system should reach steady-state behaviour when the performance is monitored over a period of time. The noise contamination percentage is considered to be ±2%, where fluctuation around the set-point within the noise band is considered to be due to noise. The dominant time constant for most of the patients is about 35 minutes which is considered to be the time limit for the convergence of the system. If the convergence time is longer than the time limit then the system is considered to have slow speed of convergence and vice versa. In the case of an occurrence of a fault, the performance monitor resets to monitor the process behaviour, but in this case shorter monitoring time should be set for the time limit since fast recovery is required when a fault occurs. Therefore the time limit for the performance monitor is set to 15 minutes.

The oscillation behaviour classification is either acceptable when no oscillation is detected, or not acceptable when an oscillatory behaviour is detected. The process behaviour is considered to be oscillatory when more than one peak is detected which should be a positive peak followed by a negative one or vice versa. A positive peak is indicated when the change in error changes from negative, to zero and then to positive, where the zero change in error should be combined by an error outside the noise band. In contrast, a negative peak is detected when the change in error changes from

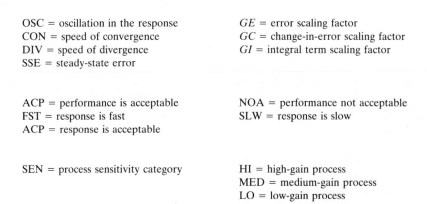

OSC = oscillation in the response
CON = speed of convergence
DIV = speed of divergence
SSE = steady-state error

GE = error scaling factor
GC = change-in-error scaling factor
GI = integral term scaling factor

ACP = performance is acceptable
FST = response is fast
ACP = response is acceptable

NOA = performance not acceptable
SLW = response is slow

SEN = process sensitivity category

HI = high-gain process
MED = medium-gain process
LO = low-gain process

Figure 5.5 *Notations used for the fuzzy quantities.*

positive, to zero and then to negative where the error should be outside the noise band when the change in error is zero. The divergence is classified as being either acceptable when the system is in its steady-state mode, or not acceptable when it diverges from the set-point. This behaviour is discussed in the fault detection section (section 5.5.7). The last behaviour is the steady-state error which is detected when the process output is steady but above or below the noise band. The fuzzy sets shapes are represented by the fuzzy number width as illustrated for each variable in Figure 5.6.

The controller tuning involves a modification to the change-in-error and the integral term scaling factors. The change-in-error scaling factor is modified when an oscillatory performance is detected or when the divergence speed is not acceptable. The integral term scaling factor is modified when a steady-state error is detected.

The amount of modification for the change-in-error scaling factor depends on the maximum change-in-error detected as follows:

$$GC(nT) = GC(nT-1) \pm \text{EMOD}(PS) \qquad (5.28)$$

where PS is the process gain category defined as follows:

low gain $(PS = 1)$ medium gain $(PS = 2)$ high gain $(PS = 3)$

and $\text{EMOD}(PS)$ is the error scaling factor modification linguistic label defined by the following:

$\text{MOD}(1) = \max CE/2.0$ $\text{MOD}(2) = \max CE/4.0$ $\text{MOD}(3) = \max CE/6.0$.

The integral term scaling factor is modified according to the classified process category as follows:

$$GI(nT) = GI(nT-1) + \text{IMOD}(PS) \qquad (5.29)$$

where $\text{IMOD}(PS)$ is the error scaling factor modification linguistic label defined by the following:

$\text{MOD}(1) = \max CE/1.0$ $\text{MOD}(2) = \max CE/0.75$ $\text{MOD}(3) = \max CE/0.5$

the correction linguistic variables represent small, medium and large respectively.

5.5.7 Fault detection and diagnosis

Three fault types are detected by the system as follows: fault in the Relaxograph, fault in the syringe drive and change in the patient dynamics.

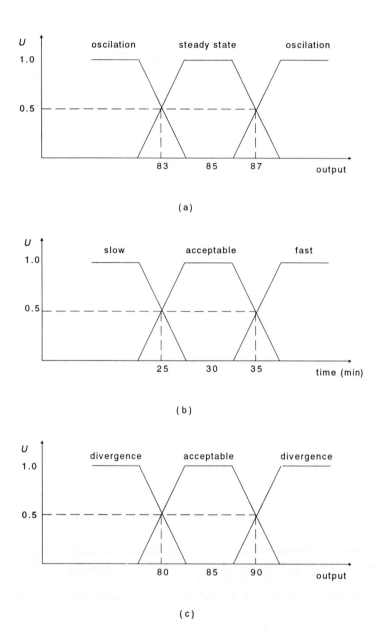

Figure 5.6 *Medical system performance monitor fuzzy rules. (a) Steady state, (b) convergence speed, (c) divergence speed.*

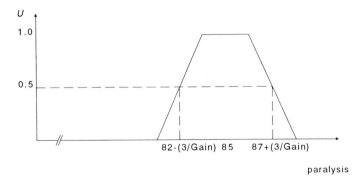

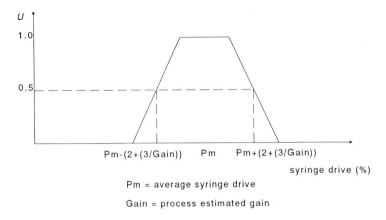

Figure 5.7 *Medical system fault detection fuzzy rules.*

A fault is detected by monitoring the input–output relationship of the patient. If divergence occurs in the output, then the fault detection and diagnosis procedure is activated. The fuzzy detection rules are shown in Figure 5.7.

A fault in the Relaxograph is recognized by a change in the device readings while the muscle relaxation is maintaining the same value. This is due to movements in the sensing probes of the Relaxograph that make the path through which the stimulus signal is passing increase its resistance. This makes the Relaxograph sense a lower relaxation level than the real value. This type of fault is detected when there is an acute sudden change in the paralysis level while keeping a steady infusion of drug.

The second type of fault is represented by a disconnection in the drug infusion tubing, or if the drug is infused into the patient but does not go inside the vein. In this case the relaxation level starts to drop while the syringe drive increases as a correction procedure via the controller.

The last type of fault is a change in the patient pharmacokinetics parameters, which is represented by a change in the patient gain due to loss of blood or other related events. In this case there will be a gradual change in the relaxation level where the controller starts to correct it by increasing the infusion rate. Therefore if the drug infusion changes while maintaining the same relaxation level, it means that there is a change in the patient dynamics. This type of fault is detected by comparing the input–output relationship in the past with the present behaviour. If there is a difference then there is a fault.

The following are linguistic rules for the defined fault detection.

1. IF there is an acute sudden change in the paralysis AND the syringe drive is steady THEN there is a fault in the Relaxograph
2. IF the paralysis is dropping AND the syringe drive is increasing THEN there is a fault in the syringe drive
3. IF there is a gradual change in the paralysis AND the syringe drive is changing THEN there is a change in the patient dynamics.

Other faults related to hardware or software errors have been described in Section 5.2.1.

The fault correction starts when there is a fault detected in the system. The first measure to be taken is to stop the rule-base modification. The next step is to diagnose the fault and a correction procedure is executed depending on the fault type. For a fault in the Relaxograph, the correction procedure will be a change in the set-point to a new paralysis level in order to keep the same amount of paralysis with respect to the shifted readings. A fault in the syringe drive will initiate an alarm to signal to the anaesthetist that he should check the system components. The last type of fault is a change in the patient dynamics. In this type of fault a correction procedure is not taken but a warning signal to the anaesthetist is initiated. Other types of faults where human interaction is required are reported to the anaesthetist. After the fault has been diagnosed and a correction procedure accomplished, the controller tuning is activated by monitoring the performance after the correction of the fault.

The alarm and warning system includes sending an alarm or warning signal via the screen or an audio signal when the fault has occurred. Also another warning signal is given when the paralysis level drops below 75% if such a level is not acceptable to the surgeon.

5.5.8 Supervisory level manager

The supervisory level manager is the part which controls all other blocks in the supervisory level. With its embedded knowledge-base it can schedule the

ance with an average drug infusion of 16.763 ml h^{-1}. The total drug consumption including the drug bolus was 99.067 mg.

The third case was the high sensitivity patient (gain = 5.0) as shown in Figure 5.8(c). A bolus of 15 mg was given to the patient at time 2 minutes, the maximum paralysis level reached being 98.14% where the patient was very sensitive and the paralysis remained in saturation for 8 minutes. The estimated gain was 4.45. The filter type selected was NRLMF. The controller was set on-line at time 36 minutes with the following settings:

> delay-in-reward = 1 min
> 15 initial rules
> $GE = 0.33 \quad GC = 10.9 \quad GI = 1.0 \quad GT = 16.66$.

No re-tuning was necessary for the controller since the performance was within the acceptable limits. The syringe drive was driven with an average of 7.01 ml h^{-1}. The total drug consumption including the initial bolus of drug was 46.14 mg.

A comparative study using manual control was undertaken for case 2 where the same parameters as for the automatic control case were used. The operation started by giving the patient a bolus of drug of 20 mg then infusing extra boluses of 3.5 mg when required as shown in Figure 5.9. Over a period of 200 minutes the total amount of drug consumed in the operation using manual control was 107.5 mg. For the same time period, the amount of drug consumed using automatic control for the same case was 81.9 mg. A reduction of 24.3% was achieved.

5.6.2 Relaxograph fault

The first type of fault considered was in the Relaxograph and was due to the movement in the patient such that a change in the sensing of the Relaxograph electrodes occurred. Such an event occurs when the Relaxograph gives a sudden change in the measured paralysis with the condition that the patient maintains the same muscle relaxation. This sudden change happens when the path in which the electronic signal sent by the two simulating electrodes and received by the recording electrodes changes its conductivity. In this case the fault is detected by monitoring the input–output relationship of the patient. When there is a sudden change in the paralysis level with steady-state drug infusion, this means that there is a fault in the Relaxograph readings. In this case the correction procedure is to change the set-point to the faulty muscle relaxation level recorded by the Relaxograph in order to keep the same level of paralysis with the faulty readings.

The fault was simulated for the three patient cases at time 100 minutes returning to the non-faulty conditions at time 150 minutes. The fault was

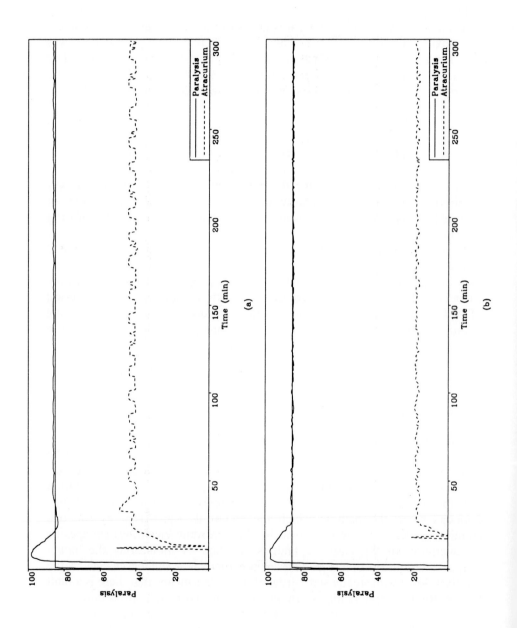

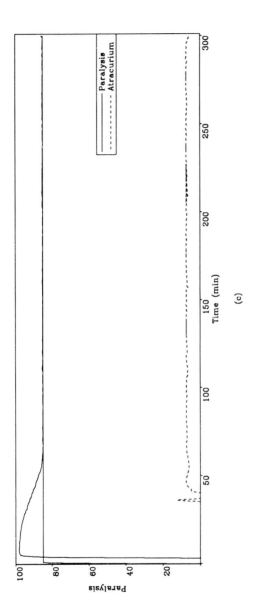

Figure 5.8 Simulation of normal operating conditions. (a) Low-sensitivity patient, (b) medium-sensitivity patient, (c) high-sensitivity patient.

162   *Intelligent Control in Biomedicine*

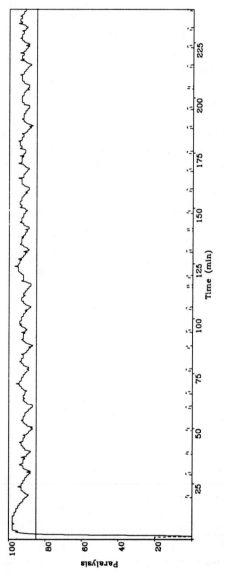

Figure 5.9 *Simulation of normal operating conditions under manual control for medium-sensitivity patient.*

simulated by changing the non-linear part of the mathematical model by introducing a shift in the non-linear curve across the X axis. This case would be satisfied by keeping the same drug plasma concentration in the blood and changing the detected paralysis. The non-faulty non-linear parameters are as follows:

$$\alpha = 2.98 \quad X_E(50) = 0.404$$

and the faulty parameters are:

$$\alpha = 2.98 \quad X_E(50) = 0.5.$$

For the first case with the low-sensitivity patient, the same settings as used for the normal conditions were used. Figure 5.10(a) shows the time response of case 1 where a fault occurred in the Relaxograph at time 100 minutes. The fault was detected and a correction procedure was undertaken by changing the set-point to 76.39%. A second fault occurred at time 150 minutes, where the patient parameters have returned to the old settings. The fault was detected and the correction procedure changed the set-point to 85.21%.

For patient case 2 with medium sensitivity, Figure 5.10(b) shows the time response. The same parameters were set the same as for the normal case, and the same procedure was undertaken over the same time. The first fault was detected and corrected by changing the set-point to 74.95%, then the second fault occurred and the correction procedure changed the set-point to 84.04%.

Simulation results for case 3 are shown in Figure 5.10(c). Similar parameters were used as for the normal case, and the fault procedure was simulated at times of 100 and 150 minutes respectively. The correction procedure for the first fault changed the set-point to 76.06%, while the second fault was corrected by changing the set-point to 84.95%.

5.6.3 Syringe drive fault

Serious faults in the syringe drive are of two types: the first is the disconnection of the drug infusion pipe, while the second is due to infusing the drug to the patient without the drug going into the veins. Both faults have the same symptoms and effects in that the patient does not receive drug infusion. The effect of such faults will be a drop in paralysis. As a correction procedure by the controller, the infusion rate will be increased in order to eliminate the error. Although the infusion rate is increasing, the paralysis level keeps dropping, and this indicates a fault in the syringe drive. At that time an alarm signal will be issued to the anaesthetist informing him of a fault in the syringe drive and in turn they have to check the system

164 Intelligent Control in Biomedicine

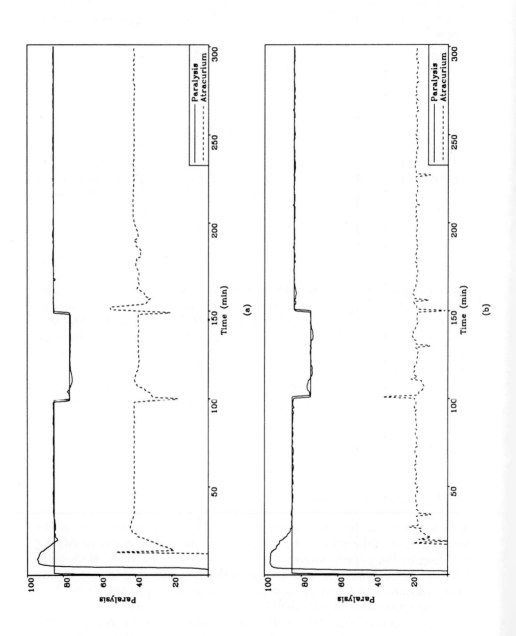

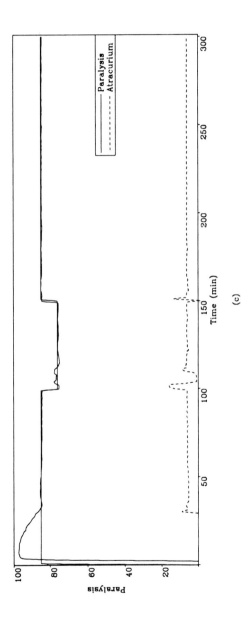

Figure 5.10 *Simulation of faults occurring in the Relaxograph.* (a) *Low-sensitivity patient,* (b) *medium-sensitivity patient,* (c) *high-sensitivity patient.*

components. In all cases the correction procedure is assumed to be taken by reconnecting the infusion line.

Simulation results are shown in Figure 5.11 for the three cases respectively. In Figure 5.11(*a*), the low-sensitivity patient was simulated. A fault in the syringe drive occurred at time 100 minutes by disconnecting the infusion line. The fault was detected at time 106 minutes and corrected. Due to the overshoot behaviour, the tuning procedure decreased GC at time 116 minutes (slow convergence).

For case 2, a medium-sensitivity patient, the fault occurred at the same time, being detected at time 119 minutes, and was corrected instantly as shown in Figure 5.11(*b*). The tuning procedure occurred at time 130 minutes where *GC* was decreased due to the overshoot behaviour (slow convergence). Figure 5.11(*c*) shows the time response of a high-sensitivity patient where the fault occurred at the same time and was detected at time 114 minutes. No tuning procedure was undertaken since the response was within the acceptable limits (convergence with acceptable speed).

5.6.4 Patient dynamics change

The last type of fault detected by the system is not a real fault in the control algorithm, or the instruments, but rather a change in the patient parameters (pharmacokinetics) which can be represented by a change in the patient gain. Such events occur when the patient loses blood, and part of the infused drug is lost with the blood, which makes the patient become less sensitive resulting in a requirement for a higher infusion rate. Other cases occur where the patient is infused with other drugs having muscle relaxation effects, such as isofluranc for general anaesthesia. If a large amount of such drugs is given to the patients, their sensitivity to the muscle relaxation drug will increase which makes them require less drug for the same paralysis level. In this case such events are detected but not considered as faults, rather, a warning signal is issued to the anaesthetists to make them aware of such an event. On the part of the controller, the control algorithm needs to be modified by changing the rule modification factor to the new gain ratio, as well as initializing the performance monitoring layer. The change in the patient sensitivity is detected by monitoring the patient input–output relation of the average drug infusion needed to maintain a certain paralysis. When the patient sensitivity changes, the controller is required either to increase or decrease the infusion rate as a correction procedure to eliminate the error. In this case the infusion rate will not be the same as the normal conditions where the fault is detected. The new gain of the patient will be estimated by calculating the ratio of the normal infusion rate and the new infusion rate.

The simulation study was carried out for the three cases as shown in Figure 5.12. The model parameters were considered to be the same for the normal case. The fault occurred at time 100 minutes by decreasing the gain by a factor of 25%, then at time 200 minutes increasing in the gain to the original normal value. Figure 5.12(a) shows the time response for the low-sensitivity case where the estimated gain was 0.74. The fault occurred at time 100 minutes and was detected at time 111 minutes, the new estimated gain being 0.57, and no tuning was necessary. The second change occurred at time 200 minutes and detected at time 209 minutes. The new estimated gain was 0.757. Again, no tuning was necessary. The second case is the medium-sensitivity 'patient' as shown in Figure 5.12(b). The estimated gain was 1.77. The first fault was detected at time 105 minutes, and the new estimated gain was 1.367. The second fault was detected at time 205 minutes, and the new estimated gain was 1.75. No parameters tuning was required. Lastly the third case, as shown in Figure 5.12(c), was for a high-sensitivity patient. The estimated gain was 4.45. At time 100 minutes the gain changed from 5.0 to 3.56 with the fault being detected at time 107 minutes, and the new estimated gain was 3.56. At time 200 minutes the gain was set back to its original value where it was detected at time 205 minutes, and the new estimated gain was 4.75. No tuning was necessary since the performance was within the acceptable measures.

5.7 Conclusions

The architecture of the supervisory system presented in this chapter incorporates a rule-based fuzzy logic controller to perform the direct control task, while the adaptive mechanism is considered to be applied to the controller in two different mechanisms: the first is the self-organizing feature which involves modifying the control rules via a performance-index measure, while the second is the self-tuning feature which involves tuning the controller scaling factors depending on the monitored performance of the system. In addition, the supervisory level has the feature of setting up the initial controller parameters, including the initial scaling factors and rule-base, based on the classified process category which is selected via the gain-scheduling procedure that estimates the process gain, depending on the initial response of the process to an input control signal.

The other control task is fault detection and diagnosis which is based on defining the physical fault in the process when its behaviour does not fall into an acceptable zone. The fault detection block incorporates fuzzy rules describing the normal conditions of the process. When a fault occurs in the process, the direct control regime is considered to correct the unacceptable behaviour until the fault is diagnosed and if possible corrected, then an adaptive control technique is applied to ensure acceptable behaviour.

In summary, the supervisory control system consists of generic control tasks for keeping the process on-line with an acceptable behaviour. If a fault

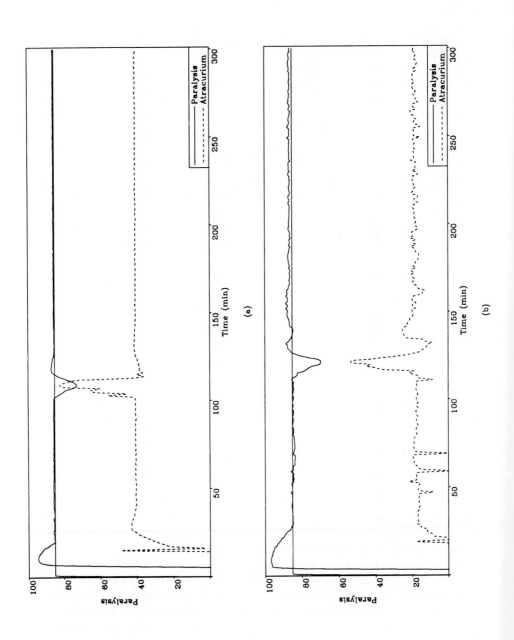

Hierarchical supervisory self-organizing fuzzy control 169

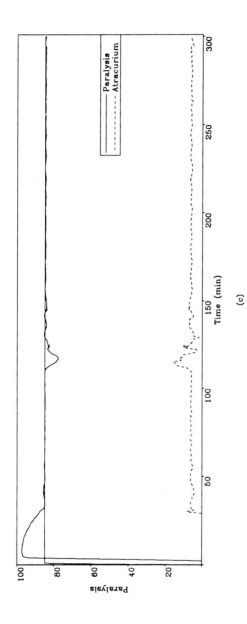

Figure 5.11 *Simulation of faults occurring in the syringe drive. (a) Low-sensitivity patient, (b) medium-sensitivity patient, (c) high-sensitivity patient.*

170   *Intelligent Control in Biomedicine*

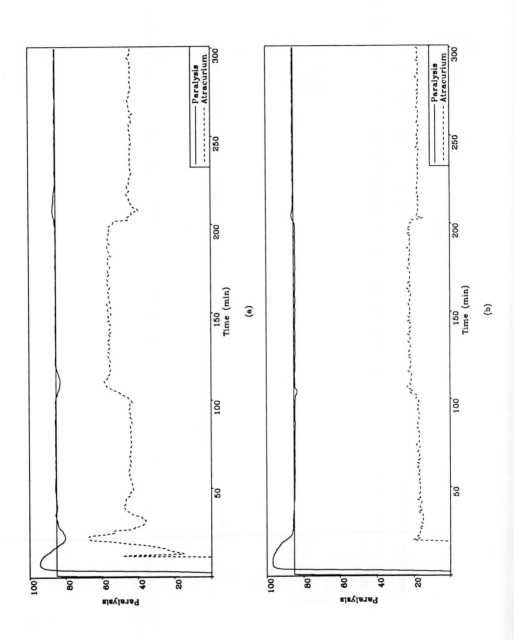

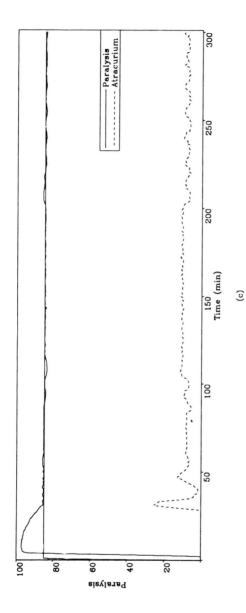

Figure 5.12 Simulation of changes in the patient conditions. (a) Low-sensitivity patient, (b) medium-sensitivity patient, (c) high-sensitivity patient.

occurs in the process, the control task passes through a primary direct control regime first, then an adaptive control regime, and finally a fault diagnosis regime, each attempting to drive the system behaviour into an acceptable zone.

The supervisory control system presented in this chapter consists of generic control tasks for keeping the process on-line within acceptable behaviour boundaries. The fact that the same architecture could be mapped between medical and industrial applications with very little change shows that it has a genericity which should encourage its use in a wider range of engineering problems. In industrial systems where a shorter sampling time is required, parallel processing techniques can be used. Therefore, a transputer-based environment has been built for the supervisory control algorithm to control an industrial-type electro-fluid system.

References

Assilian, S. and Mamdani, E.H., 1975, An experiment in linguistic synthesis with fuzzy logic controller, *International Journal of Man-Machine Systems*, **7**, 1–13.

Astola, J., Heinonen, P. and Neuvo, V., 1989, Linear median hybrid filter, *IEEE Transactions on Circuits and Systems*, **36**, 1430–8.

Daley, S. and Gill, K.F., 1986, A design study of a self-organising fuzzy logic controller, *Proceedings of the Institution of Mechanical Engineers*, **200**(C1), 59–69.

Denai, N., Linkens, D.A., Asbury, A.J., McLeod, A.D. and Gray, W.M., 1990, Self-tuning pid control of atracurium-induced muscle relaxation in surgical patients, *Proceedings of the IEE* PtD., **137**, 261–72.

deSilva, C.W. and MacFarlane, A.G.J., 1988, A knowledge-based control structure for robotic manipulators, *Proceedings of the IFAC on A.I. in Real Time Control*, pp. 143–7.

deSilva, C.W. and Macfarlane, A.G., 1989, Knowledge-based control approach for robotic manipulator, *International Journal of Control*, **50**(1), 249–73.

Kraus, T.W. and Myron, T.J., 1984, Self-tuning pid controller using pattern recognition approach, *Control Engineering*, **31**, 106–11.

Kwok, D.P., Tam, P. and Wang, P., 1990, 'Linguistic pid controller', in *Proceedings of 11th IFAC Congress*, Tallinn, USSR, pp. 192–7.

Linkens, D.A., Mahfouf, M., Asbury, A.J. and Gray, M.W., 1991, Generalized predictive control applied to muscle relaxant anaesthesia, presentation at the IEE International Conference 'Control '91', Edinburgh, Vol. 2, pp. 790–4.

Makivirta, A., Koski, E., Kari, A. and Sukuvaara, T., 1989, 'Robust signal-to-symbol transformation by using median filters', presentation at The IFAC Workshop on Decision Support for Patient Management: Measurements, Modeling and Control, pp. 91–104.

Menad, M., 1984, 'Feedback Control of Drug Administration for Muscle Relaxation', PhD thesis, Department of Automatic Control and Systems Engineering, University of Sheffield.

Miller, R.D. (Ed.), 1990, *Intravenous Anaesthetic Delivery*, 3rd Edn, New York: Churchill Livingstone.

Mizumoto, M., 1988, Fuzzy controls under various fuzzy reasoning methods, *Information Sciences*, **45**, 129–51.

Procyk, T.J., 1977, 'Self-Organizing Control for Dynamic Processes', PhD thesis, Faculty of Engineering, University of London.
Procyk, T.J. and Mamdani, E.H., 1979, A linguistic self-organising process controller, *Automatica*, **15**, 15–30.
Rasmussen, J., 1985, The role of hierarchical knowledge representation in decision making and system management, *IEEE Transactions on System, Man and Cybernetics*, **SMC-15**, 234–43.
Sutton, D.P. and Jess, I.M., 1991, A design study of a self-organizing fuzzy autopilot for ship control. *Proceedings of the Institution of Mechanical Engineers*, **205**, 35–48.
Tong, R.M., 1977, A control engineering review of fuzzy systems, *Automatica*, **13**, 559–69.
Tuckey, J.W., 1974, 'Non-linear (non superpasable) method for smoothing data', presentation at International Congress 'EASCON'74', p. 673.
Weatherley, B.C., Williams, S.G. and Neill, M., 1983, Pharmacokinetics, pharmacodynamics and dose-response relationship of atracurium administered i.v. *British Journal of Anaesthesia*, **55**, 39S–45S.
Zadeh, L.A., 1965, Fuzzy sets, *Information and Control*, **8**, 338–53.

Chapter 6
Hierarchical fuzzy modelling and fault detection for muscle relaxation anaesthesia

J. S. Shieh

6.1 Introduction

Modelling a system is very important because it is related to process characterization and design studies. In the past, it has been thought that a complicated mathematical approach could model a system more accurately, but this still has problems when ill-defined, complicated and non-linear systems are encountered. However, people can easily reach a good result when they are driving a car, playing golf, cooking a meal and so on. Although they are not aware of a mathematical description in their brain, people still perform very well from human experience.

In 1965, the fuzzy set theory proposed by L. A. Zadeh (1965) offered the possibility of creating models which function more like human thinking. Later, several authors conducted research into fuzzy modelling which can be divided into six different methods. Firstly, using verbalization or linguistics through interaction with the human operator or domain expert, the system can be modelled easily and quickly (Kickert, 1979; Kiszka *et al.*, 1985; Matsushima and Sugiyama, 1985; Peng and Wang, 1988; Shengehaog and Kreifeldt, 1989). A disadvantage of this method is that it is difficult to find suitable human operators or experts. Secondly, from logical analysis of the input and output data, the system can be modelled more accurately by a trial-and-error approach (Tong, 1978, 1980). However, with input and output data it is easy to produce a pair of rules in conflict, and a trial-and-error approach is time consuming. Thirdly, there are methods based on fuzzy implication and reasoning algorithms to identify fuzzy models (Sugeno and Kang, 1986, 1988; Sugeno *et al.*, 1989, Sugeno and Tanaka, 1991, Takagi and Sugeno, 1985). However, this involves traditional identification methods and makes the modelling system more complicated, and like conventional control theory it is difficult to apply to multivariable systems. Fourthly, using identification and self-learning algorithms for fuzzy modelling of MISO systems, the identification algorithm can produce a fuzzy model with fairly high accuracy, and the self-learning algorithm may further improve the model's accuracy (Xu and Lu, 1987, 1988; Xu and Yang, 1987), but identification and self-learning algorithms need large calculations and this makes them unsuitable for dynamic modelling. Fifthly, using learning signals to create a rule-base, the system can be modelled more generally (van der Rhee *et al.*, 1987, 1990a, 1990b). However, much research is still required to determine appropriate choices for learning signals. Lastly, by using a self-organizing fuzzy modelling algorithm to model the system via on-line input and output data, Moore (1991) has designed a fuzzy controller and applied it to an autonomous guided vehicle (AGV). However, indirect adaptive fuzzy controllers still have problems with non-minimum phase processes.

In this chapter, a knowledge-based fuzzy modelling approach is presented in an attempt to model non-linear systems in general, and to be applied in particular to model the muscle relaxation of patients in the operating theatre. The knowledge-base created by learning signals such as the pseudo-random binary sequence (PRBS) and Gaussian random noise signal (GRNS) can generate many rules and represent an almost complete knowledge structure. This has been demonstrated successfully when applied to a non-linear model process with different excitation signals. Also, it has been shown that a rule-base derived from the PRBS learning signal can model a system more accurately than with GRNS excitation.

A hierarchical self-organizing fuzzy logic control (HSOFLC) structure which includes levels of self-organizing fuzzy logic control (SOFLC), self-organizing fuzzy modelling (SOFM) and fault detection is presented in this chapter for the modelling, control and fault detection of muscle relaxation for patients in the operating theatre. Two types of fault are investigated: in a Relaxograph and in a syringe actuator during an operation. The robustness of HSOFLC has been examined by adding PRBS, GRNS, set-point changes and disturbances.

6.2. Knowledge-based fuzzy modelling for non-linear systems

The application of knowledge-based systems to the modelling process is growing, especially in the field of alarm monitoring, fault diagnosis and maintenance scheduling (Åström *et al.*, 1986). In the past, the classical approach to modelling, for instance by frequency responses or state equations, is very far from human thinking. Fuzzy set theory offers the possibility to create models which function in some ways more like humans do. Several authors who were mentioned in Section 6.1 have already conducted research into fuzzy modelling. In this section a system identification procedure, using a SOFM algorithm, is introduced and implemented as a knowledge-based model. The SOFM learns rules from observed data which are activated by learning signals. How to generate rules from observed data and calculate a fuzzy relation to obtain a fuzzy model from the SOFM algorithm will also be described in this section. The advantage of this method is that a good learning signal will result in a fairly complete knowledge structure after the learning phase. This means that all situations which may occur during an application can be derived from the knowledge structure. Hence, various learning signals can be utilized, for example step responses, sine waves, PRBSs and GRNSs; which is best will be discussed at the end of this section.

6.2.1 Self-organizing fuzzy modelling

The SOFM algorithm is derived from a SOFLC algorithm. It can automatically obtain rules from observed input and output data. Hence, SOFM consists of three main steps as shown in Figure 6.1 (Linkens and Shieh, 1992). The first step determines the rule possibilities from input and output data. The second step removes conflicting rules from the rule-base obtained from the rule possibilities. Finally, the third step constructs a fuzzy model from fuzzy set theory.

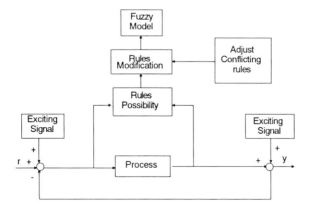

Figure 6.1 *Schematic diagram of self-organizing fuzzy modelling.*

6.2.1.1 Rule possibility

The use of input–output data from the process to estimate the rules is called logical examination and was proposed by R. M. Tong (1978). The quantization of the corresponding measured values produces a sequence of fuzzy sets, such as PB, PM and so on. For example, a single-input–single-output process might be assumed to have an output $y(t)$, which is a function of the last output, $y(t-1)$, and the last input, $u(t-1)$. On the left of Table 6.1 is a part of the input–output data from the process, while quantization of the fuzzy set values like PS or PM for $y(t)$, $y(t-1)$ and $u(t-1)$ is shown on the right side of table. Therefore, the rule $Q(u(t-1)) = PS$, $Q(y(t-1)) = PM \Rightarrow Q(y(t)) = PM$ is identified at $t = k+4$. The same procedure will be identified by different rules at $t = k+7$ and $t = k+8$. That is to say, each input and output data points have fuzzy sets and exist as a rule. Using the fuzzy set of current data compared to the previous data, it is easy to obtain the rule possibilities.

Table 6.1 *An example of logical examination*

t	$u(t)$	$y(t)$	$Q(u(t-1))$	$Q(y(t-1))$	$Q(y(t))$
.	.	.	.	.	.
.	.	.	.	.	.
$k+1$	5	2			
2	2	4			
3	1	3			
4	4	3	PS	PM	PM
5	3	2			
6	1	1			
7	5	1	PS	PS	PS
8	4	1	PB	PS	PS
.	.	.	.	.	.
.	.	.	.	.	.

t: time
$u(t)$: input data
$u(t-1)$: last input data
$y(t)$: output data
$y(t-1)$: last output data
$Q(u(t-1))$: quantization of the last input data
$Q(y(t-1))$: quantization of the last output data
$Q(y(t))$: quantization of the output data
PS: positive small
PM: positive medium
PB: positive big

6.2.1.2 Adjust conflicting rules

Using the method of logical examination, it is easy to obtain the conflicting rules. For example, one rule may be like $Q(u(t-1)) = \text{PS}$, $Q(y(t-1)) = \text{PM} \Rightarrow Q(y(t)) = \text{PM}$ and another rule is $Q(u(t-1)) = \text{PS}$, $Q(y(t-1)) = \text{PM} \Rightarrow Q(y(t)) = \text{PB}$. The two rules are in conflict. Conflicts can arise in three different ways: they may come from noisy data; they may be the result of unsuitable data quantizing; or they may mean that the proposed structure for the model is incorrect. There are two methods to solve the conflicts; one deletes all the conflicting rules; the other resolves the conflicts by choosing the rule that occurs most often. The latter method has been used in this section. With rules obtained from input and output data, one can calculate rule possibilities for each rule. If there are any conflicting rules, one can compare the rule possibilities and retain the rule with the largest possibility.

6.2.1.3 Fuzzy modelling

There are many parameters which affect the fuzzy modelling such as the choice of the input and output variables, the fuzzification strategies, the number of fuzzy modelling rules, the type of membership function and the defuzzification strategies. In fuzzy modelling for non-linear systems or biomedical systems, it is common to have a multivariable situation. A concept involving the decomposition of multivariable fuzzy systems into a set of one-dimensional systems has been proposed by Gupta et al. (1986). The input, output variable and fuzzy relations are described by the following equation:

$$Y_j = \bigwedge_{i=1}^{m}(Xi \circ Rij)$$
$$Rij = \bigvee_{k=1}^{p}[Xi(k) \wedge Yj(k)]$$

where Xi = fuzzy value of the i-input variable; Yj = fuzzy value of the j-output variable; Rij = fuzzy relations of the i-input and j-output variables; m = number of input variables; n = number of output variables; p = number of rules; $\circ$ = max–min composition; $\wedge$ = minimum operator; $\vee$ = maximum operator.

Also, the membership function is chosen so that the fuzzy labels are not too much overlapped and not isolated (Mizumoto, 1988). It is found from the computer simulations that good control results are obtained when the fuzzy sets are 25% overlapped. There are many shapes of possible membership function, such as triangular, trapezoidal and so on, which can be used in fuzzy modelling. The triangular shape is often used because it is simpler than the others. Regarding defuzzification procedures, there are two main methods: mean of maximum (MOM) and centre of area (COA)

(Braae and Rutherford, 1978). The latter procedure has been adopted because it gives smoother signals.

6.2.2 The learning signal

Before the fuzzy model can be used it must learn the process behaviour. During a certain period of time the process is activated by a signal from which the model has to learn the process behaviour. This signal is called the learning signal. In order to give the model sufficient information to provide identifiability the learning signal must be chosen to be persistently exciting. This means that all modes of interest in the process must be excited, i.e. a single step or sine wave is not generally sufficient (Gustavsson, 1975). Therefore, PRBSs have been used extensively during past years in many applications (Bohlin, 1971; Cumming, 1972; Williams and Clarke, 1968). In this section, using different learning signals such as steps, sine waves, PRBSs and GRNSs, one can test the fuzzy model for model robustness.

6.2.3 Simulation results

Simulations have been performed on a non-linear system with saturated gain as shown in Figure 6.2 to test knowledge-based fuzzy modelling. The learning signals used were steps, sine waves, PRBSs and GRNSs to decide which can construct a more complete knowledge structure. In order to obtain wider range and accuracy for fuzzy modelling, one can use separate different ranges to create a rule-base. For this system, the learning signals are set to three different values, 3, 6 and 9, to obtain knowledge-based fuzzy modelling. The number and values chosen will relate to the fuzzy model accuracy and resolution. In the modelling studies, the four input variables were chosen to be the input, change-in-input, time delay of output and change of time-delayed output, while the one output was the system output. The shape of membership function was chosen to be triangular. The rules were self-organized by data possibilities, and the defuzzification was chosen to be the centre of area. Regarding assessment of fuzzy model quality, there are three factors which are related to complexity, accuracy and uncertainty as used by R. M. Tong (1978). In this section, the assessment of fuzzy model quality was concerned with accuracy, and used the squared error given by:

$$\text{Error factor} = \frac{1}{N} \sum_{i=1}^{N} (Y_i - FM_i)^2$$

where FM_i is the fuzzy model output at the ith data point, Y_i is the process output at the ith data point, and N is the number of data points.

The different learning signals used to generate different rules without

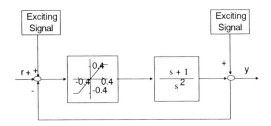

Figure 6.2 *Schematic diagram of a non-linear system.*

conflict are listed in Table 6.2. The standard deviation and mean value of the GRNS were 0.2 and 0.0; the amplitude and sequence length of the PRBS were 0.2 and 127. Also, the rule-bases obtained from different signals in Table 6.2 used 300 data points.

Comparing the four different learning signals from Table 6.2, the PRBS signal generated more rules than the other learning signals. Although the GRNS is closer to white noise, it created less rules than the PRBS. This could provide one reason why in traditional control engineering PRBSs are used to excite systems and hence obtain more process characterization (Gustavsson, 1975, Williams and Clarke, 1968). PRBSs can excite the system more strongly than GRNSs. So, we try to use a rule-base from the PRBS and GRNS, combining fuzzy set theory to model the process by adding together step responses with sine waves, PRBSs and GRNSs. Each input signal exciting the system uses five different stages, as in Figure 6.3 for a step input signal. The other exciting signals, such as sine wave, PRBSs and GRNSs always add in a step signal. The error factors are shown in Table 6.3 and the simulation results are shown in Figures 6.4–6.6. Comparing the results of Table 6.3, it can be seen that most of the error factors of the PRBS's rule-base are less than for GRNSs.

Figure 6.4 shows time responses of the fuzzy model output using PRBS and GRNS functions as the exciting signals; the amplitude and length sequence of the PRBS were 0.2 and 127; the standard deviation and mean

Table 6.2 *Rule-base from different learning signals*

Learning signal	Input signal range					
	3	6	9	3	6	9
	(original rules)			(without conflicting rules)		
Step response	20	31	33	14	19	20
Sine wave	44	32	55	31	21	35
GRNS	153	101	77	109	73	60
PRBS	173	138	122	126	99	94

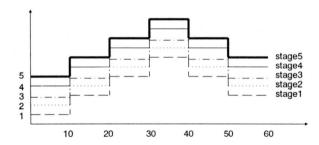

Figure 6.3 *Exciting signal of step function at five different stages.*

Table 6.3 *The error factor of different exciting signals from the PRBS's and GRNS's rule-base*

		Rule-base	
Exciting signal	Stage	GRNS (error factor)	PRBS (error factor)
Step response	1	0.19	0.30
	2	0.42	0.43
	3	0.43	0.27
	4	1.25	0.25
	5	1.24	0.28
Sine wave	1	0.34	0.25
	2	0.27	0.21
	3	0.32	0.28
	4	0.53	0.26
	5	0.82	0.34
GRNS (standard deviation = 0.1)	1	0.20	0.16
	2	0.24	0.26
	3	1.45	1.34
	4	0.69	0.25
	5	0.97	0.41
GRNS (standard deviation = 0.2)	1	2.08	1.95
	2	0.26	0.25
	3	2.08	1.94
	4	1.61	0.25
	5	1.75	0.32
PRBS (amplitude = 0.1)	1	0.41	0.24
	2	0.78	0.30
	3	3.79	0.37
	4	0.52	0.50
	5	5.39	0.66
PRBS (amplitude = 0.2)	1	0.30	0.31
	2	0.32	0.30
	3	8.52	1.08
	4	0.77	0.46
	5	1.35	0.67

value of GRNS were 0.2 and 0.0; the rule-base of the fuzzy model comes from PRBS and GRNS learning signals and the error factors were 0.46, 0.77 (for Figures 6.4(a) and (b)) and 0.25, 1.61 (for Figures 6.4(c) and (d)). Comparing the results in Figure 6.4, it can be seen that the PRBS rule-base is able to simulate more accurately and for a wider range than GRNS.

In Figure 6.5 the same process as in Figure 6.4 is shown, but the amplitude of the PRBS and standard deviation of the GRNS were 0.1 and the error factors were 0.50, 0.52 (for Figures 6.5(a) and (b)) and 0.25, 0.69 (for Figures 6.5(c) and (d)). From Figure 6.5, it can be seen that the rule-base obtained from a large amplitude and standard deviation of learning signal can simulate a process with small amplitude and standard deviation of exciting signal.

Figure 6.6 shows the time response of the fuzzy model output using a sine wave and step function as the exciting signal; the rule-base is the same as in Figure 6.4; the error factors being 0.26, 0.53 (for Figures 6.6(a) and (b)) and 0.25, 1.25 (for Figures 6.6(c) and (d)). Thus, the similar results as those obtained from Figure 6.4 show that the PRBS rule-base can model the process more accurately and with a wider range than GRNSs. Using a large rule-base created by frequently exciting learning signals like PRBS (amplitude = 0.2), one can model a process better with different exciting signals such as steps, sine waves and GRNSs.

6.3 Hierarchical self-organizing fuzzy logic control for muscle relaxation anaesthesia

The task of an anaesthetist in the operating theatre is to make sure the patient is adequately unconscious and to give pain relief during a surgical procedure. In this section, the work concerns the control of drug-induced muscle-relaxation paralysis in anaesthetized patients. Traditionally, an anaesthetist injects a bolus dose of muscle relaxant, whose size is determined by experience. However, an anaesthetist may have difficulty maintaining a steady level of paralysis which can lead to a large consumption of drug by the patient. Therefore, the development of on-line drug administration strategies in operating theatres becomes more important and also has highly safety-critical implications. Early research attempts at closed-loop control used a PI control algorithm (Linkens et al., 1982). Self-tuning PID control and a Smith predictor have been implemented in clinical trials following extensive simulation studies (Linkens et al., 1985). Generalized prediction control (Mahfouf, 1991) has been implemented for the same purpose and was successful when tested in clinical trials. More recently, supervisory hierarchical intelligent control (Linkens and Abbod, 1992) has used a fuzzy logic concept for direct and supervisory expert control of the

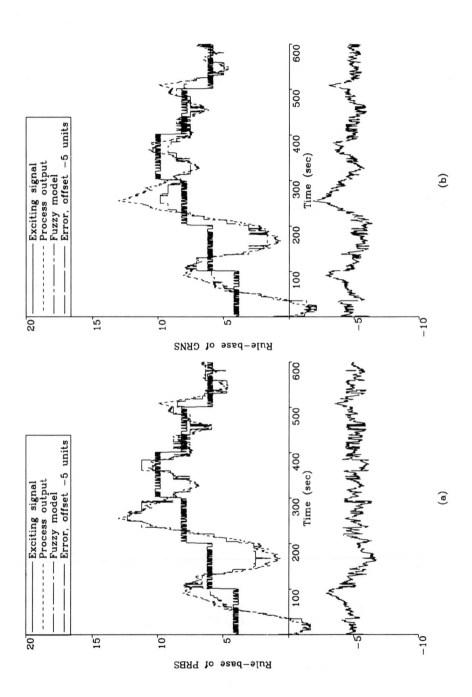

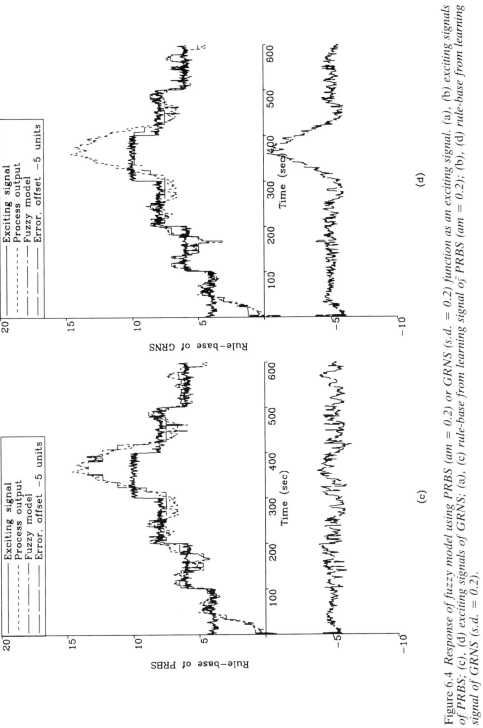

Figure 6.4 Response of fuzzy model using PRBS (am = 0.2) or GRNS (s.d. = 0.2) function as an exciting signal. (a), (b) exciting signals of PRBS; (c), (d) exciting signals of GRNS; (a), (c) rule-base from learning signal of PRBS (am = 0.2); (b), (d) rule-base from learning signal of GRNS (s.d. = 0.2).

186 *Intelligent Control in Biomedicine*

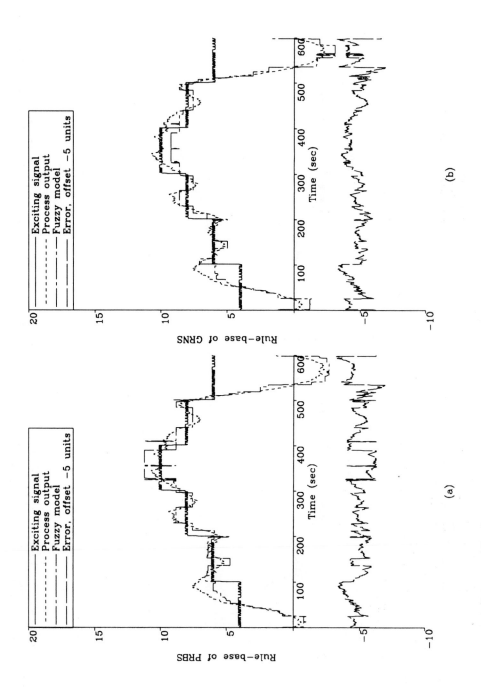

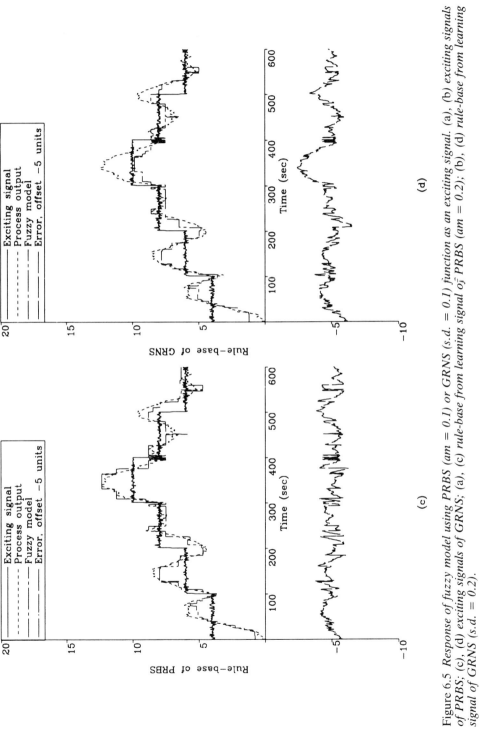

Figure 6.5 Response of fuzzy model using PRBS (am = 0.1) or GRNS (s.d. = 0.1) function as an exciting signal. (a), (b) exciting signals of PRBS; (c), (d) exciting signals of GRNS; (a), (c) rule-base from learning signal of PRBS (am = 0.2); (b), (d) rule-base from learning signal of GRNS (s.d. = 0.2).

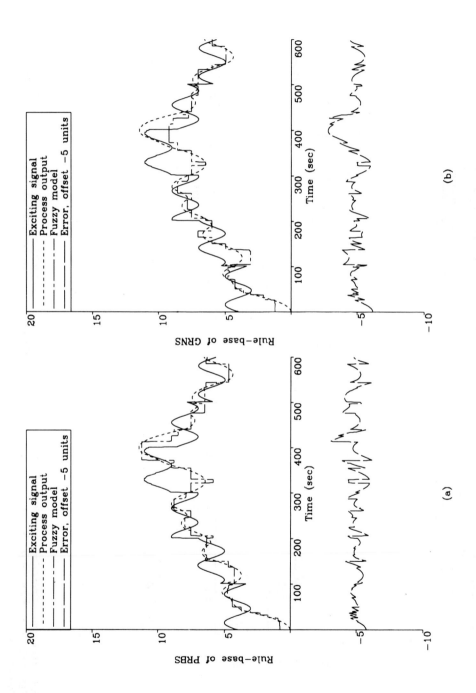

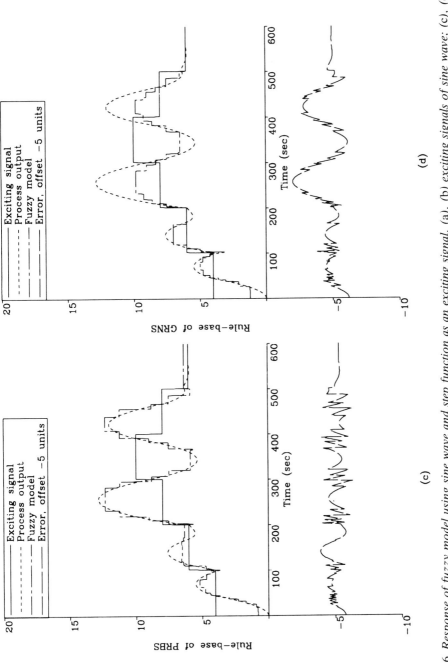

Figure 6.6 *Response of fuzzy model using sine wave and step function as an exciting signal. (a), (b) exciting signals of sine wave; (c), (d) exciting signals of step signal; (a), (c) rule-base from learning signal of PRBS (am = 6.2); (b), (d) rule-base from learning signal of GRNS (s.d. = 0.2).*

system, and has measured malfunctioning in the control system, detected a fault in the instrumentation, and given warning and alarm signals.

In this section a hierarchical self-organizing fuzzy logic control structure is introduced to simulate modelling, control and fault detection for muscle relaxation of the patient in an operating theatre.

6.3.1 Hierarchical self-organizing fuzzy logic control (HSOFLC) structure

Hierarchical self-organizing fuzzy logic control (HSOFLC) has a structure which consists of three levels as shown in Figure 6.7. The first level is a self-organizing fuzzy logic control level which is responsible for the rule generation and membership function modification. The second is a modelling level which consists of input and output data identification and self-organizing fuzzy modelling. The third is a fault detection level which obtains data from the first and second levels to monitor the operation and performance of the system, detect a fault in the instrument, and give warning and alarm signals.

6.3.1.1 Self-organizing fuzzy logic control (SOFLC)

There are many publications investigating this area of self-organizing fuzzy logic control (SOFLC) (Daley and Gill, 1986, 1987; Moore, 1991; Procyk, 1979). SOFLC is a hierarchical controller which has two levels. The basic level is a simple fuzzy logic controller and the second level is the self-organizing layer which supervises the basic level by monitoring its performance, subsequently generating and modifying the control rules. See Chapter 5 for details and diagrams about SOFLC.

6.3.1.2 Self-organizing fuzzy modelling (SOFM)

Self-organizing fuzzy modelling (SOFM) was mentioned in the previous section. In this section, some modification to on-line modelling of the system will be discussed. Firstly, in order to normalize the data to fuzzy sets, it is necessary to obtain the maximum and average value from a series of input and output data. Secondly, tuning of gains in the membership functions of fuzzy modelling will affect the sensitivity of rise time and the required steady-state accuracy of fuzzy modelling in the system. In Figure 6.8, different gains represent the range of data corresponding to membership functions of fuzzy modelling. Therefore, choosing suitable gains can lead to good transient response and small steady-state error.

Finally, in order to identify and track systems with time-varying parameters, one can consider moving a rectangular window or an exponential window (i.e. a forgetting factor) over the data (Young, 1984). There are still

Hierarchical fuzzy modelling and fault detection 191

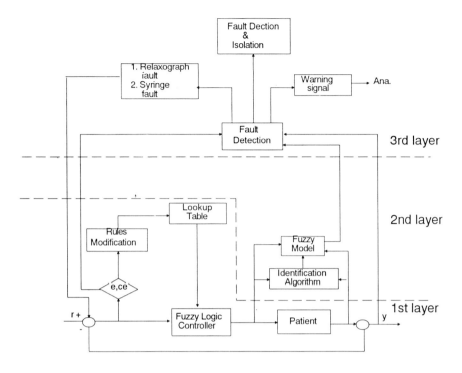

Figure 6.7 *Hierarchical self-organizing fuzzy logic control structure for muscle relaxation.*

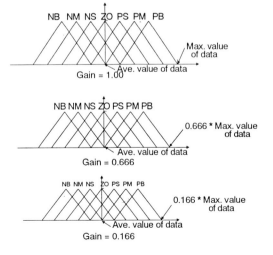

Figure 6.8 *Membership function of fuzzy model for different gains.*

some problems in choosing suitable rectangular window sample numbers and forgetting factor values.

6.3.1.3 Fault detection level

In an operating theatre, many instruments are situated around the patient for monitoring and control, in order to obtain suitable conditions for the surgical operation. Uncertainties due to patient-to-patient variability in drug sensitivity, patient movement for some operations, or the surgeon causing an electrical disturbance via diathermy will affect the surgical procedure. So, creating a good fault detection system becomes more and more important since not only can it ensure automatic control to continue but it can also help the anaesthetist to undertake some emergency action. Hence, fault detection has the task of detecting any fault occurring in the patient, the sensors, or actuators, then sends signals to inform the anaesthetist to initiate some action to minimize the danger to the patient.

There are two types of fault to be recognized during the operation, one being faults in the Relaxograph and the other faults in the syringe driver. For the Relaxograph, two faults can be recognized: firstly, when the surgeon uses a high frequency instrument to stop bleeding in the patient (which is called a diathermy effect), the electromyogram (EMG) output signal will be disturbed and often the signals reduce to zero in that situation. Secondly, a fault may occur due to movement of the patient which makes the EMG output show a sudden level change. The former fault can be detected easily, but the latter will depend on the shift in the Relaxograph readings. A possible detection procedure is to obtain the rate change of EMG output from the SOFLC level and determine a threshold which can decide when there is a sudden change of the signal. Such faults produced by the Relaxograph mean that the patient's internal state did not change but the Relaxograph gave different readings. One can replace the process output (i.e. EMG signal) with the previous fuzzy model output to avoid disturbing the controller output. When these faults disappear or are solved by the anaesthetist, the control system can switch back to the original settings and hence the patient is not disturbed.

A fault in the syringe driver can be of two kinds, either it is halted because of a mechanical problem, or the patient does not receive drug infusion which might occur when the drug line is disconnected or the drug is not infused into the veins. Such a fault could be detected from the sudden change of rule-base at the SOFM level and the gradual change of error in the SOFLC level. When this fault happens, the anaesthetist should be told quickly to change the syringe pump or adjust the drug line to infuse the drug into the patient's veins. If this does not work, the automatic control system must be changed to manual control by the anaesthetist to keep the patient in a safe condition.

6.3.2 Implementation

The hierarchical structure can be implemented at different levels. The first level of SOFLC always controls the system according to the patient output and predefined paralysis set-point. The second level of SOFM identifies and models the system depending on the system input and output data. These two levels work by on-line self-organizing rules to control and model the system at all times. When faulty behaviour is detected from the first- and second-level information, a diagnosis procedure is executed by the third level which forces the first and second levels to change to compensate for the fault and send a warning message to the anaesthetist.

6.3.3 Simulation results

Simulations have been performed on a patient model which is for a pancuronium bromide muscle relaxant drug model, as shown in Figure 6.9, to test this hierarchical self-organizing fuzzy logic control structure. The set-point value was 80% muscle relaxation for a 200 minute operation using pancuronium bromide. Figure 6.10(*a*) shows normal operation under closed-loop control with no faults occurring. In Figure 6.10(*b*), a fault in the Relaxograph was simulated at time 80 minutes where the status was changed due to a movement of the patient. When the HSOFLC structure detected this fault, it replaced the patient output with the previous fuzzy model output and informed the anaesthetist to move the patient back to the original conditions. After one step the patient was returned to his previous condition, and the controller output maintained a steady level. At time 100 minutes, a fault in the syringe driver was simulated by assuming that no drug was infused to the patient, and as a result the patient's paralysis started to drop. After three or four steps, the fault was detected and the anaesthetist was prompted to solve this problem. Assuming that the fault was corrected, the controller took over again to bring the patient back to the required status as shown in Figure 6.10(*b*). At time 150 minutes, a fault in the Relaxograph was simulated where the status was changed due to a diathermy disturbance. When this fault had been detected, by using the previous fuzzy model output instead of the patient output HSOFLC was

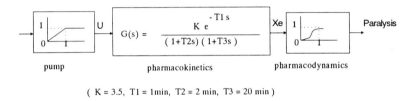

(K = 3.5, T1 = 1min, T2 = 2 min, T3 = 20 min)

Figure 6.9 *Pancuronium bromide drug muscle relaxant model.*

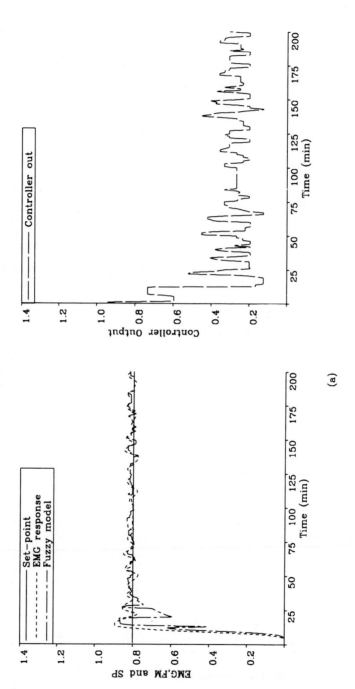

(a)

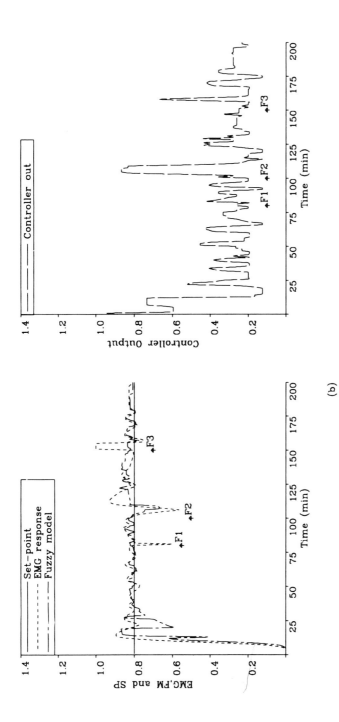

Figure 6.10 *HSOFLC control of muscle relaxation (a) with no faults occurring; (b) with three faults occurring; F1: a fault in the Relaxograph due to a movement of the patient; F2: a fault in the syringe driver; F3: a fault in the Relaxograph due to a diathermy disturbance.*

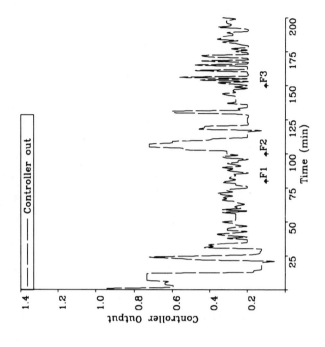
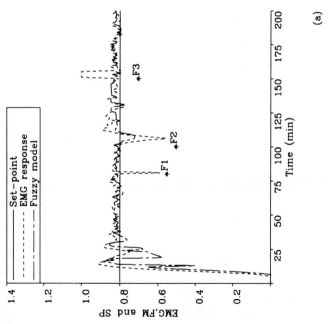

(a)

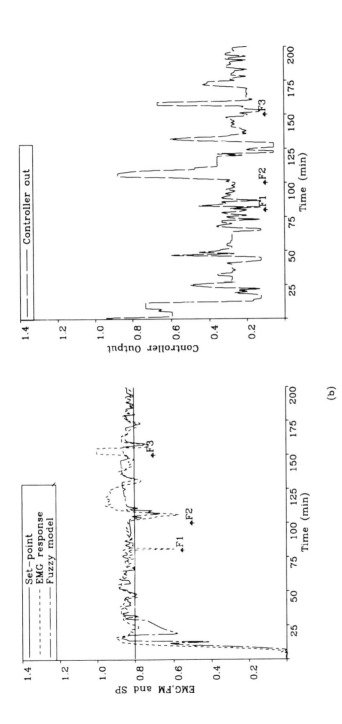

Figure 6.11 HSOFLC control of muscle relaxation (a) with three faults occurring and added GRNS noise; (b) with three faults occurring and added PRBS noise; (c) added disturbance and step change with no faults occurring; F1, F2 and F3 are the same faults as in Figure 6.10; S1, S2: muscle relaxation change of 10% and −10% from the set-point, D1, D2: disturbance with amplitude −0.05 and 0.05 added to the process.

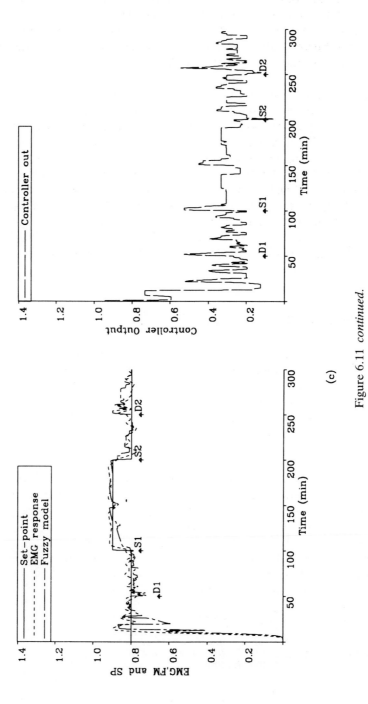

Figure 6.11 continued.

able to continue controlling the process. As the fuzzy model considers a one-step delay in the patient output, one can use the model to predict the process output in this case by performing a one-step-ahead prediction. Hence, from Figure 6.10(*b*), one can see the deviation of the fuzzy model and the patient output after the diathermy effect had finished at 155 minutes.

In Figure 6.11(*a*) the same process as in Figure 6.10(*b*) is shown, but PRBS noise with amplitude 0.01 and a sequence length of 127 has been added to the output. The same procedure is shown in Figure 6.11(*b*) except that PRBS has been replaced by GRNS with a standard deviation of 0.01 and a mean of 0.0. From Figures 6.11(*a*) and (*b*), it can be seen that HSOFLC can detect faults of the same type as those shown in Figure 6.10(*b*) although PRBS or GRNS signals were being added. Finally, in Figure 6.11(*c*), two disturbances with amplitude -0.05 and 0.05 were added to the process at time 50 and 250 minutes, and muscle relaxation changes of $\pm 10\%$ from the set-point were made at time 100 and 200 minutes. The results show that disturbance and set-point changes do not affect the fault detection level if there are no faults occurring.

6.4 Conclusions

In this chapter, a knowledge-based fuzzy modelling approach has been presented to model non-linear systems for application in modelling muscle relaxation for patients in the operating theatre. In addition, a hierarchical self-organizing fuzzy logic control structure has been presented for modelling, control and fault detection in muscle relaxation. The results can be summarized by the following.

1. The knowledge-base created by learning signals such as PRBSs and GRNSs can generate more rules and obtain more complete knowledge structure than the other two learning signals such as step response and sine wave, and has been demonstrated successfully when applied to a non-linear model process with different exciting signals.
2. The rule-base derived from a PRBS learning signal can model a system more accurately and with a wider range than that of a GRNS rule-base.
3. The results of modelling, control and fault detection for muscle relaxation by applying a hierarchical self-organizing fuzzy logic control structure are very promising.
4. PRBS, GRNS, set-point changes and disturbances added to the system to demonstrate the HSOFLC structure robustness have been successful.

Currently of particular interest is the control of the depth of anaesthesia (unconsciousness) during an operation. However, the depth of anaesthesia cannot be detected directly. According to anaesthetists' experience, the depth of anaesthesia is evaluated by measuring blood pressure, heart rate and clinical signs such as pupil response, tears, sweating and movement. A hierarchical rule-based fuzzy logic control structure for depth of anaesthesia is being studied. The first level is focused on measuring blood pressure and heart rate. The second level is focused on clinical signs such as sweating, tears, pupil response and movement. The rules of primary depth of anaesthesia come from anaesthetists' experience and machine-learning from clinical trials. The results of these two different rule-bases to decide primary depth of anaesthesia are very similar and can be used to design a drug controller. Furthermore, using the first-level results, the design of a second level of depth of anaesthesia is being investigated, which will include how to decide the depth of anaesthesia from clinical signs and how to adjust the drug administered at the first level.

References

Åström, K.J., Anton, J.J. and Arzen, K.E., 1986, Expert control, *Automatica*, **22**, 277–86.
Bohlin, T., 1971, On the problem of ambiguities in maximum likelihood identification, *Automatica*, **7**, 199–210.
Braae, M. and Rutherford, D.A., 1978, Fuzzy relation in a control setting, *Kybernetes*, **7**, 185–88.
Cumming, I.G., 1972, On line computer control of a cold rolling mill, *Automatica*, **8**, 531–41.
Daley, S. and Gill, K.F., 1986, A design study of a self-organizing fuzzy logic controller, *Proceedings of the Institution of Mechanical Engineers*, **200**, 59–69.
Daley, S. and Gill, K.F., 1987, Attitude control of spacecraft using an extended self-organizing fuzzy logic controller, *Proceedings of the Institution of Mechanical Engineers*, **201**, 97–106.
Gupta, M.M., Kiszka, J.B. and Trojan, G.M., 1986, Multivariable structure of fuzzy control systems, *IEEE Transactions on Systems, Man, and Cybernetics*, **SMC-16**, 638–56.
Gustavsson, I., 1975, Survey of applications of identification in chemical and physical processes, *Automatica*, **11**, 3–24.
Kickert, J.M., 1979, An example of linguistic modeling: the case of Mulder's theory of power, in Ragade, R.K., Gupta, M.M. and Yager, R.R. (Eds) *Advances in Fuzzy Set Theory and Application*, pp. 519–40, Amsterdam: North-Holland.
Kiszka, J.B., Kochanska, M.E. and Sliwinska, D.S., 1985, The influence of some parameters on the accuracy of a fuzzy model, in Sugeno, M. (Ed.) *Industrial Application of Fuzzy Control*, pp. 187–230, Amsterdam: Elsevier Science/North-Holland.
Linkens, D.A. and Abbod, M.F., 1992, 'Supervisory hierarchical intelligent control for medical and individual systems', presentation at the ISA Conference and Exhibition on Industrial Automation, Montreal, Canada, pp. 1.21–1.24.
Linkens, D.A., Asbury, A.J., Rimmer, S.J. and Menad, M., 1982, Identification and control of muscle-relaxant anaesthesia, *Proceedings of the IEE, Pt D, Control Theory and Application*, **129**, 136–41.

Linkens, D.A., Menad, M. and Asbury, A.J., 1985, Smith predictor and self-tuning control of muscle-relaxant drug administration, *Proceedings of the IEE, Pt D, Control Theory and Application*, **132**, 212–8.

Linkens, D.A. and Shieh, J.S., 1992, 'Self-organising fuzzy modelling for nonlinear system control', in Proceedings of the 1992 IEEE International Symposium on Intelligent Control, Glasgow, UK, pp. 210–5.

Mahfouf, M., 1991, 'Adaptive control and identification for on-line drug infusion in anaesthesia', PhD thesis, Department of Automatic Control and Systems Engineering, University of Sheffield.

Matsushima, K. and Sugiyama, H., 1985, 'Human operator's fuzzy model in man-machine system with a nonlinear controlled object', in Sugeno, M. (Ed.), *Industrial Application of Fuzzy Control*, pp. 175–85, Amsterdam: Elsevier Science/North-Holland.

Mizumoto, M., 1988, Fuzzy controls under various fuzzy reasoning methods, *Information Sciences*, **45**, 129–51.

Moore, C., 1991, 'Indirect adaptive fuzzy controllers', PhD thesis, Department of Aeronautics and Astronautics, University of Southampton.

Peng, X.T. and Wang, P.Z., 1988, 'On generating linguistic rules for fuzzy models', in Proceedings of the 2nd International Conference on Information Processing and Management of Uncertainty in Knowledge Based Systems, Italy, pp. 185–92.

Procyk, T.J., 1977, 'Self-organizing control for dynamic processes', PhD Thesis, Queen Mary College, London, UK.

Shengehaog, L. and Kreifeldt, J.G., 1989, 'Human fuzzy control model and its application to fuzzy control system design', in Proceedings of the 4th IFAC Man-Machine Systems Conference, China, pp. 99–102.

Sugeno, M. and Kang, G.T., 1986, Fuzzy modeling and control of multilayer incinerator. *Fuzzy Sets and Systems*, **18**, 329–46.

Sugeno, M. and Kang, G.T., 1988, Structure identification of fuzzy model, *Fuzzy Sets and Systems*, **28**, 15–33.

Sugeno, M. and Tanaka, K., 1991, Successive identification of a fuzzy model and its applications to prediction of a complex system, *Fuzzy Sets and Systems*, **42**, 315–34.

Sugeno, M., Morofushi, T., Mori, T., Tatematsu, T. and Tanaka, J., 1989, Fuzzy algorithmic control of a model car by oral instructions, *Fuzzy Sets and Systems*, **32**, 207–19.

Takagi, T. and Sugeno, M., 1985, Fuzzy identification of systems and its application to modeling and control, *IEEE Transactions on Systems, Man, and Cybernetics*, **SMC-20**, 116–32.

Tong, R.M., 1978, Synthesis of fuzzy models for industrial processes—some recent results, *International Journal of General Systems*, **4**, 143–62.

Tong, R.M., 1980, The evaluation of fuzzy models derived from experimental data, *Fuzzy Sets and Systems*, **4**, 1–12.

van der Rhee, F., van Nautaa Lemke, H.R. and Dijkman, J.G., 1987, 'Applying fuzzy set theory to modeling processes', in *Proceedings of the 10th IFAC Triennial World Congress*, Munich, Germany, pp. 343–8.

van der Rhee, F., van Nautaa Lemke, H.R. and Dijkman, J.G., 1990a, Knowledge based fuzzy control of systems, *IEEE Transactions on Automatic Control*, **35**, 148–55.

van der Rhee, F., van Nautaa Lemke, H.R. and Dijkman, J.G., 1990b, 'Knowledge based fuzzy modelling of systems', in Proceedings of the 11th IFAC Triennial World Congress, Tallinn, Estonia, USSR, pp. 199–204.

Williams, B.J. and Clarke, D.W., 1968, Plant modelling from p.r.b.s. experiments, *Control*, **12**, 856–60.

Xu, C.W. and Lu, Y.Z., 1987, Fuzzy model identification and self-learning for dynamic systems, *IEEE Transactions on Systems, Man, and Cybernetics*, **SMC-17**, 683–9.

Xu, C.W. and Lu, Y.Z., 1988, Identification and self-learning of fuzzy models for dynamic systems, *Acta Automation Sinica*, **14**(2).

Xu, C.W. and Yang, Z.Y., 1987, On approach of designing a self-tuning regulator based on the fuzzy model, *Acta Automation Sinica*, **13**(3).

Young, P.C., 1984, Recursive estimation and time-series analysis, Berlin: Springer.

Zadeh, L.A., 1965, Fuzzy sets, *Information and Control*, **8**, 338–53.

Chapter 7
Unified fuzzy reasoning and blood pressure management

Junhong Nie

7.1 Introduction

Rule-based fuzzy control has been considered as an efficient method to control complicated and ill-defined processes. This results primarily from the fact that no explicit mathematical model governing the controlled process is needed to design the controller. The most distinct difference between a fuzzy controller and a conventional adaptive or non-adaptive controller is that the former tries to model the human's control experience or knowledge using qualitative language, whereas the latter attempts to model the process being controlled by means of a quantitative approach. Therefore they can be regarded as knowledge-based control and model-based control respectively. When difficulties arise using traditional control methods, because of the lack of mathematical models for the process being controlled, rule-based fuzzy control may be adequate because no exact and explicit process models are required. This is a common situation in biomedical engineering. Both the theory and the application of fuzzy control are extensively reviewed by several researchers, for example Tong (1984, 1985), Sugeno (1985), Efstathiou (1988) and, more recently, Lee (1990).

Despite the fact that there are many successful examples found in industrial process control, only a few applications of rule-based control (not necessarily fuzzy) have been reported in biomedical and clinical situations. These situations are very complex, non-linear and time-varying, and should be suitable candidates for fuzzy control. Vishnoi and Gingrich (1987) constructed a fuzzy logic controller for the delivery of gaseous anaesthesia based on vital signs. Isaka *et al.* (1988, 1989) applied a fuzzy control method to regulate mean arterial blood pressure in a noisy environment. Den Brok *et al.* (1987) built a rule-based supervisory expert system to control a patient's blood pressure, in which the expert system was used to tune the parameters of a PID controller based on the analysis of step responses. A hybrid controller for drug delivery was proposed by Neat *et al.* (1989), and consists of a fuzzy controller, a multiple-model controller and a model reference controller. The expert system is used to adjust the structure of the whole controller in accordance with the dynamic plant. Ying *et al.* (1988) and Yamashita (1988) have applied fuzzy control methods to arterial pressure control by single drug infusion. Linkens *et al.* (1986) and Linkens and Mahfouf (1988) describe an application of fuzzy control to unconsciousness and muscle relaxation during surgery.

All the work reviewed above involved the automated infusion of a single drug, which therefore represents a single-input–single-output problem. Not surprisingly, these single drug delivery systems have been investigated for some years although the control strategies used have primarily been traditional control algorithms. In contrast, multivariable drug delivery systems have received little attention, and have been studied only recently by some researchers for blood pressure control (Serna *et al.*, 1983; McInnis *et al.*, 1985; Voss *et al.*, 1987; Linkens and Mansour, 1989). The control algorithms adopted have been either traditional adaptive schemes or self-tuning control methods.

This chapter deals with the problem of multivariable control of blood pressure which is the same system as used in the work reported by Mansour and Linkens (1990), but here a rule-based fuzzy control method is employed. The problem involves a two-input–two-output multivariable control situation. There are two cases considered in this chapter. The first case is to control arterial pressure and systemic venous pressure by means of heart rate and systemic resistance. The second one is to regulate simultaneously arterial pressure and cardiac output using a vasoactive drug (sodium nitroprusside (SNP)) and an inotropic drug (dopamine (DOP)). Significant interactions exist between the two drugs, which present a difficult control problem.

A control architecture has been developed which consists mainly of a rule-based fuzzy controller plus a simple pre-compensator. The reasoning algorithms used by the fuzzy controller are based on the unified approximate reasoning model derived in Linkens and Nie (1992a). The proposed control method and the reasoning models are investigated via a number of simulations. The simulation model is based on the cardiovascular system dynamics developed by Moller *et al.* (1983). The simulation is aimed at not only demonstrating the feasibility of the proposed method when applied to a relatively complicated situation, but also at evaluating a number of reasoning schemes. Eight reasoning algorithms are chosen for comparison using the following two approaches. The first is to compare the control performance measured by integral of error criteria when the parameters of the controlled model are fixed. The second is to investigate the robustness of the algorithms with respect to variations in each process model parameter. The parameters include pure time delay, time constants, gains and compensation factors. A number of simulations have shown that blood pressure can be controlled successfully using the proposed algorithms. In addition, some useful conclusions about the selection of reasoning algorithms have been drawn from analysis of the comparative studies.

7.2 Statement of the problems

7.2.1 Moller's model of the cardiovascular system

Over the years, a variety of mathematical models of the cardiovascular system (CVS) have been developed (Mansour, 1988), some of which are pulsatile and are suitable for investigating phenomena that can change in a fraction of a heart beat. Models for studying long-term effects are usually non-pulsatile. Blood circulation is described in terms of non-pulsatile pressures, flows and volumes. The model used in this study is a non-pulsatile model developed by Moller *et al.* (1983). A two-pump circulatory model was postulated and the basic relationship governing the physiologically closed cardiovascular system was derived. The two parts of the heart are represented by flow sources *QL* and *QR* for left and right ventricles respectively. The systemic circulation is represented by the arterial systemic compliance *CAS*, the systemic peripheral resistance *RA*, and the venous systemic distensible capacity *CVS*. Similarly, the pulmonary circulation consists of the arteriopulmonary compliance *CAP*, the pulmonary resistance *RP*, and the venopulmonary distensible capacity *CVP*. The cardiovascular system dynamics governing the relationship between the blood pressures and flow sources can be described by the following differential vector equation

$$\frac{d\mathbf{X}}{dt} = \mathbf{AX} + \mathbf{BV} \tag{7.1}$$

where $\mathbf{X} = [PAS, PVS, PAP, PVP]^T$ with *PAS*, *PVS*, *PAP* and *PVP* being the systemic arterial pressure, systemic venous pressure, pulmonary arterial pressure and pulmonary venous pressure respectively; $\mathbf{V} = [QL, QR]^T$, and

$$\mathbf{A} = \begin{bmatrix} (-CAS \cdot RA)^{-1} & (CAS \cdot RA)^{-1} & 0 & 0 \\ (CVS \cdot RA)^{-1} & (-CVS \cdot RA)^{-1} & 0 & 0 \\ 0 & 0 & (-CAP \cdot RP)^{-1} & (CAP \cdot RP)^{-1} \\ 0 & 0 & (CVP \cdot RP)^{-1} & (-CVP \cdot RP)^{-1} \end{bmatrix}$$
(7.2)

$$\mathbf{B} = \begin{bmatrix} \dfrac{1}{CAS} & 0 \\ 0 & \dfrac{-1}{CVP} \\ 0 & \dfrac{1}{CAP} \\ \dfrac{-1}{CVP} & 0 \end{bmatrix}. \tag{7.3}$$

Equation (7.1) is a non-linear vector equation because the resistances and the compliances are non-linear functions of the pressure. Furthermore, the inputs QL and QR are also pressure-dependent, that is,

$$QL = SV_L \cdot HR \quad QR = SV_R \cdot HR \tag{7.4}$$

where HR stands for the heart rate, and SV_L and SV_R are the stroke volumes of left and right ventricles respectively. SV can be related to arterial and venous pressures by a complicated non-linear algebraic function (Moller et al., 1983).

If the compliances and the resistances are treated as pressure-independent, (7.1) represents a linear state-space model with QL and QR as independent system inputs. By selecting the heart rate HR and resistance RA as the system inputs, Moller et al. derived a linear model near the stationary state $PAS_0 = 117.5\,\text{mmHg}$, $PVS_0 = 7.15\,\text{mmHg}$, $PAP_0 = 17.18\,\text{mmHg}$ and $PVP_0 = 10.87\,\text{mmHg}$, which is given by

$$\frac{d\Delta\mathbf{X}}{dt} = \mathbf{A}_l \Delta\mathbf{X} + \mathbf{B}_l \Delta\mathbf{U} \tag{7.5}$$

where $\Delta\mathbf{X} = [\Delta PAS, \Delta PVS, \Delta PAP, \Delta PVP]^\mathrm{T}$, $\Delta\mathbf{U} = [\Delta HR, \Delta RA]^\mathrm{T}$ and

$$\mathbf{A}_l = \begin{bmatrix} -3.4370 & 1.8475 & 0.0 & 18.7584 \\ 0.01834 & -0.3015 & 0.06855 & 0.0 \\ 0.0 & 7.3514 & -10.1131 & 8.3333 \\ 0.2049 & 0.0 & 4.1667 & -6.5846 \end{bmatrix} \tag{7.6}$$

$$\mathbf{B}_l = \begin{bmatrix} 125.8 & 194.3 \\ -0.5048 & -1.929 \\ 13.1058 & 0.0 \\ -16.2125 & 0.0 \end{bmatrix}. \tag{7.7}$$

Equation (7.5) indicates that the processes can be controlled with a fast response time by manipulating heart rate and systemic resistance. It should be noted that the activation of *HR* is currently feasible through direct electrical stimulation of the heart, but activation is not yet available directly for *RA*.

7.2.2 Model of drug dynamics

Simultaneous regulation of blood pressure and cardiac output (*CO*) is needed in some clinical situations, for instance congestive heart failure. It is desirable to maintain or increase *CO* and, at the same time, to decrease the blood pressure. This goal can be achieved by simultaneous infusions of a positive inotropic agent, which increases the heart's contractility and cardiac output, and with a vasodilator which dilates the vasoclature and lowers the arterial pressure. Two frequently used drugs in clinical practice are the inotropic drug DOP and the vasoactive drug SNP. It is worth noting that the inputs are interactive with respect to the controlled variables *CO* and mean arterial pressure (*MAP*). The inotropic agent increases *CO* and thus *MAP*, whereas the vasoactive agent decreases *MAP* and increases *CO*.

An accurate dynamical model associating *CO* and *MAP* with DOP and SNP is not available to date. However, Serna *et al.* (1983) derived a first-order model for which different time constants and time delays in each loop were obtained. The steady-state gains in the model were obtained from Miller's study (1977). The dynamics in the *s*-domain are given by

$$\begin{bmatrix} \Delta CO_d \\ \Delta RA_d \end{bmatrix} = \begin{bmatrix} \dfrac{k_{11} e^{-\tau_1 s}}{s T_1 + 1} & \dfrac{k_{12} e^{-\tau_2 s}}{s T_1 + 1} \\ \dfrac{k_{21} e^{-\tau_2 s}}{s T_2 + 1} & \dfrac{k_{22} e^{-\tau_2 s}}{s T_2 + 1} \end{bmatrix} \begin{bmatrix} I_1 \\ I_2 \end{bmatrix} \qquad (7.8)$$

where ΔCO_d (ml s^{-1}) is the change in *CO* due to I_1 and I_2, ΔRA_d (mmHg s ml^{-1}) is the change in *RA* due to I_1 and I_2; I_1 (μg kg^{-1} min^{-1}) is the infusion rate of DOP; I_2 (ml h^{-1}) is the infusion rate of SNP; k_{11}, k_{12}, k_{21} and k_{22} are steady-state gains with typical values of 8.44, 5.275, −0.09 and −0.15 respectively; τ_1 and τ_2 represent two time delays with typical values of $\tau_1 = 60$ s and $\tau_2 = 30$ s; T_1 and T_2 are time constants typified by the values of 84.1 s and 58.75 s respectively. The model parameters presented above will be varied during the simulations in order to evaluate the robustness of the proposed controller.

Because the accessible measurable variables are *MAP* and *CO*, a model which relates the ΔCO_d and ΔRA_d due to drug infusions is needed. Moller's cardiovascular model can be used for this purpose. Note that the cardiovascular dynamics are much faster than the drug dynamics. Consequently, it is reasonable to neglect the cardiovascular dynamics, and only retain the steady-state gains in the CVS model. With this consideration, Mansour and Linkens (1990) derived a simulation model from Moller's CVS model and the drug dynamics, which is given by

$$\begin{bmatrix} \Delta CO \\ \Delta MAP \end{bmatrix} = \begin{bmatrix} 1.0 & -24.76 \\ 0.6636 & 76.38 \end{bmatrix} \begin{bmatrix} \dfrac{k_{11}e^{-\tau_1 s}}{sT_1+1} & \dfrac{k_{12}e^{-\tau_2 s}}{sT_1+1} \\ \dfrac{k_{21}e^{-\tau_2 s}}{sT_2+1} & \dfrac{k_{22}e^{-\tau_2 s}}{sT_2+1} \end{bmatrix} \begin{bmatrix} I_1 \\ I_2 \end{bmatrix}. \quad (7.9)$$

7.3 Unified fuzzy reasoning algorithm

Fuzzy reasoning plays a fundamental role in rule-based fuzzy logic control, where the main task of the fuzzy controller is to infer the present control output from the present input based on the control rules. This process, by which a set of imprecise conclusions is deduced from a collection of imprecise premises, implies two important features possessed by the method. First, the information involved in the system is linguistic, and thus usually imprecise. Secondly, an approximate conclusion can be reached even though the incoming data do not match any rule's premise exactly. The reasoning algorithm involves two issues, the mathematical representation of the rules and the inference implementation. Most existing fuzzy controllers adopt the relation equation method to translate the rules into a matrix and employ Zadeh's inference rule of composition to reach a conclusion. Alternatively, in this work a unified fuzzy reasoning model (Linkens and Nie, 1992a) will be used.

Assume that there are M rules in the rule-base which are connected by the connective ALSO:

$$R^1 \text{ ALSO } R^2 \text{ ALSO } \ldots \text{ ALSO } R^M$$

each of which is represented in the form of an IF ... THEN statement with n input variables connected by the connective AND and one output variable with the form:

IF X_1 is A_1^j AND X_2 is A_2^j AND ... AND X_n is A_n^j THEN Y is B^j.

Furthermore, assume that the present input is

X_1 is C_1 AND C_2 is A_2 AND ... AND X_n is C_n

where X_i and Y are variables whose values are taken from the universes of discourse U_i and V respectively. A_i^j, C_i and B^j are fuzzy subsets defined on the corresponding universes and represent fuzzy concepts such as *big*, *medium*, *small*, etc.

Relevant problems are how to represent linguistic rules numerically, how to define linguistic connectives mathematically, and how to infer an approximate action (output) in response to a novel situation (input). One solution is to follow the inferencing procedures used by traditional data-driven reasoning systems and take the fuzzy variable into account. By using possibility theory (Zadeh, 1978) as a representational tool, we obtained a unified reasoning algorithm in terms of the present output '*Y* is *D*', represented by its membership function $D(u)$, which is given by

$$D(v) = \Theta_{j=1}^{j=m} \{[\Xi_{i=1}^{i=n} \beta_i^j] \Phi B^j(v)\} = \Theta_{j=1}^{j=m} \beta^j \Phi B^j(v) \quad (7.10)$$

where Θ, Ξ and Φ stand for linguistic connectives ALSO, AND and IF . . . THEN respectively, and β_i^j denotes the possibility measure between $C_i(u_i)$ and $A_i^j(u_i)$ which is defined by

$$\beta_i^j = \text{Poss}(C_i/A_i^j) = \text{Sup}_{u_i \in U_i} \text{Min}[C_i(u_i), A_i^j(u_i)]. \quad (7.11)$$

The above reasoning algorithm can be interpreted as follows. First, the possibility measure between the present input and each rule is calculated. Then the THEN part of each rule is modified to $\beta^j \Phi B^j$. Finally, the m results derived from M rules are combined according to the definition of ALSO to produce the global result.

Various reasoning algorithms can be obtained by selecting different mathematical definitions for the linguistic connectives ALSO, AND and IF-THEN. There exist a number of possibilities but the four which are used in this chapter are presented below:

$$D(v) = \bigvee_{j=1}^{m} \left[\left(\bigwedge_{i=1}^{n} \beta_i^j \right) \wedge B^j(v) \right] \quad (7.12)$$

$$D(v) = \bigvee_{j=1}^{m} \left[\left(\prod_{i=1}^{n} \beta_i^j \right) * B^j(v) \right] \quad (7.13)$$

$$D(v) = \bigwedge_{j=1}^{m} \left\{ 1 \wedge \left[1 - \left(\bigwedge_{i=1}^{n} \beta_i^j \right) + B^j(v) \right] \right\} \quad (7.14)$$

$$D(v) = \bigwedge_{j=1}^{m} \begin{cases} 1 & \text{if } [\wedge_{i=1}^{n} \beta_i^j] \leq B^j(v) \\ B^j(v) & \text{if } [\wedge_{i=1}^{n} \beta_i^j] > B^j(v) \end{cases} \quad (7.15)$$

where $\vee$, $\wedge$, and Π correspond to maximum, minimum, and algebraic product operators respectively.

7.4 Architecture of multivariable fuzzy control

The majority of work reported in the literature on fuzzy control involves single-input–single-output processes (SISO), although some researchers have investigated the multivariable case, but it is much more difficult to control because of the interactions that occur between input–output variables. Gupta *et al.* (1986) put forward, from a theoretical point of view, a multivariable fuzzy control structure based on decomposition of the relation equations. Ray *et al.* (1985) implemented a fuzzy controller for a multivariable non-linear process by decomposing the process into several non-interacting processes and then treating them independently.

From the design viewpoint, the existing multivariable fuzzy control algorithms, such as proposed in Gupta *et al.* (1986), are difficult to apply. The difficulty stems not from the algorithm implementation, but from building the rule-base. Suppose that the process being controlled is a two-input–two-output process with u_1 and u_2 as the inputs and y_1 and y_2 as the outputs. Furthermore, suppose the control goal is to maintain y_1 and y_2 at a desired level by adjusting u_1 and u_2. Then the fuzzy controller will have four input variables and two output variables if a fully cross-coupled multivariable controller is to be used, and if both error and the change-in-error for each controlled variable are taken into consideration. Correspondingly, a control rule must take the form of IF V_1 and V_2 AND V_3 AND V_4 THEN U_{c1} AND U_{c2}. It will be difficult to obtain this kind of rule from ordinary domain operators. This is because it is very hard for operators to express their control strategies when so many variables interact with each

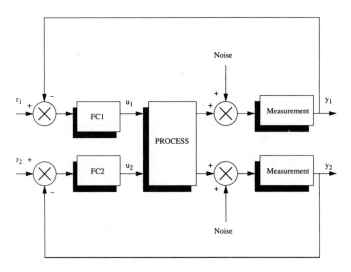

Figure 7.1 *System structure for multivariable fuzzy control.*

other, even though they may be capable of manually controlling the process satisfactorily.

In order to handle the above difficulty, an architecture for a multivariable fuzzy controller is suggested as shown in Figure 7.1. The system comprises two independent fuzzy controllers FC_1 and FC_2, a compensator unit, and the process. The main idea is to adopt a decentralized control strategy which treats the multivariable process as two separated single-input–single-output processes provided that the input/output pairs are properly selected according to some criteria. The interacting effects are partly removed by introducing a simple compensation procedure which consists of two factors calculated from the approximate steady-state gains of the process. It is also expected that the interaction effect on one loop produced by the other loop, if viewed as a perturbation, can be compensated to some extent by the robustness property possessed by the fuzzy controller. The details concerning the design and implementation are presented below.

7.4.1 Fuzzy control algorithms

The two fuzzy controllers shown in Figure 7.1 have structures depicted in Figure 7.2. They consist of a fuzzification unit, a rule-base, a reasoning algorithm and a defuzzification unit. The fuzzification procedure converts the measured numerical values into fuzzy subsets. The reasoning algorithm infers the corresponding output, which is a fuzzy subset, which is subsequently converted into a real numerical control signal by the defuzzification procedure.

Referring to Figure 7.2, suppose that E, C and U are variables taking their values on the universes of discourse $\bar{E}$, $\bar{C}$ and $\bar{U}$ respectively. Then a typical rule in the rule-base has the form of 'IF E is G_1 AND C is G_2 THEN U is D', where G_1, G_2 and D are the fuzzy subsets defined over the universes of discourse $\bar{E}$, $\bar{C}$ and $\bar{U}$ respectively. They represent some fuzzy concepts such as positive-big, negative-small and zero, etc, and are

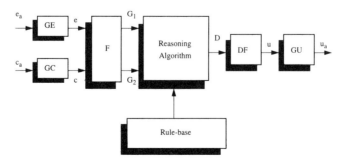

Figure 7.2 *Single-loop fuzzy controller.*

numerically characterized by the corresponding membership function $G_1(e)$, $G_2(c)$ and $D(u)$, that is, $G_1(e)$: $\bar{E} \to [0,1]$, $G_1(c)$: $\bar{C} \to [0,1]$ and $D(u)$: $\bar{U} \to [0,1]$. The rule-form mentioned above is a mathematical translation of a linguistic statement derived from domain experts. The IF-THEN clause states the relationship between the observed *condition* of the controlled process and the control *action* employed by the expert. An example of this statement might be 'IF the error is positive-big AND IF the change-in-error is negative-small, THEN the change-in-control output is positive-medium'.

Assuming that we have obtained a set of linguistic rules relating error and change-in-error to a control action, then the computational process from a measurement e_a and a change-in-error c_a to the controller output u_a can be described as follows.

First, measured numerical values e_a and c_a at sample instant nT are mapped into $e \in \bar{E}$ and $c \in \bar{C}$ respectively, that is,

$$\begin{cases} e = GE \cdot e_a(nT) \\ c = GC \cdot [e_a(nT) - e_a(nT - T)] \end{cases} \quad (7.16)$$

where T is the sample period, $e_a(nT)$ = set-point $r(nT)$ − process output $y(nT)$, and GE and GC are scaling factors which are selected so that all possible measured values of e_a and c_a will fall into the corresponding universes $\bar{E}$ and $\bar{C}$.

Secondly, the fuzzification unit fuzzifies e and c into fuzzy subsets G_1 and G_2 that will be singletons characterized by

$$G_1(e) = \begin{cases} 1 & \text{if } e = e(nT) \\ 0 & \text{otherwise} \end{cases} \quad (7.17)$$

$$G_2(c) = \begin{cases} 1 & \text{if } c = c(nT) \\ 0 & \text{otherwise} \end{cases} \quad (7.18)$$

where $e \in \bar{E}$ and $c \in \bar{C}$.

At this point the input data with respect to the reasoning model are of the standard form 'E is G_1 and C is G_2'. Based on this data, the controller output 'U is D' can be inferred by means of one of the algorithms presented in equations (7.12)–(7.15).

The value D obtained from the reasoning stage is a fuzzy subset defined on $\bar{U}$. To implement the control action, a real numerical value is required. This will be done by utilizing a defuzzification stage. In general, there are two popular algorithms called the mean of maxima and the centre of gravity given by (7.19) and (7.20) respectively.

- The mean of maxima (MOM)

$$u = \frac{1}{L}\sum_{l=1}^{L} u_l \qquad (7.19)$$

where u_l satisfies $D(u_l) = \text{Max}_{u \in U} D(u)$.

- The centre of gravity (COG)

$$u = \frac{\sum_{k=1}^{K} u_k D(u_k)}{\sum_{k=1}^{K} D(u_k)} \quad u_k \in \bar{U} \text{ for all } k \qquad (7.20)$$

where K is the element number in $\bar{U}$, i.e. Card $(\bar{U}) = K$.

The final step in the calculation is to convert the integer value $u \in \bar{U}$ computed from one of the above equations into an appropriate control signal u_a by multiplying u by a scaling factor GU.

Up to now, the whole computational procedure within a sample period T is carried out if the single-input–single-output process is involved, with the understanding that u_a is the change in control. The procedure, however, is not completed when a multivariable process is considered. This will be discussed in the next section.

7.4.2 Compensation procedure

As mentioned previously, the interactive effects between the variables should be taken into account. A simple compensator is connected to the outputs of two fuzzy controllers to cope with this problem. It should be emphasized that this scheme does not aim to eliminate the interaction completely. Rather, it is intended to reduce it to acceptable levels using a simple structure.

It is impossible to design a controller, no matter what principle it is based on, without knowing something about the controlled process. The process information needed, however, may be more/less, explicit/implicit, qualitative/quantitative, or exact/vague, depending on the design strategies used. For instance, no explicit and exact process model is needed for designing a rule-based fuzzy controller, because all of the information about the process is fused and embodied into the control rule-base in a qualitative manner. We want to use as little information about the process as possible. It is argued by Grosdidier *et al.* (1985) that steady-state information can be obtained for open-loop stable systems and is often the only information available. The steady-state gains in a multivariable system may be represented by a matrix denoted as **G**. In some cases, **G** can be obtained readily by undertaking experiments on the system considered, or by questioning skilful domain experts.

If, on the other hand, the process is characterized by a set of differential equations (not necessarily linear), **G** may be derived using the following procedures. Suppose the system is described by

$$\frac{dx}{dt} = f(x, u) \tag{7.21}$$

$$y = Cx \tag{7.22}$$

where f is the function vector, $x \in R^n$ is the state vector, $u \in R^m$ is the control vector, $y \in R^m$ is the output vector and **C** is a $m \times n$ constant matrix. An incremental model near the nominal states may be obtained by means of the first-order approximation of the Taylor series, which is given by

$$\frac{d\Delta x}{dt} = A\,\Delta x + B\,\Delta u \tag{7.23}$$

$$\Delta y = C\,\Delta x \tag{7.24}$$

where $\mathbf{A} = \partial f/\partial x \in R^{n \times n}$ and $\mathbf{B} = \partial f/\partial u \in R^{n \times m}$ are constant Jacobian matrices with the elements being partial derivatives evaluated at the nominal states. Then the steady-state equation can be written as

$$A\,\Delta x + B\,\Delta u = 0 \tag{7.25}$$

or

$$\Delta x = -A^{-1} B\,\Delta u. \tag{7.26}$$

Thus the steady-state output equation is given by

$$\Delta y = -CA^{-1} B\,\Delta u. \tag{7.27}$$

The above equation indicates an incremental relationship between the small inputs Δu and the corresponding small outputs Δy about the nominal states under steady-state conditions. It is clear that the steady-state matrix $G_{m \times m} = -CA^{-1}B$. A special case occurs when the system is governed by a linear state vector equation

$$\frac{dx}{dt} = A_l x + B_l u \quad y = C_l x. \tag{7.28}$$

The gain matrix will then be $\mathbf{G} = -C_l A_l^{-1} B_l$. Equivalently, in the linear case, the matrix **G** is simply equal to **H**(0) if the transfer function matrix **H**(s) is given.

There are many useful closed-loop properties which can be extracted from the open-loop steady-state gain matrix (Grosdidier et al., 1985). For instance, the interaction effects can be measured by the relative gain array (RGA) which is defined from the gain matrix. The relative gain γ_{ij} between an input u_j and an output y_i is the ratio of two steady-state gains: gain g_{ij} between u_j and y_i when all loops are open and the gain $\bar{g}_{ij}$ when all outputs except the ith output are tightly controlled. The RGA can be calculated using only the steady-state gain matrix **G**. More specifically, γ_{ij}, the (i,j)th element of the RGA matrix Γ, is expressed in terms of g_{ij} as

$$\gamma_{ij} = g_{ij}\hat{g}_{ji} \tag{7.29}$$

where g_{ij} is the (i,j)th element of **G** and $\hat{g}_{ji}$ denotes the (j,i)th element of the matrix $\mathbf{G}^{-1}$, the inverse of **G**. For a 2×2 system with a steady-state gain matrix **G**

$$\mathbf{G} = \begin{bmatrix} g_{11} & g_{12} \\ g_{21} & g_{22} \end{bmatrix} \tag{7.30}$$

the corresponding RGA matrix Γ is given by

$$\Gamma = \begin{bmatrix} \gamma_{11} & \gamma_{12} \\ \gamma_{21} & \gamma_{22} \end{bmatrix} = \begin{bmatrix} \dfrac{g_{11}g_{22}}{\Delta} & \dfrac{-g_{12}g_{21}}{\Delta} \\ \dfrac{-g_{12}g_{21}}{\Delta} & \dfrac{g_{11}g_{22}}{\Delta} \end{bmatrix} \tag{7.31}$$

where $\Delta = g_{11}g_{22} - g_{12}g_{21}$.

The RGA, introduced as a measurement of interaction, provides guidelines for pairing input/output variables and for predicting when interactions are significant. The input/output pairing is of significant importance if a decentralized control structure is required. This is due to the fact that satisfactory control would be unattainable if an input were to be paired with an output over which the input has little or no influence. Therefore it is desirable to pair the input/output in such a way that the input has as strong an influence as possible over the output. This goal can be achieved by pairing those variables whose relative gain is positive and as close to unity as possible. Also, if any γ_{ij} is much larger than one or less than zero, pairing the corresponding variables will result in a loop that is difficult to control.

Suppose that the system considered is a 2×2 system and a steady-state gain matrix **G** is available. Furthermore, assume that the input/output pairs are appropriately selected and two feedback control loops are constructed.

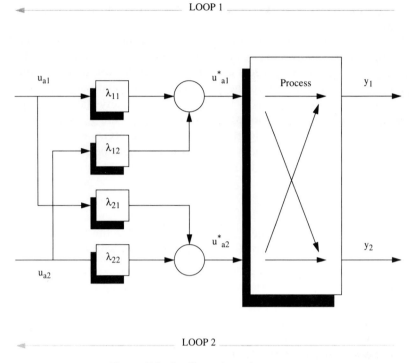

Figure 7.3 *Configuration of compensator.*

Then the configuration of the proposed compensator is that shown in Figure 7.3. The relationship between the inputs and outputs of the compensator is given by

$$\begin{bmatrix} u_{a1}^* \\ u_{a2}^* \end{bmatrix} = \begin{bmatrix} \lambda_{11} & \lambda_{12} \\ \lambda_{21} & \lambda_{22} \end{bmatrix} \begin{bmatrix} u_{a1} \\ u_{a2} \end{bmatrix}$$

$$= \begin{bmatrix} 1 & -\dfrac{g_{12}}{g_{11}} \\ -\dfrac{g_{21}}{g_{11}} & 1 \end{bmatrix} \begin{bmatrix} u_{a1} \\ u_{a2} \end{bmatrix} \quad (7.32)$$

where the 2×2 matrix $\boldsymbol{\Lambda}$ is called the compensation matrix.

The basic operation of the compensator may be stated as follows. When there is a change in the first controller output u_{a1}, it not only produces a change in the input of loop 1, but also presents a change in the input of loop 2 with an amount $\lambda_{21} u_{a1}$ so that when the interaction from loop 1 to loop 2 occurs, it will be compensated by the change in the input of loop 2. As a result, the effect caused by the interaction in y_2 will be reduced. The same behaviour will take place with respect to the change of the second controller output u_{a2}.

The reason for selecting $\lambda_{11} = \lambda_{22} = 1$ is apparent from above discussion, whereas the determination of λ_{12} and λ_{21} is based on the following concept. Suppose that there is a change in y_1, denoted as Δy_1, caused by interaction, due to the change of u_2, denoted as Δu_2. Δy_1 would be approximately equal to $\Delta u_2 g_{12}$. This Δy_1 may be equivalently caused by $g_{11} \Delta u_1$, assuming that only u_1 is applied to loop 1. Thus to prevent interaction we have

$$g_{11} \Delta u_1 = -\Delta u_2 g_{12} \tag{7.33}$$

or

$$\Delta u_1 = \left(-\frac{g_{12}}{g_{11}}\right) \Delta u_2 = \lambda_{12} \Delta u_2. \tag{7.34}$$

Therefore, λ_{12}, in fact, is the ratio of two inputs provided that only loop 1 is concerned. It indicates what percentage of Δu_2 should be applied to the input of loop 1 in order to compensate for the perturbation caused by Δu_2. Likewise, λ_{21} can be determined by the same consideration. It is noticed that the above result derived from a conceptual consideration can also be verified easily by a simple calculation.

It is clear that the two components λ_{12} and λ_{21} are essentially two feedforward control elements, the compensation action taking place before the perturbation produced by the other input enters the loop being considered. It should be stressed that because the parameters of the compensator are derived only from the steady-state gains we never expect the interaction to be removed completely in both transient and steady states. Instead, what we want is to reduce the effects partly by means of a simple and realizable structure. The rest of the effects are intended to be compensated by the robustness of the fuzzy controller with respect to the perturbation.

7.5 Simulation results

There are eight algorithms if we combine the four reasoning methods presented in equations (7.12)–(7.15) with the two defuzzification algorithms given in equations (7.19) and (7.20). All the algorithms will be investigated in this study. For simplicity, each algorithm is denoted by one of the following abbreviations: *mmm*, *mmc*, *ppm*, *ppc*, *mzm*, *mzc*, *mgm* and *mgc*, in which the first letter stands for the operation of AND with *m* being minimum and *p* algebraic product; the second letter denotes the operation of IF-THEN with *m* being minimum, *p* algebraic product, *z* Zadeh's

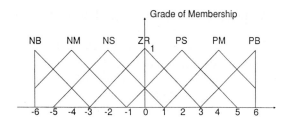

Figure 7.4 *Definition of the membership function.*

implication operator (7.14) and *g* Godel's implication operator (7.15); the third letter designates the method of defuzzification with *m* being the mean of maxima and *c* the centre of gravity. For instance, *mgc* indicates a combination of (7.15) with (7.20).

The variables E, C and U take values on the same finite and discrete universes of discourse, that is, $\bar{E} = \bar{C} = \bar{U} = \{-6, -5, -4, -3, -2, -1, 0, 1, 2, 3, 4, 5, 6\}$. There are seven fuzzy subsets for each variable. They are NB, NM, NS, ZR, PS, PM and PB representing negative-big, negative-medium, negative-small, zero, positive-small, positive-medium and positive-big respectively. The definitions of the grade of membership for these fuzzy sets on the three universes $\bar{E}$, $\bar{C}$ and $\bar{U}$ are taken to be the same. Figure 7.4 shows one of them. The same definitions will be used in all simulation cases.

Although it is usually a difficult task to build a good rule-base for a general expert system, the control rules involving a single-input–single-output process may be obtained from some common control experience and knowledge. Assuming that the SISO process has a monotonic input–output relationship (not necessarily linear), the control goal is to maintain a controlled variable at a desired level, and the response of the system will not be ideal due to the inertial property possessed by the process, Yamazaki and Sugeno (1985) obtained a group of control rules that are summarized in Table 7.1, where variables E, C and U stand for error, the change-in-error and the change-in-control respectively. There are 33 rules in the table with

Table 7.1 *Control rules*

E \ C	NB	NM	NS	ZR	PS	PM	PB
NB		NB		NM	NM	NS	
NM	NB		NM		NS		PS
NS		NM	NS	NS	ZR	PS	PM
ZR	NB		NS	ZR	PS		PB
PS	NM	NS	ZR	PS	PS	PM	
PM	NS		PS		PM		PB
PB		PS	PM	PM		PB	

each entry being read as a rule. 'IF E is G_1 AND C is G_2 THEN U is D'. It has been found, from both physiological and mathematical model studies, that the two cases we are dealing with, blood pressure control with and without the drug infusions, approximately satisfy the assumptions made in deriving the rules as summarized in Table 7.1. Therefore, this rule-base will be employed throughout our studies.

The objectives of the simulation were to demonstrate the feasibility of the proposed controller when applied to multivariable biomedical situations and to compare various reasoning schemes from a practical viewpoint. The comparative studies were carried out in two senses. One was a comparison of performance, meaning that the controlled responses under various reasoning algorithms were investigated assuming that both controller parameters and process parameters are fixed. The performances were evaluated by two frequently used error integral criteria, i.e. integral of square of the error (ISE) and integral of time and absolute error product (ITAE), which are defined as

$$\text{ISE} = \int_0^\infty e_a^2(t)\,dt \tag{7.35}$$

$$\text{ITAE} = \int_0^\infty t|e_a(t)|\,dt \tag{7.36}$$

where $e_a(t)$ is the measured error. The calculation in the studies was implemented by substituting an algebraic sum for the integrals. The other comparison was via performance robustness, where the aim was to study the robustness property of the proposed controller with respect to variations in the parameters of the process.

7.5.1 *PAS* and *PVS* control

The Moller linearized model given in equation (7.5) was used to simulate the cardiovascular system. It was implemented by using a fourth-order Runge–Kutta routine with an integration interval of 0.001 s. The controlled variables were *PAS* and *PVS* and the manipulated variables were heart rate *HR* and systemic resistance *RA*.

The steady-state gain matrix **G** was obtained by using (7.5) and (7.27) with outputs being ΔPAS and ΔPVS, that is

$$\begin{bmatrix} \Delta PAS \\ \Delta PVS \end{bmatrix} = \begin{bmatrix} 26.69 & 77.25 \\ -0.117 & -1.16 \end{bmatrix} \begin{bmatrix} \Delta HR \\ \Delta RA \end{bmatrix}. \tag{7.37}$$

220   *Intelligent Control in Biomedicine*

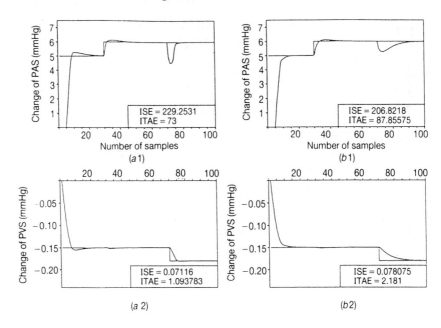

Figure 7.5 *Fuzzy control of* PAS *and* PVS: *(a)* mmm *method;* (b) mmc *method.*

The RGA matrix Γ can be calculated from the **G** matrix as

$$\Gamma = \begin{bmatrix} 1.41 & -0.41 \\ -0.41 & 1.41 \end{bmatrix}. \tag{7.38}$$

Because $\gamma_{12}(\gamma_{21})$ is negative and $\gamma_{11}(\gamma_{22})$ is positive, proper pairing can be made with *HR/PAS* and *RA/PVS*. Thus two decentralized control loops can be constructed. In addition, the compensation factors are obtained from the **G** matrix according to (7.32).

Taking a sampling period of 0.1 s, the output responses obtained under each approximate reasoning scheme are shown in Figures 7.5–7.8. In the figures, the set-points of ΔPAS and ΔPVS were changed at time zero from 0 to 5 mmHg and from 0 to −0.15 mmHg respectively. In order to demonstrate the interactive effects in one loop upon the other and to show the controller's compensating ability, the set-point of ΔPAS was increased at the 30th sample instant whereas the set-point of ΔPVS was unchanged. Furthermore, the set-point of ΔPVS was decreased at the 70th sample instant whereas the set-point of ΔPAS remained at its previous level.

It can be seen that *PAS* and *PVS* were successfully controlled using the various reasoning approaches. However, there are some differences between the algorithms. While smoother responses with slower tracking speeds were produced by the Godel IF-THEN operator (*mgm* and *mgc*), opposite results

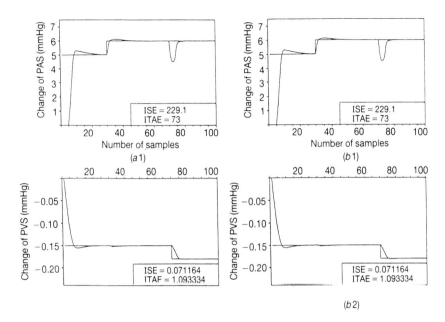

Figure 7.6 *Fuzzy control of* PAS *and* PVS: *(a)* ppm *method; (b)* ppc *method.*

were obtained by the minimum and Zadeh implication operators with the use of the mean of maxima defuzzification method. As expected, the centre of gravity defuzzification strategy usually gave a much smoother transient response than for the mean of maxima. An exception is in the case of employing the *ppm* and *ppc* algorithms (Figure 7.6), in which algebraic product operators were used for both AND and IF-THEN connectives. It appears that there is no significant difference between the two defuzzification methods in the sense of control performance.

The interactive effects between the two loops are evident in the figures. They appeared at the 30th sampling instant in the *PVS* response and at the 70th sampling instant in the *PAS* response. It can be seen that the proposed controller was able to handle the interaction problem satisfactorily. Note that the two effects were different in amplitude. The change of set-point for *PVS* had a much greater influence on the *PAS* loop than did the change in *PAS*. This is primarily due to the fact that *RA* had a stronger cross-coupling effect on *PAS* than that produced by *HR* on *PVS*.

7.5.2 Simultaneous control of *CO* and *MAP*

As discussed previously, it is necessary to increase *CO* while *MAP* is lowered. Equation (7.9) is an approximate model, consisting of the *CVS* and

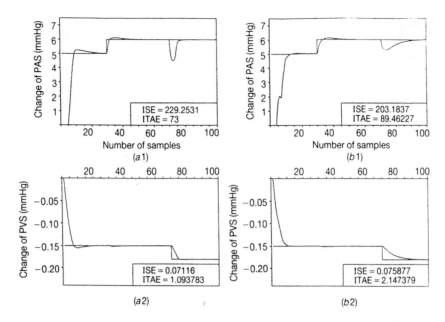

Figure 7.7 *Fuzzy control of* PAS *and* PVS: (a) mzm *method;* (b) mzc *method.*

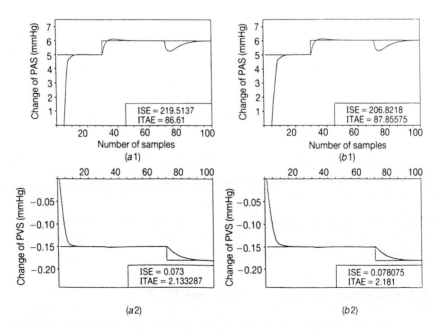

Figure 7.8 *Fuzzy control of* PAS *and* PVS: (a) mgm *method;* (b) mgc *method.*

the drug dynamics, which relates *CO* and *MAP* to the infusions of DOP and SNP. When k, τ and T are set to the typical values given in Section 7.2.2, the steady-state gain matrix can be calculated as

$$\mathbf{G} = \begin{bmatrix} 1.0 & -24.76 \\ 0.6635 & 76.38 \end{bmatrix} \begin{bmatrix} 8.44 & 5.275 \\ -0.09 & -0.15 \end{bmatrix} \tag{7.39}$$

and the RGA matrix Γ is given by

$$\Gamma = \begin{bmatrix} 1.559 & -0.1559 \\ -0.1559 & 1.559 \end{bmatrix}. \tag{7.40}$$

Considering the elements of Γ, we conclude that the loops should be constructed by pairing *CO*/DOP and *MAP*/SNP. It is worth noting that this conclusion agrees with the conceptual consideration in which DOP is primarily used to increase *CO*, and SNP is mainly aimed at lowering *MAP*.

The same controller parameters were used as in the previous simulations, except for the scaling factors and compensator elements. In the first place, the parameters of the simulated drug dynamic model were fixed at typical values. Again, eight algorithms were investigated. The sampling period was chosen to be 30 s. The results obtained are shown in Figures 7.9–7.12. In each figure two groups of results (*a*) and (*b*) are displayed which were obtained by using two different algorithms in which the defuzzification method was different whereas the reasoning scheme remained the same. The set-points for *CO* and *MAP* were square-like but with different times of change in order to show the interactive effects and to demonstrate the compensating ability possessed by the proposed controller.

It is clear that all the eight algorithms could be used to control the process. Comparing these figures, it can be seen that there are no large differences within the reasoning algorithms although the integral indices are slightly different. However, different transient responses were exhibited if the defuzzification method was different under the same reasoning scheme. This can be seen by comparing the two responses in the same figure. A smoother response was given by the centre of gravity method.

Next, uniformly distributed background noise was added to the simulation model. The amplitude of the noise was about 20 per cent of the set-points. Because of space limitation, only one of the results is shown in Figure 7.13. This was obtained by using *mmm* and *mmc* algorithms. The result indicates the feasibility of the controller within a noise-contaminated environment. Basically, the output responses could follow the change of the set-point and provide good regulation despite the presence of the noise. The performance of the system would be improved further if the noise-contaminated measurement data were filtered before being used for feedback.

224   *Intelligent Control in Biomedicine*

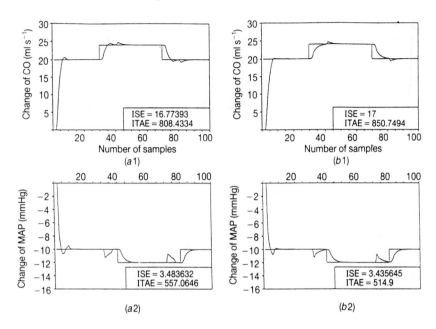

Figure 7.9 *Fuzzy control of* CO *and* MAP: *(*a*)* mmm *method;* (b) mmc *method.*

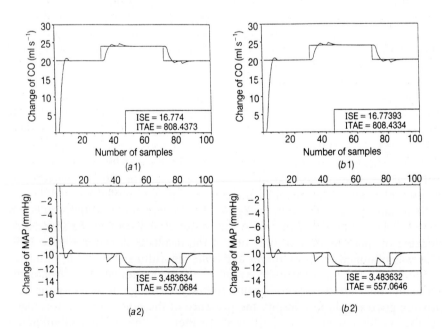

Figure 7.10 *Fuzzy control of* CO *and* MAP: *(*a*)* ppm *method;* (b) ppc *method.*

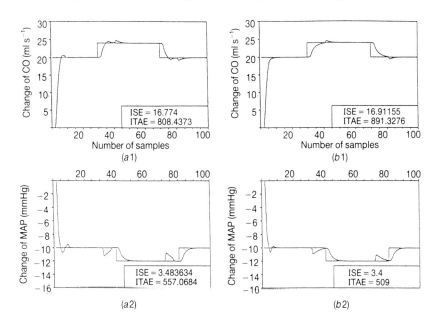

Figure 7.11 *Fuzzy control of* CO *and* MAP: (a) mzm *method;* (b) mzc *method.*

Finally, the robustness of specific reasoning algorithms with respect to changes in the process parameters was investigated. Here the robustness is referred to as performance robustness. Comparative studies on eight algorithms were performed according to the following steps. First, a set of typical process parameters was selected known as the reference parameter set $\Omega_r \in \Omega = \{T_1, T_2, \tau_1, \tau_2, g_{11}, g_{12}, g_{21}, g_{22}\}$ with T, τ and g being the time constants, the transport delays and the gains. Secondly, eight algorithms were employed in turn with the controller parameters taken to be the same for all algorithms. The results produced were evaluated by a set of indices known as the reference index set $\Psi_r \in \Psi = \{$CISE, PISE, CITAE, PITAE, SISE, SITAE$\}$, where the first letter in each element stands for the different response, that is, C is for *CO*, P for *MAP* and S for the sum of the corresponding two indices (SISE = CISE + PISE). Note that in this way eight reference index sets were generated. Then one of the process parameters was varied, and the eight algorithms were applied again without changing any controller parameters. Thus eight index sets were obtained which will be compared with the corresponding reference index set.

Let us define the relative variation with respect to a specific process parameter $\omega \in \Omega$ as

$$\Delta \tilde{\omega} = \frac{\Delta \omega}{\omega_r} = \frac{|\omega - \omega_r|}{\omega_r} \qquad (7.41)$$

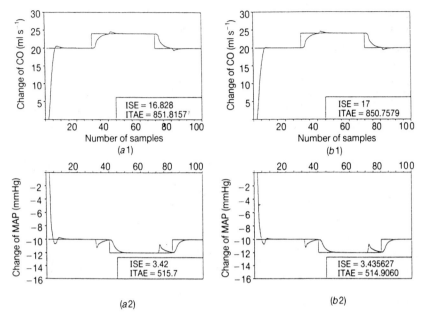

Figure 7.12 *Fuzzy control of* CO *and* MAP: (a) mgm *method;* (b) mgc *method.*

with $\omega_r \in \Omega_r$ and relative variation with respect to a specific control index $\psi \in \Psi_r$ as

$$\Delta \tilde{\psi} = \frac{\Delta \psi}{\psi_r} = \frac{|\psi - \psi_r|}{\psi_r} \qquad (7.42)$$

with $\psi_r \in \Psi_r$.

It is evident that the smaller the ratio of $\Delta \tilde{\psi} / \Delta \tilde{\omega}$, the more robust is the corresponding reasoning algorithm with respect to this parameter, based on this performance index.

Figure 7.14 shows the results obtained when the gains of the drug dynamic model represented by (7.9), k_{11}, k_{12}, k_{21} and k_{22}, were varied by 10 per cent from their typical values. The horizontal axis represents eight reasoning algorithms whereas the vertical axis corresponds to one of the six relative indices defined by (7.42). Actual responses are not presented here because of the huge number of simulation results and space limitation. Generally, the responses were acceptable, especially for transient behaviour. It should be noted, however, that sometimes a non-zero steady-state error appeared which resulted in a relatively large ITAE.

It appears that the COG defuzzification method is less robust than the MOM. This can be seen from the figures. The same reasoning algorithm with the COG method usually produced larger index variations than with

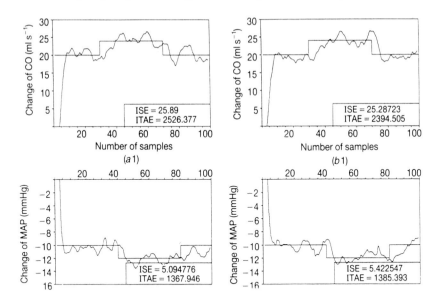

Figure 7.13 *Fuzzy control of CO and MAP with background noise:* (a) ppm *method;* (b) ppc *method.*

the MOM method. This may be explained by the fact that the former pays more attention to details of the inferred fuzzy subset than the latter.

We can deduce, by careful observation and comparison, that Mamdani's and Larsen's IF . . . THEN operators (minimum and algebraic product) are usually less sensitive to gain variation than Zadeh's and Godel's IF . . . THEN operators. It should be noted that an exception is the *mmc* algorithm which usually gave much worse response and therefore larger error indices than the others. It is also worth noting that almost all of the algorithms were less robust with respect to variation in the gains k_{21} and k_{22} than for the gains k_{11} and k_{12}. In other words, not all gains have equal influence on the robustness property of the algorithms.

The comparative results when variations in the time constants and the pure time delays were made are shown in Figure 7.15. The time constants T_1 and T_2 and time delays τ_1 (d_1 in Figure 7.15) and τ_2 (d_2 in Figure 7.15) were changed by 10 per cent from their typical values. It seems that most conclusions for the case of gain variation with respect to the algorithms are applicable also to this situation. However, we notice that changing the time constants gave rise to a small variation in the indices. In contrast, changing the time delays usually resulted in a large change in the indices, thus demonstrating large sensitivity to these parameters.

The final simulation results involved the investigation of effects caused by changes in the compensator factors, namely λ_{12} and λ_{21} in (7.32). The

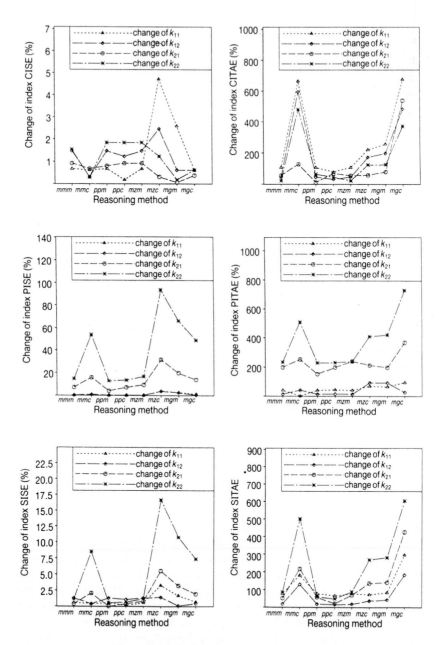

Figure 7.14 *Robustness to change in the gains.*

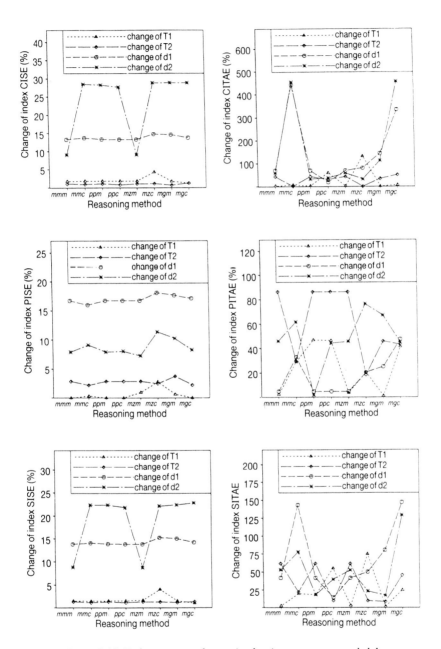

Figure 7.15 *Robustness to change in the time constants and delays.*

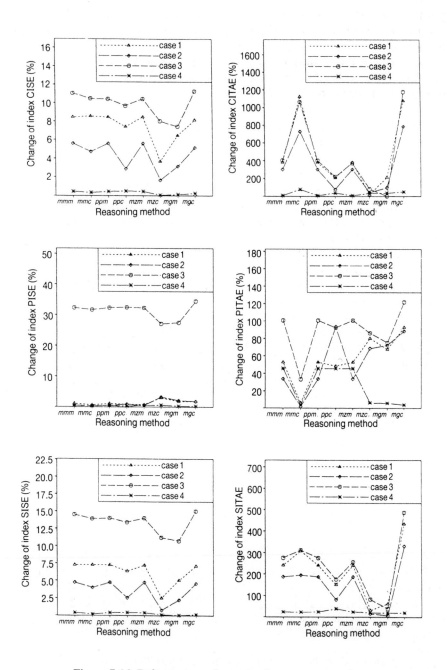

Figure 7.16 *Robustness to change in the compensator factors.*

purpose was to evaluate how robust the proposed multivariable fuzzy controller is with respect to the compensator factors, as indicated by the error integral indices. We considered four cases, in each of which λ_{12} and λ_{21} were changed by a different amount. If the nominal values of λ_{12} and λ_{21} are denoted as λ_{12}^* and λ_{21}^* and their changed values are λ_{c12} and λ_{c21}, then four cases were considered as follows:

$$\text{case 1: } \lambda_{c12} = 1.5\lambda_{12}^* \quad \lambda_{c21} = 0.5\lambda_{21}^*$$
$$\text{case 2: } \lambda_{c12} = 0.5\lambda_{12}^* \quad \lambda_{c21} = 1.5\lambda_{21}^*$$
$$\text{case 3: } \lambda_{c12} = 0.0\lambda_{12}^* \quad \lambda_{c21} = 0.0\lambda_{21}^*$$
$$\text{case 4: } \lambda_{c12} = 0.75\lambda_{12}^* \quad \lambda_{c21} = 0.75\lambda_{21}^*.$$

It should be noted that the variations of λ_{12} and λ_{21} are due to changes in the steady-state gains. Therefore the cases we are considering are, in fact, intended to show the robustness performance of the compensator factors with respect to the variation of the steady-state gains. This variation may reflect inconsistency between the estimated and actual gains.

The simulation results are shown in Figure 7.16. It is clear that the worst situation occurred when case 3 was tried. In this case there is no compensation action applied to the system and, as expected, the interactive effects within the two loops are responsible for the poor performance. In contrast, the 25 per cent changes in λ_{12} and λ_{21} (case 4) produced only a small variation in the indices and the responses were acceptable. It appears reasonable to conclude that the introduction of the compensator does eliminate the interactive effects effectively, and therefore the control performance can be improved by this simple scheme. In addition, the performance of the system is not affected greatly when a mild change is made in the factors, which indicates that useful robustness properties are possessed by the compensator.

7.6 Conclusion

The simulation results have demonstrated the feasibility of the proposed multivariable fuzzy controller when it is applied to the different processes under consideration. In our case, both fast and slow human blood pressure dynamic processes have been controlled successfully. Comparative simulation results have revealed that the selection of the reasoning algorithms should not be too crucial. However, from the robustness and simplicity point of view, it seems that *mmm*, *ppm* and *ppc* algorithms are good candidates to be selected for real-time control applications.

The decentralized control strategy simplifies the design procedures and overcomes the difficulty in constructing the rule-base. In this study, a common-sense rule-base has been used to control two different processes.

The interactive effects between the variables are partly handled by introducing a simple compensation scheme, whose realization is based on the process steady-state gains. The simulation results showed that the scheme is necessary and efficient in compensating the cross-coupling effects and, perhaps more importantly, that the compensator possesses useful robustness properties against variation in the gains.

The proposed multivariable fuzzy controller is applicable only if the steady-state gains of the controlled process are available, although they do not need to be known accurately. If this is not the case, a fully cross-coupling fuzzy controller must be adopted which gives rise to the difficulty of building a rule-base consisting of rules with multiple-premises. This will be the main concern of the following two chapters where self-learning strategies are studied.

References

Den Brok, M.W.N.M. et al., 1987, 'A rule-based blood pressure controller', in Proceedings of the Second European Workshop on Fault Diagnostics, Reliability and Related Knowledge-based Approaches, pp. 67–74.

Efstathiou, J., 1988, Expert systems, fuzzy logic and rule-based control explained at last, *Transactions of the Institute of Measurement and Control*, **10**, 198–206.

Grosdidier, P. et al., 1985, Closed-loop properties from steady-state gain information. *Industrial and Engineering Chemistry Fundamentals*, **24**, 221–35.

Gupta, M.M. et al., 1986, Multivariable structure of fuzzy control systems, *IEEE Transactions on Systems Man, and Cybernetics*, **16**, 638–56.

Isaka, S. et al., 1988, 'On the design and performance evaluation of an adaptive fuzzy controller', in Proceedings of the IEEE the 27th conference on decision and control, pp. 1068–9.

Isaka, S. et al., 1989, 'An adaptive fuzzy controller for blood pressure regulation', in Proceedings of the IEEE Engineering in Medicine and Biology Society 11th Annual International Conference, pp. 1763–4.

Jensen, N. et al., 1986, Interaction analysis in multivariable control systems, *AIChE Journal*, **32**, 959–70.

Lee, C.C., 1990, Fuzzy logic in control systems: fuzzy logic controller—part one and part two, *IEEE Transactions on Systems Man, and Cybernetics*, **20**, 404–35.

Linkens, D.A. and Mahfouf, M., 1988, 'Fuzzy logic knowledge-based control for muscle relaxant anaesthesia', in Proceedings of IFAC Modelling and Control in Medicine, pp. 185–90.

Linkens, D.A. and Mahfouf, M., 1991, 'Multivariable generalized predictive control for anaesthesia', European Control Conference, Grenoble.

Linkens, D.A. and Mansour, N.-E., 1989, Pole-placement self-tuning control of blood pressure in post-operative patients: a simulation study, *IEE proceedings*, Pt D, **136**, 1–11.

Linkens, D.A. and Nie, J., 1992a, A unified real time approximate reasoning approach for use in intelligent control. Part 1: theoretical development, *International Journal of Control*, **56**, 334–63.

Linkens, D.A. and Nie, J., 1992b, A unified real time approximate reasoning approach for use in intelligent control. Part 2: application to multivariable blood pressure control, *International Journal of Control*, **56**, 365–97.

Linkens, D.A., Greenhow, S.G., and Asbury, A.J., 1986, An expert system for the control of depth of anaesthesia, *Biomedical Measurement Information Control*, **1**, 223–8.
Mansour, N.-E., 1988, 'Adaptive control of blood pressure', PhD thesis, Department of Control Engineering, University of Sheffield.
Mansour, N.-E. and Linkens, D.A., 1990, Self-tuning pole-placement multivariable control of blood pressure for post-operative patients: a model-based study, *IEE Proceedings*, Pt D, **137**, 13–29.
McInnis, B.C. et al., 1985, Automatic control of blood pressure with multiple drug inputs, *Annals of Biomedical Engineering*, **13**, 217–25.
Miller, R.R. et al., 1977, Combined dopamine and nitroprusside therapy in congestive heart failure, *Circulation*, **55**, 881.
Moller, D. et al., 1983, Modelling, simulation and parameter-estimation of the human cardiovascular system, in *Advances in Control Systems and Signal Processing*, Vol. 4.
Neat, G.W. et al., 1989, Expert adaptive control for drug delivery systems, *IEEE Control Systems Magazine*, June, 20–3.
Ray, K.S. et al., 1985, 'Structure of an intelligent fuzzy logic controller and its behaviour', in *Approximate Reasoning in Expert Systems*, 553–61.
Serna, V. et al., 1983, 'Adaptive control of multiple drug infusion', in Proceedings of JACC Conference, pp. 22–6.
Sugeno, M., 1985, An introductory survey of fuzzy control, *Information Science*, **36**, 59–83.
Tong, R.M., 1984, A retrospective view of fuzzy control systems, *Fuzzy Sets and Systems*, **14**, 199–210.
Tong, R.M., 1985, An annotated bibliography of fuzzy control, in *Industrial Application of Fuzzy Control*, pp. 249–69.
Vishnoi, R. and Gingrich, K.J., 1987, 'Fuzzy controller for gaseous anaesthesia delivery using vital signs', in Proceedings of the IEEE 26th Conference on Decision and Control, pp. 346–7.
Voss, G. et al., 1987, Adaptive multivariable drug delivery control of arterial pressure and cardiac output in anaesthetised dogs, *IEEE Transactions*, **BME 134**, 617–23.
Yamashita, Y. et al., 1988, Fuzzy control of blood pressure by drug infusion, *Journal of Chemical Engineering of Japan*, **21**, 541–3.
Yamazaki, T. and Sugeno, M., 1985, 'A microprocessor based fuzzy controller for industrial purposes', in *Industrial Application of Fuzzy Control*, pp. 231–9.
Ying, H. et al., 1988, Expert-system-based fuzzy control of arterial pressure by drug infusion, *Medical Progress Through Technology*, **13**, 203–15.
Zadeh, L.A., 1978, Fuzzy sets as a basis for a theory of possibility, *Fuzzy Sets and Systems*, **1**, 3–28.

Chapter 8
Learning-based fuzzy and neural control for blood pressure management

Junhong Nie

8.1 Introduction

An obvious and fundamental question arising from the real implementation of rule-based control systems is how a set of control rules can be derived. The success and performance of rule-based control systems depend largely on the availability and the performance of the rule-base. Basically, there are two approaches for building the rule-base, namely, either from human experts and/or from the process being controlled. The former method, which is common in general expert systems, has a heuristic and qualitative nature. A number of successful engineering control applications have been reported based on this approach (Sugeno, 1985; Lee, 1990). It is evident that this approach relies on the availability of domain experts. When there are no experts or skilled operators available at hand to supply necessary knowledge or to be used as an identified model, it would be desirable to construct the rule-base by directly operating the process being controlled. It is also desirable to refine and improve the rough rule-base derived from experts which may be incomplete, inconsistent or even partly incorrect, especially when the operating condition is changed.

In recent years there have been some efforts towards this direction within the fuzzy rule-based control realm. The development of this approach is mainly along two lines: model-based and learning-based. The former is more closely related to the traditional adaptive control strategy, whereas the latter has some connection with machine learning and intelligence. The basic principle of the model-based method is that the relationships governing the process inputs and outputs are represented by a set of IF . . . THEN rules (Takagi and Sugeno, 1985) or a relational equation (Pedrycz, 1985) termed a fuzzy model of the process. After the fuzzy model is identified, a set of control rules or a controller relational equation can be created based on the identified model. In contrast, the learning-based approach tries to emulate the human learning ability by means of operating the process repeatedly, and thus the process behaviour is not explicitly taken into account.

Procyk and Mamdani (1979) developed a so-called linguistic self-organizing controller (SOC) in which a performance loop was added to a basic fuzzy controller. Measured performance indicated by a performance index table was used to create or modify the rule-base. Following this, some improved algorithms as well as some applications have been reported (Scharf and Mandic, 1985; Daley and Gill, 1986; Shao, 1988; Linkens and Abbod, 1992).

By noting that it is possible to construct a rule-base with the rules having less linguistic meaning but having an IF . . . THEN statement form, this chapter proposes a methodology that can be used to construct such a rule-base for multivariable fuzzy controllers via self-learning. We consider two approaches to implementing the fuzzy controller, i.e. fuzzy algorithm-based and neural network-based implementations. As an application and feasibility demonstration of the proposed system, the problem of multivariable control of blood pressure is studied by means of simulation. By defining several evaluation measures, learning ability relating to change of performance specifications and variation of process parameters is investigated. Reproducibility of the fuzzy controller, utilizing the rule-base extracted from the learning control, is also evaluated in terms of relative accuracy with respect to the learning results. In addition, the issue of learning speed, which is affected by learning gains, initial controls and different learning laws, is explored.

8.2 Fuzzy controller implementation

One of the remarkable features possessed by fuzzy systems is their inferencing capability from a set of imprecise, incomplete, and even only partially reliable premises and incoming data. Such inferential ability comes mainly from the power of approximate reasoning. Although the reasoning scheme is usually carried out at a linguistic level (even for numerical applications such as fuzzy control), it is possible and sometimes desirable to perform approximate reasoning strategies at a numerical level, thereby establishing a numerical environment for use of fuzzy control where the inputs and outputs of the controller are numerical. In particular, such a reasoning scheme will require a rule-base to be numerically oriented, which may be derived directly from the process being controlled. In what follows, we describe two possible approaches to performing the task of approximate reasoning at a numerical level.

8.2.1 Fuzzy algorithm implementation

In this subsection, we assume that the multivariable system is fully decoupled in the sense that two independent control loops can be built with the corresponding rule-bases derived by using the learning scheme described in the following section. A method for achieving this has been described in Chapter 7. Therefore it is sufficient to discuss only one control loop.

Assume that the input variables to the fuzzy controller are error E and change-in-error C which take their values on universes of discourse $\bar{E}$ and $\bar{C}$ respectively. We define $\bar{E}$ and $\bar{C}$ as finite, discrete and symmetric about zero, that is,

$$\bar{E} = \{-v_N, -v_{N-1}, \ldots, -v_1, 0, v_1, \ldots, v_{N-1}, v_N\} \quad \text{Card}[\bar{E}] = 2N+1$$

$$\bar{C} = \{-w_M, -w_{M-1}, \ldots, -w_1, 0, w_1, \ldots, w_{M-1}, w_M\} \quad \text{Card}[\bar{C}] = 2M+1$$

where $v_i, i \in [1, N]$ and $w_j, j \in [1, M]$ are positive and are assumed to be equally spaced on the real line.

The output of the fuzzy controller is a control action U which takes its value in $\bar{U}$. Here $\bar{U} = [u_{\min}, u_{\max}]$ is a closed and continuous interval with $u_{\min}$ and $u_{\max}$ being minimum and maximum admissible control values.

Suppose that there are N_f fuzzy sets $A_i, i \in [1, N_f]$ defined over $\bar{E}$, and M_f fuzzy sets $B_j, j \in [1, M_f]$ defined over $\bar{C}$. A_i and B_j may represent some fuzzy concepts such as positive-large and negative-small, etc, and their membership functions $A_i(\bar{e})$ and $B_j(\bar{c})$ are of triangular form and possess some properties such as normality, interval monotonicity and symmetry about $\bar{e}_i^*$ and $\bar{c}_j^*$. More specifically, the membership function of a fuzzy set is characterized by $\bar{e}_i^*(\bar{c}_j^*)$ and $\delta_i^e(\delta_j^c)$, where $\bar{e}_i^*(\bar{c}_j^*)$ represents the central value of the corresponding support set at which maximum grade 1 is assigned and $\delta_i^e(\delta_j^c)$ designates the half-width of the support set. Hereafter, a given fuzzy set will be expressed by its central value with an implicit support width, i.e. $A_i = \bar{e}_i^*$ and $B_j = \bar{c}_j^*$. Linguistically, the above expression may be interpreted as *about* $\bar{e}_i^*(\bar{c}_j^*)$ in which *about* is constrained by the width value $\delta_i^e(\delta_j^c)$ of the corresponding support set.

Suppose that there are K rules in the rule-base denoted as

$$R_1 \text{ ALSO } R_2 \text{ ALSO}, \ldots, \text{ALSO } R_K.$$

Each rule R_k has the form of

$$R_k: \text{IF } \bar{e}_k^* \text{ AND } \bar{c}_k^* \text{ THEN } u_k \quad k \in [1, K] \tag{8.1}$$

where $\bar{e}_k^*$ is the central value corresponding to one of the predefined fuzzy sets $A_i, i \in [1, N_f], \bar{c}_k^*$ is the central value in accordance with one of the predefined fuzzy sets $B_j, j \in [1, M_f]$, and u_k is a real number in $\bar{U}$. Here no linguistic label is attached to the THEN part of the rule.

If we consider $\bar{e}_k^*$ and $\bar{c}_k^*$ as a two-dimensional vector $r_k = (\bar{e}_k^*, \bar{c}_k^*)$, then r_k will create a rectangle in the $\bar{E} \times \bar{C}$ plane taking $(\bar{e}_k^*, \bar{c}_k^*)$ as its central point and $2\delta_k^e$ and $2\delta_k^c$ as its sides. Therefore, K rules partition the $\bar{E} \times \bar{C}$ plane into K subplanes. Similarly, current inputs $\bar{e}_I$ and $\bar{c}_I$ mapped from measured values $\bar{e}_m$ and $\bar{c}_m$ by scaling factors GE and GC can be expressed as a two-dimensional vector $(\bar{e}_I, \bar{c}_I)$ in the $\bar{E} \times \bar{C}$ plane.

The control algorithm can be viewed as a process in which an appropriate control action is deduced from a current input $(\bar{e}_I, \bar{c}_I)$ and K rules according to some prespecified reasoning algorithms. In this study, the reasoning procedure consists of two steps: pattern matching and weighted averaging. The first operation deals with the IF part for all rules, whereas the second one involves an operation on the THEN part of the rules.

It is convenient to view the IF part of a rule and an input as patterns to be called a rule pattern and an input pattern respectively. In this view, the first step in the reasoning algorithm is to compute the matching degree between the input pattern and the rule patterns. Here we adopt the following Hamming distance algorithm.

Let

$$l_k = (l_k^1, l_k^2) = (|\bar{e}_k^* - \bar{e}_I|, |\bar{c}_k^* - \bar{c}_I|) \tag{8.2}$$

be a minus vector. Then the relative Hamming distance $d_k \in [0, 1]$ from input pattern $(\bar{e}_I, \bar{c}_I)$ to the kth rule pattern is given by

$$d_k = \frac{l_k^1 + l_k^2}{\delta_k^e + \delta_k^c} \tag{8.3}$$

where $l_k^1 \leq \delta_k^e$ and $l_k^2 \leq \delta_k^c$.

The matching degree $s_k \in [0, 1]$ is calculated by

$$s_k = 1 - d_k. \tag{8.4}$$

It is evident from (8.3) and (8.4) that if the input pattern is fully matched with the kth rule pattern, meaning that the input vector is exactly the same as the central value vector of the kth rule, then $d_k = 0$ and $s_k = 1$, and if they are completely unmatched, implying that the input vector is on one of the corners of the rectangle created by the kth rule pattern, then $d_k = 1$ and $s_k = 0$; otherwise $0 < s_k < 1$, indicating that there exists some similarity between the two patterns. Note that if the input pattern falls outside the kth rectangle, we define $s_k = 0$.

Suppose that for a specified input a set of matching degrees s_k are obtained using the above algorithm. Then the present control value is given by

$$u = \frac{\sum_{q=1}^{Q} s_q \cdot u_q}{\sum_{q=1}^{Q} s_q}. \tag{8.5}$$

8.2.2 Neural network implementation

As mentioned previously, two key issues concerning the implementation of the fuzzy controller are knowledge representation and associated inferencing schemes. Traditionally they are carried out from a logical point of view by performing some fuzzy logic calculations. Recently the author has made an attempt to implement the approximate reasoning by means of back-propagation neural networks (BNN) (Nie and Linkens, 1992). The underlying principles lie in the fact that by viewing the given rule-base as defining a global linguistic association constrained by fuzzy sets, a functional mapping from the fuzzy logic-based algorithm to the network-based approach can be established and approximate reasoning is implemented by a BNN with the aid of the fuzzy set theory.

A block diagram of the proposed BNN-based fuzzy control system is depicted in Figure 8.1. It is a feedback control system with a similar structure to that for a traditional fuzzy control system. However, the system here works in two distinct modes: training and operation. Assuming that the rule-base is given, the BNN network is trained off-line by presenting all rules sequentially to the network. Then the successfully trained network (in terms of having a sufficient accuracy) can be inserted in the control loop for on-line operation.

Depending on the methods for converting qualitative (linguistic) labels into quantitative (numerical) values, the structures of the resulting controllers are significantly different. There are at least two possibilities for doing this, namely, fuzzy set interpretation, characterized by graded membership

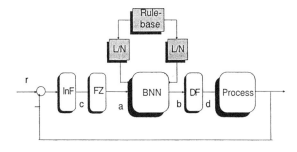

Figure 8.1 *A diagram of BNN-based fuzzy control system.*

functions, and fuzzy number translation, featured typically by central values and spread widths. In the former case, the linguistic labels in the rules are interpreted as fuzzy sets and therefore the inputs and the outputs of the BNN net are graded membership functions during the training stage. To use such a trained network during the operational stage, the measured crisp controller inputs must be fuzzified and the outputs of the BNN must be defuzzified so as to establish a compatible operating environment for use of both modes. An immediate effect of this is that the size of the resulting neural network will be large depending on the number of process inputs/outputs, the number of elements in the corresponding universes, and also the number of hidden units. For example, for a 2×2 process with errors and change-in-errors as inputs and with 13 elements in each of the universes, there will be $2 \times 2 \times 13 = 52$ input units and $2 \times 13 = 26$ output units in the BNN. Obviously such a realization would be extremely inefficient, in terms of training time and computer storage, and even impossible due to the BNN's limited tractability of dealing with a large-scale problem.

However, if we were able to make the environment of the training mode adapt to that of the operational mode instead of vice versa as above, the situation would be changed dramatically. This is possible because if we think of c and d as the input and output points of the system as indicated in Figure 8.1, then no fuzzy signals are involved, but rather they are completely determined. Thus what we need to do is to enable the BNN to work at the signal level instead of the graded membership level. This can be done by interpreting the linguistic labels via fuzzy numbers as described below.

A fuzzy number is typically characterized by a central value with an interval around the centre. The central value is most representative of the fuzzy number and the width of the associated interval determines the degree of fuzziness, a wider interval indicating more fuzziness. In this perspective, the underlying realization of the BNN-based fuzzy controller can be restated as follows. By explicitly embedding the meaning of the linguistic labels, the control rule relating n inputs to m outputs can be rewritten as

IF X_1 is $(\hat{u}_1^j, \delta_1^j)$ AND X_2 is $(\hat{u}_2^j, \delta_2^j)$ ..., AND X_n is $(\hat{u}_n^j, \delta_n^j)$

THEN Y_1 is $(\hat{v}_1^j, \gamma_1^j)$ AND Y_2 is $(\hat{v}_2^j, \gamma_2^j)$ ..., AND Y_m is $(\hat{v}_m^j, \gamma_m^j)$

or more compactly

$$\text{IF } X \text{ is } (\hat{u}^j, \delta^j) \text{ THEN } Y \text{ is } (\hat{v}^j, \gamma^j) \qquad (8.6)$$

where $\hat{u}^j = [\hat{u}_1^j, \hat{u}_2^j, \ldots, \hat{u}_n^j]$, $\hat{u}_i^j \in U_i$, and $\hat{v}^j = [\hat{v}_1^j, \hat{v}_2^j, \ldots, \hat{v}_m^j]$, $\hat{v}_k^j \in V_k$ are the input and output central value vectors in the jth rule, $\delta^j = [\delta_1^j, \delta_2^j, \ldots, \delta_n^j]$ and $\gamma^j = [\gamma_1^j, \gamma_2^j, \ldots, \gamma_m^j]$ are the input and output width vectors in the jth rule. Now it is possible to train the BNN with only the central value vectors, i.e. $(\hat{u}^j, \hat{v}^j)$ pairs while leaving the width vectors untreated explicitly. One may ask the question of how the fuzzy concept is handled in such a paradigm. The answer is, as concluded in the author's previous study (Nie and Linkens, 1992), that the BNN network inherently possesses some fuzziness which is exhibited in the form of interpolation over new situations. This desirable property, obtained primarily from the distributiveness of the BNN, is precisely the one an approximate reasoning system seeks to achieve.

Once the functional equivalence between fuzziness and distributiveness is acknowledged, the structural complexity of the BNN can be reduced greatly. This can be attributed to the fact that both fuzzification and defuzzification procedures are no longer necessary, and more importantly the number of input and output units are dramatically decreased to being equal to n and m respectively. Taking the same example as before, only four input units and two output units are needed in this case compared with 54 and 26 in the previous situation. Needless to say, the computational efficiency would be greatly increased in both training and operational stages, and more importantly this interpretation provides a basis for learning and extracting rules directly from the controlled environment as described in the next section. It is worth noting that the values of the inputs and the outputs of the BNN are no longer bounded in $[0,1]$, but are within the range of the corresponding universes.

8.3 Learning

One of the principal objectives in this chapter is to develop a fuzzy control system not only satisfying the desired control performances, but also requiring only little prior knowledge about the controlled process. In particular, we assume that the control rules or teacher signals are unavailable. Obviously a procedure for deriving the needed rules must be determined. Here we propose a scheme capable of achieving the above objectives and requirements. By introducing a learning mechanism (Linkens and Nie, 1993a), the required teacher signals are obtained first and then in turn processed to provide extraction of a set of rules which are suitable for use in either an algorithm-based or a network-based fuzzy controller as described in the last section. In the latter case, the rules are used as training examples during the training stage. The details concerning the learning processes are described below.

Figure 8.2 shows a block diagram of the learning system consisting of the reference model, the learning algorithm, the rule-base formation mechanism, and the controlled process, which is assumed to have two inputs and two outputs. Corresponding to this process, it is assumed that the fuzzy controller is of a decentralized structure and is composed of two independent controllers. Notice that the approach that will be described below is also applicable to the situation where a centralized controller is required.

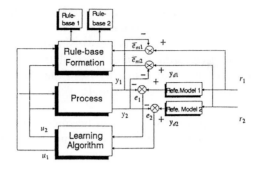

Figure 8.2 *System structure for constructing rule-bases.*

This will be seen in Section 8.5 in which the BNN-based controller has a centralized structure. By operating the learning mechanism iteratively, the desired control performances specified by the reference model subject to the command signals are gradually achieved and the desired control trajectory denoted by u_d is obtained. At the same time, the controller input vectors are constructed and, together with the learned control u_d, are stored in ordered pairs which are subsequently used as the basis for extracting rules. In addition, the learning algorithm learns appropriate scaling factors that are subsequently used for fuzzy control. It should be noted that there are two types of error in Figure 8.2, namely learning errors e_1 and e_2 and control errors $\bar{e}_{m1}$ and $\bar{e}_{m2}$. The former are defined as the difference between the output of the reference model y_d and the output of the process y, whereas the latter are defined as the discrepancy between the output of the command signal r and the output of the process y.

8.3.1 Reference model

The reference model with inputs $r = [r_1, r_2]^T$ and outputs $y_d = [y_{d1}, y_{d2}]^T$ is used to designate the desired performance. Notice that although the process may have strong interaction effects between the two inputs, the desired performance for the two output variables can be represented by two independent models, each of which has an appropriately chosen input. In other words, the reference model is non-interacting. The model can be a low-order linear one described by either a transfer function or a state equation. For example, the transfer functions of first-order and second-order systems with pure time delay are given by

$$H_r(s) = \frac{K_r e^{-\tau_r s}}{T_r s + 1} \tag{8.7}$$

and

$$H_r(s) = \frac{\omega_{nr}^2 e^{-\tau_r s}}{s^2 + 2\xi_r \omega_{nr} s + \omega_{nr}^2}. \tag{8.8}$$

The parameters in the model are determined by the desired time domain indices such as overshoot, settling time and steady-state error, or alternatively by the desired pole position in the s plane. Thus the outputs of the models represent the desired outputs.

8.3.2 Learning algorithm

Once the desired response y_d is specified, the next step is to determine the process input u_d with which the corresponding response y of the controlled process will be close enough to y_d. With the assumption of little prior knowledge about the process being available, obtaining such a u_d is by no means trivial. Here we adopt a simple but efficient approach which is usually referred to as *iterative learning control* (Arimoto, 1990; Linkens and Nie, 1993a). Although the algorithm was primarily designed for robotic tracking applications, we have suggested some modifications which make it capable of learning a set of control actions for multivariable systems with time delays in control. While the details of the algorithms and associated convergence proofs can be found in Linkens and Nie (1993a), the basic principle and a general learning algorithm are briefly outlined below.

The main function of the learning algorithm is to obtain the correct control signal $u_d = [u_1, u_2]^T$ corresponding to the desired output y_d. The error $e = [e_1, e_2]^T$, called the learning error, is used as a learning signal. It is expected that e will asymptotically approach zero or a predefined small region with increase in the trial number. It is worth noting that this asymptotic property is along the iteration direction not along the time direction. More specifically, we require that $\|e_k(t)\| \to 0$ or $\|e_k(t)\| < \gamma$ in $t \in [0, T]$ as $k \to \infty$, where k denotes the iteration number, $\gamma > 0$ is a predefined error tolerance and $\|\cdot\|$ stands for the norm. Thus convergence occurs uniformly in the time interval of interest $[0, T]$. Obviously, the desired control u_d is learned at this time.

According to the learning goal described above, the corresponding learning laws are given as follows.

- Error correction algorithm:

$$u_{1,k+1}(t) = u_{1,k}(t) + g_1 e_{1,k}(t + \lambda_1)$$
$$u_{2,k+1}(t) = u_{2,k}(t) + g_2 e_{2,k}(t + \lambda_2). \tag{8.9}$$

- Cross-error correction algorithm:

$$u_{1,k+1}(t) = u_{1,k}(t) + g_{11} e_{1,k}(t + \lambda_1) + g_{12} e_{2,k}(t + \lambda_2)$$
$$u_{2,k+1}(t) = u_{2,k}(t) + g_{22} e_{2,k}(t + \lambda_2) + g_{21} e_{1,k}(t + \lambda_1). \quad (8.10)$$

- Error and derivative correction algorithm:

$$u_{1,k+1}(t) = u_{1,k}(t) + p_1 e_{1,k}(t + \lambda_1) + q_1 \dot{e}_{1,k}(t + \lambda_1)$$
$$u_{2,k+1}(t) = u_{2,k}(t) + p_2 e_{2,k}(t + \lambda_2) + q_2 \dot{e}_{2,k}(t + \lambda_2). \quad (8.11)$$

where $\dot{e}$ denotes the derivative of e with respect to time, k denotes iteration number, λ_i, $i = 1, 2$ is time advance and g, p, q are learning gains.

If we assume that $\lambda_1 = \lambda_2 = \lambda$, then the above algorithms may be represented in a compact form given by

$$u_{k+1}(t) = u_k(t) + \mathbf{P} e_k(t + \lambda) + \mathbf{Q} \dot{e}_k(t + \lambda) \quad (8.12)$$

where $\mathbf{P}$ and $\mathbf{Q}$ are learning matrices. It is clear that (8.9), (8.10) and (8.11) can be derived from (8.12) if $\mathbf{P}$ and $\mathbf{Q}$ are suitably chosen. However, we keep the algorithms separated in order to stress the loop effects upon the learning process and to show how the algorithm can be intuitively derived from common control knowledge as discussed later.

The discrete versions of the above algorithms are given in a compact form by

$$u_{k+1}(n) = u_k(n) + \mathbf{P} e_k(n + \mu) + \mathbf{Q} c_k(n + \mu) \quad (8.13)$$

where n denotes the nth sampling instant, μ is an integer representing the advance sampling number and $c_k(n)$ is change-in-error defined by $c_k(n) = e_k(n+1) - e_k(n)$. When $\mathbf{P} = \text{diag}\{p_1, p_2\}$ and $\mathbf{Q} = 0$ the discrete version corresponding to (8.9) is obtained. Likewise $\mathbf{Q} = 0$ corresponds to (8.10) and $\mathbf{P} = \text{diag}\{p_1, p_2\}$ with $\mathbf{Q} = \text{diag}\{q_1, q_2\}$ corresponds to (8.11).

8.4 Rule extracting

Parallel to learning, the rule-base formation mechanism at each trial creates two sets of control rules for two input/output pairs. Notice that although the multivariable process may possess strong interaction between the two inputs, the control rules can be set up independently since interaction effects are suitably and implicitly embedded into the learned u_d. Each rule relates the measured control error $\bar{e}_m$ and change-in-error $\bar{c}_m$ to the control action

u. It is worth noting that the rules are purely value-based in the sense that there is no time relationship embedded in the rule variables. The rule-bases are memoryless meaning that they are updated at each trial and rely only on the values of $\bar{e}$, $\bar{c}$ and u obtained in the present trial. It should be pointed out that $\bar{e}_m$ always undergoes a time course at each iteration, consisting of a transient stage and a steady-state stage. The details of the approach are described next.

8.4.1 Measurement of variables

Suppose that, at the kth learning iteration, correct control actions $u_1(iT_s)$ and $u_2(iT_s)$ are learned with which the desired output responses specified by the reference models are achieved, where T_s is sampling period and $i \in [0, L]$ with L being the maximum sampling number. At the same time, two sets of inputs, $(\bar{e}_{m1}(iT_s), \bar{c}_{m1}(iT_s))$ and $(\bar{e}_{m2}(iT_s), \bar{c}_{m2}(iT_s))$, for two control loops are recorded. Here,

$$\begin{cases} \bar{e}_{m1}(iT_s) = SP_1 - y_1(iT_s) \\ \bar{c}_{m1}(iT_s) = \bar{e}_{m1}(iT_s) - \bar{e}_{m1}(iT_s - T_s) \\ \bar{e}_{m2}(iT_s) = SP_2 - y_2(iT_s) \\ \bar{c}_{m2}(iT_s) = \bar{e}_{m2}(iT_s) - \bar{e}_{m2}(iT_s - T_s) \end{cases} \quad (8.14)$$

for $i = 0, 1, 2, \ldots, L$, where SP_1 and SP_2 denote set-points for loop 1 and loop 2 respectively.

With corresponding $u_1(iT_s)$ and $u_2(iT_s)$, two sets of input–output pairs relating the input to the control action can be constructed in order as follows.

$$\begin{cases} \{(\bar{e}_{m1}(iT_s), \bar{c}_{m1}(iT_s))\} \Rightarrow \{u_1(iT_s)\} \\ \{(\bar{e}_{m2}(iT_s), \bar{c}_{m2}(iT_s))\} \Rightarrow \{u_2(iT_s)\} \end{cases} \quad (8.15)$$

for $i = 0, 1, 2, \ldots, L$, where $u_1(iT_s) \in [u_{min1}, u_{max1}]$ and $u_2(iT_s) \in [u_{min2}, u_{max2}]$.

8.4.2 Scaling process

Define two sets of scaling factors (GE_1, GC_1) and (GE_2, GC_2) so that the following is satisfied

$$\begin{cases} (\bar{e}_1(iT_s), \bar{c}_1(iT_s)) \in \bar{E}_1 \times \bar{C}_1 \\ (\bar{e}_2(iT_s), \bar{c}_2(iT_s)) \in \bar{E}_2 \times \bar{C}_2 \end{cases} \quad (8.16)$$

where $\bar{E}$ and $\bar{C}$ are the universes of discourse defined by Equation (8.1), and

$$\begin{cases} \bar{e}_1(iT_s) = S[\bar{e}_{m1}(iT_s) \cdot GE_1] \\ \bar{c}_1(iT_s) = S[\bar{c}_{m1}(iT_s) \cdot GC_1] \\ \bar{e}_2(iT_s) = S[\bar{e}_{m2}(iT_s) \cdot GE_2] \\ \bar{c}_2(iT_s) = S[\bar{c}_{m2}(iT_s) \cdot GC_2] \end{cases} \quad (8.17)$$

where S denotes an operation with which the scaled values are set to the nearest elements in $\bar{E}$ or $\bar{C}$.

Now, we have the following ordered pairs.

$$\begin{cases} \{(\bar{e}_1(iT_s), \bar{c}_1(iT_s))\} \Rightarrow \{u_1(iT_s)\} \\ \{(\bar{e}_2(iT_s), \bar{c}_2(iT_s))\} \Rightarrow \{u_2(iT_s)\} \end{cases} \quad (8.18)$$

for $i = 0, 1, \ldots, L$. In what follows, we will drop subscripts 1 and 2 and deal only with one set of the data given in (8.16).

8.4.3 Conflict resolution

In order to create rules similar to the form of (8.1), it is necessary to transform these $L+1$ *time-ordered* data into a set of *value-based* input–output data in which there is no time index iT_s involved.

First, $L+1$ data pairs are rearranged into J groups according to their vector values $(\bar{e}(iT_s), \bar{c}(iT_s))$ denoted as follows:

$$\Gamma_j: \begin{cases} (\bar{e}, \bar{c})_{\Gamma_j} \Rightarrow u^1_{\Gamma_j} \\ (\bar{e}, \bar{c})_{\Gamma_j} \Rightarrow u^2_{\Gamma_j} \\ \cdot \\ \cdot \\ \cdot \\ (\bar{e}, \bar{c})_{\Gamma_j} \Rightarrow u^P_{\Gamma_j} \end{cases} \quad (8.19)$$

where $j = 1, 2, \ldots, J$. Notice that a single vector $(\bar{e}, \bar{c})$ may be associated with several different control values, $u^1_{\Gamma_j}, u^2_{\Gamma_j}, \ldots, u^P_{\Gamma_j}$. A data group Γ_j, $j = 1, 2, \ldots, J$, is said to be in conflict if $P \neq 1$. We need to solve this conflict problem and it is referred to as conflict resolution.

A simple and reasonable method for solution is to take the average of $u^1_{\Gamma_j}, u^2_{\Gamma_j}, \ldots, u^P_{\Gamma_j}$ as their typical value provided that the properties possessed by these data are not taken into consideration, that is

$$u_{\Gamma_j} = \frac{1}{P} \sum_{p=1}^{P} u^p_{\Gamma_j}. \quad (8.20)$$

However, by observing and inspecting the error response subject to the step command signal, we can conclude that the conflict is most likely to occur at both the beginning of the transient response stage and at the steady-state stage. Two reasons for this can be given. The pure time delay h in control possessed by the controlled process is responsible for the former due to the fact that the error and change-in-error remain unchanged in the time interval $[0, hT_s]$, although the control action in $[0, hT_s]$ may take different values during the learning phase. In contrast, the discrete property of $\bar{E}$ and $\bar{C}$ and continuous characteristic of $\bar{U}$ cause conflict during the steady state. It is evident that the average scheme is suitable for handling the latter situation because control action $u_{\Gamma_j}^p$ during steady state can be viewed as some fluctuation above the average. However, the transient performance of the output will be degraded if this scheme is applied to the former case. An alternative method is to exclude $u(0), u(1), \ldots, u(h)$ from the data set (8.15) and to use them directly as a set of initial control values when the fuzzy control algorithm is applied.

8.4.4 Rule-base formation

Now, after the conflict resolution process, we obtain J distinct data pairs:

$$\begin{cases} \Gamma_1 : (\bar{e}_{\Gamma_1}, \bar{c}_{\Gamma_1}) \Rightarrow u_{\Gamma_1} \\ \Gamma_2 : (\bar{e}_{\Gamma_2}, \bar{c}_{\Gamma_2}) \Rightarrow u_{\Gamma_2} \\ \vdots \\ \Gamma_J : (\bar{e}_{\Gamma_J}, \bar{c}_{\Gamma_J}) \Rightarrow u_{\Gamma_J} \end{cases} \quad (8.21)$$

Note that $u_{\Gamma_j}, j = 1, 2, \ldots, J$, need not be distinct. If we assign some appropriate fuzzy sets predefined over $\bar{E}$ and $\bar{C}$ to $\bar{e}_{\Gamma_1}$ and $\bar{c}_{\Gamma_1}$, with $\bar{e}_{\Gamma_1}$ and $\bar{c}_{\Gamma_1}$ being corresponding central values, then the above data pairs can be thought of as a set of control rules with the understanding that the half-width $\delta_j^e(\delta_j^c)$ is embedded implicitly.

Thus we obtain J control rules denoted as follows:

$$\begin{cases} R_1 : \text{IF } (\bar{e}_{\Gamma_1}^*, \bar{c}_{\Gamma_1}^*) \text{ THEN } u_{\Gamma_1} \\ R_2 : \text{IF } (\bar{e}_{\Gamma_2}^*, \bar{c}_{\Gamma_2}^*) \text{ THEN } u_{\Gamma_2} \\ \vdots \\ R_J : \text{IF } (\bar{e}_{\Gamma_J}^*, \bar{c}_{\Gamma_J}^*) \text{ THEN } u_{\Gamma_J} \end{cases} \quad (8.22)$$

where the symbol * is added to emphasize that $\bar{e}^*$ and $\bar{c}^*$ are fuzzy sets.

Notice that the present J control rules are derived from either a positive or negative step command input. If it is assumed that the process being controlled has a skew symmetric input–output property about an operating point, that is, if the following equation is satisfied

$$f(\hat{u} + \Delta u) - f(\hat{u}) = f(\hat{u}) - f(\hat{u} - \Delta u) \tag{8.23}$$

where $f(\cdot)$ denotes the process input–output function, $f(\hat{u})$ is the operating point and $\Delta u \in [u_{\min}, u_{\max}]$ is an increment around $\hat{u}$, then it is expected that, in accordance with an opposite sign step input, a set of data pairs having the same absolute values as in (8.18) but with opposite signs would be obtained. Taking into account the symmetric property of $\bar{E}$ and $\bar{C}$ and the assumption about the process made above, we derive another set of rules given by

$$\tilde{R}_j : \text{IF } (-\bar{e}^*_{\Gamma_j}, -\bar{c}^*_{\Gamma_j}) \text{ THEN } -u_{\Gamma_j} \tag{8.24}$$

for $j = 1, 2, \ldots, J$.

Therefore, corresponding to the positive and negative step commands, two sets of rules are built into the rule-base with the number of rules being $2J$.

8.4.5 Rule-base verification

The rule-base constructed following the procedures presented above must be verified to make sure that it is trustworthy. There are a number of specifications employed to evaluate its quality. Here some of them are discussed.

8.4.5.1 Completeness

Completeness means that there always exists at least one rule which will be fired for any possible input data, implying that rules should be well distributed on the rule plane $\bar{E} \times \bar{C}$. In particular, given any input pattern $(\bar{e}_I, \bar{c}_I) \in \bar{E} \times \bar{C}$, there must exist at least one rule pattern, say $(\bar{e}^*_k, \bar{c}^*_k) \in \bar{E} \times \bar{C}$, in the rule-base with which the matching degree between those two patterns is more than zero, i.e. $0 < s_k \leq 1$. This requirement is of potential importance for an algorithm-based fuzzy controller because non-completeness of the rule-base may result in a situation in which no control action is taken during some control cycles. However, it should be emphasized that completeness for a fuzzy rule-base does not mean that there must exist a rule for all possible combinations of fuzzy sets defined over $\bar{E}$ and $\bar{C}$.

8.4.5.2 Correctness

This requirement mainly involves the THEN part of the rule. It is guaranteed by the fact that the control action (THEN part) is derived by learning and is considered to be correct.

8.4.5.3 Consistency

The conflict resolution procedure discussed earlier ensures that inconsistent data pairs are excluded from the constructed rule-base. Unlike non-fuzzy reasoning systems, in our case it is allowed that one input pattern should fire several rules at the same time and this situation is not regarded as being inconsistent.

8.4.5.4 Complexity

Here complexity simply refers to the number of rules in the rule-base. It depends primarily upon the definition of the universes of discourse $\bar{E}$ and $\bar{C}$, more specifically upon the cardinalities of $\bar{E}$ and $\bar{C}$, i.e. $2N+1$ and $2M+1$ respectively. The larger $N(M)$ is, the larger the rule-base size and hence more complicated the rule-base. In addition, the rule number is affected by the transient performance specified during the learning stage. The learning mechanism with different requirements will produce different data sets which are the basis for building the rule-base. For example, more rules will be created if the overshoot index is larger because in this case more rule patterns have to be excited in the rule plane.

8.4.5.5 Reproducibility

Recall that, in the learning stage, the system performance specified by the reference models are the objectives for the learning system to achieve. The term reproducibility is used to indicate the capacity of the learned rule-based fuzzy controller to reproduce this performance. This ability depends not only on the rule-base, but also on the fuzzy control algorithm employed.

8.5 Application to blood pressure control

The problem of simultaneous regulation of blood pressure (more specifically, mean arterial pressure (MAP)) and cardiac output (CO) has been studied using the proposed method. Before presenting the simulation results using the model given in Chapter 7, the performance measures are defined next.

8.5.1 Performance assessment

The results of the learning control and the fuzzy control can be evaluated in a number of ways. Besides directly inspecting the output response curves, this chapter defines some numerical measures used to assess the performance.

First, we define the following errors.

$$\varepsilon_d = SP - y_d$$
$$\varepsilon_f = SP - y_f \qquad (8.25)$$
$$\varepsilon_l^k = SP - y_l^k$$

where y_d, y_f and y_l^k denote the desired, the fuzzy controlled and the kth learned process output responses, with y being referred to either y_{CO} or y_{MAP}. Notice that, by the definition, $\varepsilon_f = \bar{e}_m$, the measured control error, and $\varepsilon_l^k - \varepsilon_d = e$, the learning error.

Secondly, two frequently used error integral criteria are defined as

$$\text{ISE} = \int_0^\infty \varepsilon^2(t)\,dt$$
$$\text{ITAE} = \int_0^\infty t \cdot |\varepsilon(t)|\,dt \qquad (8.26)$$

where ε can be one of the errors defined in (8.25).

Finally, denoting

$$\Phi_d = \{\text{ISE}_{COd}, \text{ITAE}_{COd}, \text{ISE}_{MAPd}, \text{ITAE}_{MAPd}\}$$
$$\Phi_f = \{\text{ISE}_{COf}, \text{ITAE}_{COf}, \text{ISE}_{MAPf}, \text{ITAE}_{MAPf}\} \qquad (8.27)$$
$$\Phi_l^k = \{\text{ISE}_{COl}^k, \text{ITAE}_{COl}^k, \text{ISE}_{MAPl}^k, \text{ITAE}_{MAPl}^k\}$$

where Φ_d, Φ_f, and Φ_l^k denote the desired, the fuzzy controlled and the kth learned indices, the following performance measures are defined:

(1) Absolute and relative differences between the learned and the desired performances (AD and RD)

$$AD_i^k = |\phi_{li}^k - \phi_{di}^k|$$
$$RD_i^k = \frac{|\phi_{li}^k - \phi_{di}^k|}{\phi_{di}^k} \qquad (8.28)$$

where $i = 1,2,3,4$, $\phi_{li}^k \in \Phi_l^k$, and $\phi_{di} \in \Phi_d$.

AD and RD are primarily used to compare the learning speed in terms of the performance errors when the different learning gains, initial controls and learning algorithms are performed.

(2) Performance improvement factor (*IP*)

$$IP_i^k = 1 - \frac{|\phi_{di} - \phi_{li}^k|}{|\phi_{di} - \phi_{li}^1|} \qquad (8.29)$$

where $i = 1, 2, 3, 4$, $\phi_{li}^k \in \Phi_l^k$, $\phi_{di} \in \Phi_d$, and $\phi_{li}^1 \in \Phi_l^1$ is the index produced at the first iteration.

IP is employed to measure the learning ability with respect to a variety of situations such as the change of process parameters and the change of the desired responses.

(3) The relative difference between the rule-based fuzzy controlled and the learned responses (*FRD*).

$$FRD_i = \frac{|\phi_{li}^k - \phi_{fi}|}{\phi_{li}^k} \qquad (8.30)$$

where $i = 1, 2, 3, 4$, $\phi_{fi} \in \Phi_f$ and $\phi_{li}^k \in \Phi_l^k$ with k being the iteration number at which the rule-base is constructed.

FRD is adopted to assess the reproducibility of the fuzzy controller in which the rule-base is built from the *k*th learned control actions.

8.5.2 Simulation results

The situations concerned in this simulation study are divided into three main groups. The first group of simulations is aimed at testing the adaptability of the learning algorithm with respect to the variation of the desired response, the process parameters, and a noisy environment, whereas the intention of the second group is to investigate how the convergency rate of the learning system is affected by the learning gains, initial control actions and different learning update laws. Along with all simulation cases, reproducibility of the resultant algorithm-based fuzzy control system in terms of the control performances is evaluated. The purpose of the last group of simulations is to examine the performance of the network-based controller.

Basically, the computational process consists of three main steps: applying the learning algorithm, constructing rule-bases, and operating the fuzzy control system by using the derived rule-bases. However, when the network-based controller is used, the network must be trained using the rule-bases before on-line operation.

The following values are used throughout the simulations:

- sampling period $T_s = 30$ s,
- learning interval $L = 100$,
- maximum iteration number $K = 15$,
- initial condition $y_{CO}^k(0) = y_{MAP}^k(0) = 0$,
- normal value of CO: $CO_0 = 100$ ml s^{-1},
- normal value of MAP: $MAP_0 = 120$ mmHg,
- set-point for CO: $SP_{CO} = 20$ ml s^{-1},
- set-point for MAP: $SP_{MAP} = -10$ mmHg,
- time delay in the reference model: $\tau_{CO} = \tau_{MAP} = 3T_s$.

In addition, it is assumed that the rule-base is constructed based on the data obtained at the tenth iteration, and that CO/DOP and MAP/SNP are paired, comprising two control loops.

8.5.2.1 Learning ability/reproducibility

Throughout this group of simulations, the following is assumed: only the error correction learning law is used; initial control actions u_{CO}^0, u_{MAP}^0 are set to zero; the estimated time delay number μ in the learning law is chosen to be 5; and the learning gains are set to $g_1 = 0.06$ and $g_2 = -0.07$.

(1) *The second-order specifications.* When the desired responses are specified by the second-order reference models, three cases were considered:

$$\begin{aligned}
\xi_{CO} &= 0.8 \quad t_{sCO} = 240 \text{ s} \quad \xi_{MAP} = 0.8 \quad t_{sMAP} = 240 \text{ s} \\
\xi_{CO} &= 0.9 \quad t_{sCO} = 240 \text{ s} \quad \xi_{MAP} = 0.7 \quad t_{sMAP} = 300 \text{ s} \\
\xi_{CO} &= 0.7 \quad t_{sCO} = 300 \text{ s} \quad \xi_{MAP} = 0.8 \quad t_{sMAP} = 240 \text{ s}
\end{aligned} \quad (8.31)$$

where t_s denotes the settling time. It is noted that flexible transient responses can be experienced by selecting the values of ξ and $t_s(\omega_n)$. Small ξ will result in a faster rise time and a larger overshoot. A good selection of ξ is about 0.7.

By taking the parameters mentioned above, three sets of simulations were performed. Figure 8.3 shows one of the results corresponding to the first case. The desired, learned (at the 1st, 5th and 10th iterations) and fuzzy controlled y_{CO} and y_{MAP} are displayed in the figure. It can be seen that the learned response asymptotically approached the desired one with increase of the iteration number. Interaction effects within the two control loops are well handled by the learned individual control actions u_{DOP} and u_{SNP} which are also illustrated in Figure 8.3.

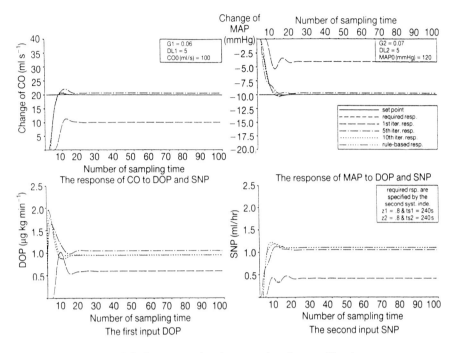

Figure 8.3 *Responses for the second-order specifications.*

Learning ability is also demonstrated in Figure 8.4 by the fact that the improvement factors (here only the results corresponding to *CO* are given) under different desired specifications approach unity after a few iterations. It can be seen from the figures that the transient responses (indicated by ISE) improved more quickly than the steady-state responses (indicated by ITAE). However, after a few iterations not much improvement in the transient responses took place, while the steady-state responses were improved further.

Reproducibility of the resultant fuzzy controller can be verified by comparing the learned response at the 10th iteration with the fuzzy controlled response in Figure 8.3. The relative differences in FRD_i defined in the last subsection corresponding to Figure 8.3 are presented in Table 8.1 where small values imply that a higher accuracy is possessed by the constructed rule-bases with respect to the learned control actions. The number of rules for loop 1 and loop 2 with the iteration number are shown in Table 8.2. It can be seen that the number of rules remained stable after about seven iterations.

(2) *Variation of process parameters.* In order to investigate the adaptability of the learning system with respect to the different process parameters, process gains and time constants were changed from their typical values by

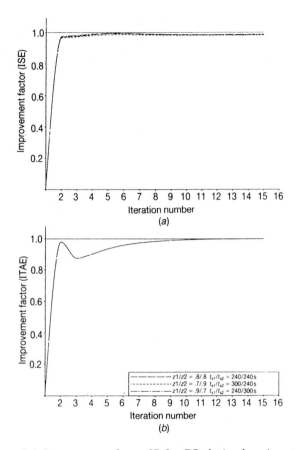

Figure 8.4 *Improvement factor IP for CO during learning stage.*

up to 20% increase or decrease. Here again, the learning gains were the same as before, i.e. $g_1 = 0.06$ and $g_2 = -0.07$. In addition, the desired responses were specified by the second-order models with $\xi_{CO} = \xi_{MAP} = 0.8$ and $t_{sCO} = t_{sMAP} = 240$. Although simulations for all of the gains and the time constants were performed, we show only one of them for illustration. Figure 8.5 shows the process outputs and inputs when gain k_{22} increased by 20% from its typical value. It appears that the learning system is capable of tracking the desired responses in spite of large variations of the process parameters. By comparing the results, we find that all the output responses with different process parameters are similar to each other but the learned control actions are substantially different implying that the learning scheme is very efficient at dealing with different processes.

The results of the fuzzy control indicated in Figure 8.5 once again demonstrate that the rule-based controller established from the learning

Table 8.1 *Reproducibility of fuzzy controller measured by FRD*

Fig. No.	$FRD_1 \times 100$	$FRD_2 \times 100$	$FRD_3 \times 100$	$FRD_4 \times 100$
Figure 8.3	0.00	1.73	0.00	0.44
Figure 8.5	0.50	1.75	0.00	0.11
†	0.05	5.17	0.16	1.07
‡	0.00	1.74	0.25	0.47

†change of k_{11}.
‡change of T_2.

Table 8.2 *Rule numbers in rule-base 1 and 2*

Loop number	Iteration number										Corresponding Fig. No.
	1	2	3	4	5	6	7	8	9	10	
1	14	20	24	24	18	16	16	16	16	16	Figure 8.3
2	20	26	18	12	12	12	10	12	12	14	
Sum	34	46	42	36	30	28	26	28	28	30	
1	14	22	24	20	16	14	16	16	16	16	Figure 8.5
2	24	32	14	12	12	12	12	12	12	14	
Sum	38	54	38	32	28	26	28	28	28	30	
1	14	22	22	18	16	16	16	16	16	16	†
2	18	30	14	10	10	10	12	12	12	12	
Sum	32	52	36	28	26	26	28	28	28	28	
1	16	20	24	24	20	16	16	16	14	14	‡
2	18	22	16	14	14	12	12	12	12	12	
Sum	34	42	40	38	34	28	28	28	26	26	

†change of k_{11}.
‡change of T_2.

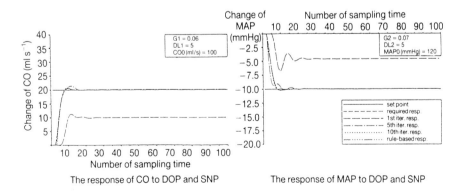

Figure 8.5 *Responses of the learning and fuzzy control with the process gain changed.*

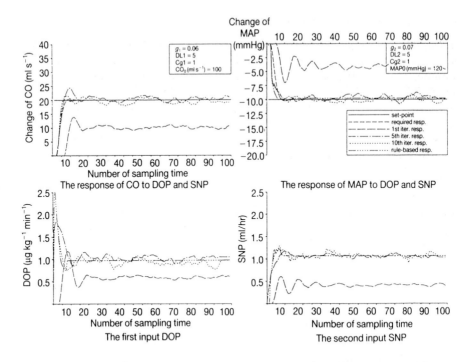

Figure 8.6 *Responses of learning and fuzzy control with noisy learning signals.*

system is capable of producing a performance as good as the learning system. *FRD* measures and rule numbers created corresponding to Figure 8.5 (the change of k_{22}), to the change of k_{11}, and to the change of T_2 are presented in Tables 8.1 and 8.2 respectively.

(3) *Noisy environment.* Finally, we examine the effects caused by noise-contaminated data. Intuitively, the learning performance will be degraded to some extent if the measured outputs, and hence the learning errors, are heavily contaminated by noise. A uniformly distributed noise signal with zero mean value and an amplitude of 5% about the set-point was added to the outputs y^k_{CO} and y^k_{MAP}. Figure 8.6 shows the simulation result. It can be seen that convergence to the desired response within a small deviation was achieved despite the presence of the noisy learning signals.

Note that we deliberately let the outputs of the fuzzy controller be noise-free in order to display the ability of the proposed method to build the rule-base in a noisy environment. Although the learned control signals fluctuated in the steady-state, the fuzzy control signal remained constant. This is due to the conflict resolution procedure involved during the rule formation stage which ensures that not too many rules are extracted. In fact, 18 and 16 rules were obtained for two loops in this case, which are only slightly more than those in the noise-free case.

8.5.2.2 Learning speed/reproducibility

This group of studies attempted to explore this issue by means of numerical simulations. Here the learning speed is defined as the required iteration number at which the desired performance measured by AD and RD defined in (8.28) is achieved. In general, there are three factors affecting the learning speed, namely, learning gains, initial control actions and learning update laws. In what follows, no detailed comments on reproducibility will be made because a number of simulations have suggested that this ability can almost always be ensured.

(1) *Learning gains.* Learning gains are perhaps the main factors in determining the learning speed. Assume that the desired responses are specified by second-order models with $\xi_{CO} = \xi_{MAP} = 0.8$ and $t_{sCO} = t_{sMAP} = 240$ and the error correction update law is used. The following three gain sets were chosen for the simulations:

$$g_1 = 0.06 \quad g_2 = -0.07$$
$$g_1 = 0.04 \quad g_2 = -0.05$$
$$g_1 = 0.08 \quad g_2 = -0.09.$$

For the purpose of a clear comparison, Figure 8.7 shows only a detailed version of the performance measures AD against the iteration number, starting from the third iteration. Note that the three curves are comparable because they are, by definition, either absolute (for ITAE) or relative (for ISE) differences with respect to the same quantity, desired ITAE or ISE. As expected, larger gains result in a steeper curve indicating a faster convergence speed in terms of performance measures. For instance, convergence takes place more quickly in the case of $g_1 = 0.08$, $g_2 = -0.09$ than that for $g_1 = 0.04$, $g_2 = -0.05$.

(2) *Initial control actions.* Since, during the learning process, there is no apparent basis for setting the values of initial control $u_{DOP}^0(i)$ and $u_{SNP}^0(i)$, $i = 1, 2, \ldots, L$, they were simply set to zero in all the simulations undertaken. Obviously, reasonable initial control values may bring the learning process to convergency more rapidly. First, a simple rule-base derived from common control knowledge as adopted in Chapter 7 was used to produce two sets of initial control $u_{DOP}^0(i)$ and $u_{SNP}^0(i)$. Afterwards, the same learning procedures as used before were applied. By choosing two different scaling factors in producing the initial control, two sets of results were obtained. The results have indicated that a faster convergency speed could be achieved if initial control values were appropriately chosen. This can be seen clearly by inspecting AD or RD curves as shown in Figure 8.8. Here only a detailed version of ITAE is presented. AD measures of the non-zero initial control approach zero much more quickly than those of zero

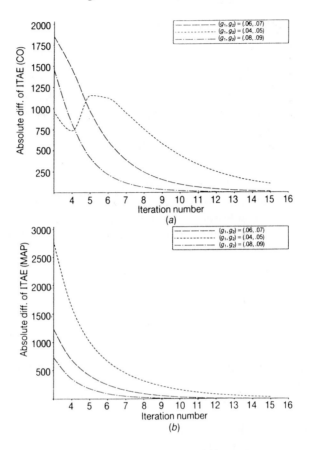

Figure 8.7 *Detailed version of AD with different learning gains.*

initial control, suggesting that fewer iterations are needed in the former case.

(3) *Different update laws.* The above simulations involve only the error correction update law in which the control update in each loop is based only on the learning error produced by its own loop. We note that it is not easy to compare directly the learning speed within three schemes in a meaningful way because of the difficulty arising from determining the learning gains to be used for comparisons. It makes sense only if the comparisons are made under the condition that optimal gains for each algorithm are employed. Here rather than seeking the optimal gains, we simply make a comparison in the sense of the contributed correcting proportion of one loop's error to the other part (change-in-error of one loop or the other loop's error). *AD* performance measures are shown in Figure 8.9, where the three curves correspond to Figure 8.3 (proportions of 1 to 0), to the case of proportions

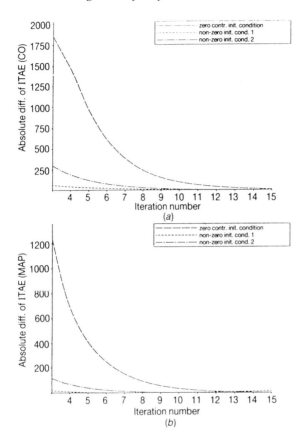

Figure 8.8 *Detailed performance measures AD with non-zero initial control.*

of 0.8 to 0.2 in the change-in-error algorithm, and to that of proportions of 0.8 to 0.2 in the error-cross correction algorithm. We see that the convergence speeds of both the cross-error and the change-in-error correction algorithms are slower than that of the error correction algorithm. It should be emphasized that it is not clear whether this statement can be applied generally. However, it seems that a faster speed is achieved in the cross-error algorithm than in the change-in-error correction algorithm.

8.5.2.3 Results on the network-based controller

The aim of the simulation is to examine the control performances of the BNN-based fuzzy controller which is built on the basis of the learned rules. Instead of using two separate control loops for two controlled variables CO and MAP as adopted in the algorithm-based case, here only one BNN was used, meaning that a centralized controller was employed. Accordingly, the

260   Intelligent Control in Biomedicine

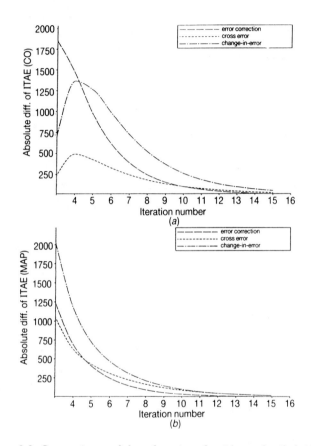

Figure 8.9 *Comparisons of three learning algorithms: detailed AD.*

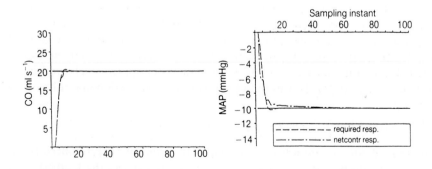

Figure 8.10 *Outputs of the process with BNN-based controller.*

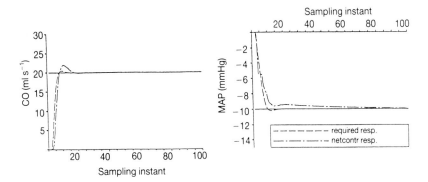

Figure 8.11 *Outputs of the process with BNN-based controller: the process delay changed.*

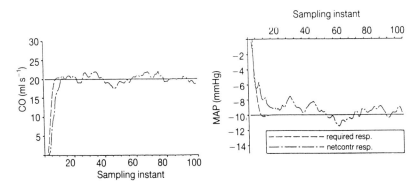

Figure 8.12 *Outputs of the process with BNN-based controller in a noisy environment.*

BNN had four input units (errors and change-in-errors for *CO* and *MAP*) and two output units (DOP and SNP). One hidden layer was used with 15 hidden units. The output units were linear whereas the hidden units were non-linear with sigmoid functions. After learning and extracting, the network was trained using derived rules as input and output samples and the standard back-propagation training algorithm (Rumelhart *et al.*, 1986) was adopted.

By setting parameters ξ_{CO}, ξ_{MAP}, t_{CO}, and t_{MAP} in the reference models to be 0.8, 0.8, 240, and 240 respectively, nine rules were obtained, where the error correction update law was employed with learning gains being 0.06 and -0.07. After the training stage was completed, the BNN-based controller was operated on-line. Figure 8.10 shows the desired and actual output responses of the process with actual responses being obtained by using the trained network. It can be seen that the network-based controller is able to reproduce similar control performance to that produced during the learning procedure. By comparing Figures 8.10 and 8.3, we conclude that similar performances can be achieved despite very different controller paradigms being involved. To examine the robust capability of the trained controller with respect to variations of the process parameters during the operational stage, we carried out a set of simulations using the above trained network but with different process parameters. Figure 8.11 shows one of the results, where the process pure time-delay τ_1 was changed from 60 to 90 seconds. The controller was also operated in a noisy environment as shown in Figure 8.12. The results indicate that the BNN-based controller possesses certain robustness or generalization properties with respect to some novel situations.

8.6 Conclusions

We have presented a methodology that is capable of learning and extracting rules automatically from the controlled environment for use with either algorithm-based or network-based fuzzy controllers. The proposed system has been applied to the problem of multivariable control of blood pressure which is characterized by strong interactions and pure time-delays in controls. A variety of simulation studies have revealed that the blood pressure system can be controlled satisfactorily and that the proposed method is feasible. Some important conclusions can be drawn from the simulation studies. For example, the desired transient requirement for each controlled variable can be specified separately; the learning system possesses a high adaptability with respect to various operating conditions such as variations of the desired response and the process parameters; the reproducibility of the rule-based fuzzy control can almost always be guaranteed; and the learning system is relatively robust with respect to variations in the estimated time-delay and noisy measurement data.

References

Arimoto, S., 1990, Learning control theory for robotic motion, *International Journal of Adaptive Control and Signal Processing*, **4**, 543–64.
Daley, S. and Gill, K.F., 1986, A design study of a self-organizing fuzzy logic controller, *Proceedings of the Institution of Mechanical Engineers*, **200**, 59–69.
Lee, C.C., 1990, Fuzzy logic in control systems: fuzzy logic controller. Part 1 and Part 2, *IEEE Transactions on Systems, Man, and Cybernetics*, **20**, 404–35.
Linkens, D.A. and Abbod, M.F., 1992, Self-organizing fuzzy logic control and the selection of its scaling factors, *Transactions of the Institute of MC*, **14**, 114–25.
Linkens, D.A. and Nie, J., 1993a, Constructing rule-bases for multivariable fuzzy control by self-learning. Part 1: system structure and learning algorithms, *International Journal of System Science*, **24**, 111–27.

Nie, J. and Linkens, D.A., 1992, Neural network-based approximate reasoning: principles and implementation, *International Journal of Control*, **56**, 399–414.

Pedrycz, W., 1985, 'Design of fuzzy control algorithms with the aid of fuzzy model', in Sugeno, M. (Ed.) *Industrial Applications of Fuzzy Control*, Amsterdam: North-Holland.

Procyk, T.J. and Mamdani, E.H., 1979, A linguistic self-organizing process controller, *Automatica*, **15**, 15–30.

Rumelhart, D., Hinton, G.E. and Williams, R.J., 1986, 'Learning internal representation by error propagation', in Rumelhart, D.E. and McClelland, J.L. (Eds) *Parallel Distributed Processing*, Vol. 1, Cambridge, MA: MIT Press.

Scharf, E.M. and Mandic, N.J., 1985, 'The application of a fuzzy controller to the control of a multi-degree-freedom robot arm', in Sugeno, M. (Ed.), *Industrial Applications of Fuzzy Control*, Amsterdam: North-Holland.

Shao, S., 1988, Fuzzy self-organizing controller and its application for dynamic processes, *Fuzzy Sets and Systems*, **26**, 151–64.

Sugeno, M. (Ed.), 1985, *Industrial Applications of Fuzzy Control*, Amsterdam: North-Holland.

Takagi, T. and Sugeno, M., 1985, Fuzzy identification of systems and its application to modeling and control, *IEEE Transactions on Systems, Man, and Cybernetics*, **15**, 116–32.

Chapter 9
Self-organizing fuzzy-neural control for blood pressure management

Junhong Nie

9.1 Introduction

While the method of combining neural networks with fuzzy control described in the last chapter focused primarily on the functional mapping between an approximate reasoning algorithm and a neural network approach, this chapter is concerned mainly with the structural mapping between those two paradigms. However, the basic issues we address remain the same regardless of the methods adopted, that is, rule-base acquisition, computational representation, and approximate reasoning. The objective is to deal with these issues under a unified framework of neural networks in such a way that the rule-base can be constructed automatically, also the fuzzy reasoning mechanism can be implemented easily, and the required prior knowledge about the controlled environment should be as little as possible. We present here a novel approach capable of fulfilling the objectives specified above. In particular, we describe a simple and efficient scheme capable of self-organizing and self-learning the required control knowledge in a real-time manner under multivariable controlled environments. The starting point of the approach is to structurally map a simplified fuzzy control algorithm (SFCA) (Nie, 1987, 1989) into a counter-propagation network (CPN) as developed by Hecht-Nielsen (1987, 1988, 1990). The CPN is of a very simple structure, but is often overlooked, and is used here in such a way that the control knowledge is explicitly represented in the form of connection weights of the nets. Then, by introducing a valid radius into the Kohonen layer and providing an on-line learning teacher to the Grossberg layer, the control rule-base, initially empty, is gradually self-organized and self-constructed to achieve fulfilment of the prespecified performance requirements. Finally, the approximate reasoning is carried out by replacing a winner-take-all competitive scheme with a soft matching cooperative strategy.

The next section introduces a simplified fuzzy control algorithm suitable for sensor data-base control environments. Section 9.3 is devoted to mapping the fuzzy control algorithm to the CPN network relevant to the issues of representation and reasoning. The underlying principles concerning self-organizing and self-learning are described in Section 9.4. As a demonstration example, a problem of multivariable control of blood pressure is studied in Section 9.5 and the chapter ends with some concluding remarks in Section 9.6.

9.2 Simplified fuzzy control algorithms (SFCA)

The operation of a fuzzy controller typically involves the following main stages within one sampling instant: sampling the measured inputs, fuzzifying the non-fuzzy inputs into fuzzy sets, inferencing the current controller fuzzy outputs, and finally defuzzifying the inferred fuzzy outputs into non-fuzzy values and sending them to the process being controlled. Among these, the reasoning stage usually comprises three further substages, namely, computing the matching degrees between the current fuzzy inputs with respect to each rule's IF part, determining which rules should be fired, and combining these fired rules' THEN parts with different strengths into final fuzzy sets. It can be observed that it is the incompatible property of the numerical (or non-fuzzy) control environment with the linguistic (or fuzzy) reasoning algorithm that makes the operation complex in terms of requiring two interfaces to connect the external non-fuzzy environment with a fuzzy inference engine which is developed normally within a fuzzy environment. In our view, it is possible to simplify the above process by taking the non-fuzzy property regarding the input/output of the fuzzy controller into account. We have derived a very simple but efficient MISO fuzzy control algorithm SFCA which consists of only two main steps, pattern matching and weighted averaging, thereby eliminating the necessity for fuzzifying and defuzzifying procedures (Nie, 1987, 1989). The basic idea is to make the approximate reasoning strategy usually derived for linguistic variables suitable directly for use with numerical variables by introducing notions of pattern and pattern matching. The algorithm can be extended to the MIMO case in a straightforward way and is described below.

INPUT AND OUTPUT
Assume that the controlled process is multivariable with m inputs and m outputs. The inputs to the fuzzy controller are various combinations of

Self-organizing fuzzy-neural control for blood pressure management

control error, change-in-error, and sum of error. Suppose that the measured control error at time lT_s with T_s sampling period is denoted as $e_{c1}(lT_s)$, $e_{c2}(lT_s)$, ..., $e_{cm}(lT_s)$ corresponding to m process outputs, i.e. $e_{ci}(lT_s) = r_i(lT_s) - y_{p,i}(lT_s)$, where r, $y_p \in R^m$ are set-point and process output vectors respectively. Each $e_c(lT_s)$ is extended into three elements: $e_c(lT_s)$, $c_c(lT_s)$, and $s_c(lT_s)$, where

$$c_c(lT_s) = e_c(lT_s) - e_c((l-1)T_s) \qquad (9.1)$$

is the change-in-error and

$$s_c(lT_s) = \sum_{i=1}^{l} e_c(iT_s) \qquad (9.2)$$

is the sum of error. Thus in light of different combinations, three possible controller input modes can be constructed, i.e.

(a) input variables: $e_{c1}, c_{c1}, e_{c2}, c_{c2}, \ldots, e_{cm}, c_{cm}$
(b) input variables: $e_{c1}, s_{c1}, e_{c2}, s_{c2}, \ldots, e_{cm}, s_{cm}$
(c) input variables: $e_{c1}, c_{c1}, s_{c1}, e_{c2}, c_{c2}, s_{c2}, \ldots, e_{cm}, c_{cm}, s_{cm}$.

We refer to the input types (a), (b) and (c) as EC, ES, and ECS respectively, In what follows, it is assumed that the controller mode is one of these types and is composed of n variables, each of which is denoted by u_i. The output of the fuzzy controller consists of m variables, each of which is denoted by v_k. Thus, an $n \times m$ controller is used to control an $m \times m$ process with $n > m$ in general.

RULE PATTERN AND INPUT PATTERN

Assume that there are P rules in the rule-base, each of which has the form:

IF U_1 is A_1^j AND U_2 is A_2^j AND ... AND U_n is A_n^j
THEN V_1 is B_1^j AND V_2 is B_2^j AND ..., AND V_m is B_m^j

where U_i and V_k are linguistic variables corresponding to the numerical variables u_i and v_k, A_i^j and B_k^j are fuzzy subsets representing some linguistic terms and defined on the corresponding universes of discourse $\bar{U}_i$ and $\bar{V}_k$ which are assumed to be compact on R. Fuzzy subsets A_i^j and B_k^j are characterized by the corresponding membership functions $A_i^j(u_i): \bar{U}_i \to [0, 1]$, and $B_k^j(v_k): \bar{V}_k \to [0, 1]$. More precisely, let A_i^j and B_k^j be normalized fuzzy subsets whose membership functions are defined uniquely as

$$A_i^j(u_i) = \begin{cases} 1 - \left[\dfrac{|M_{u,i}^j - u_i|}{\delta_{u,i}^j}\right] & \text{if } |M_{u,i}^j - u_i| \leq \delta_{u,i}^j \\ 0 & \text{if } |M_{u,i}^j - u_i| > \delta_{u,i}^j \end{cases} \quad (9.3)$$

$$A_i^j(v_i) = \begin{cases} 1 - \left[\dfrac{|M_{v,i}^j - v_i|}{\delta_{v,i}^j}\right] & \text{if } |M_{v,i}^j - v_i| \leq \delta_{v,i}^j \\ 0 & \text{if } |M_{v,i}^j - v_i| > \delta_{v,i}^j \end{cases} \quad (9.4)$$

where $M_{u,i}^j \in \bar{U}_i$, $M_{v,k}^j \in \bar{V}_k$, $\delta_{u,i}^j > 0$, and $\delta_{v,k}^j > 0$.

Observe that each of the membership functions in (9.3) and (9.4) is characterized only by two parameters, $M_{u,i}^j$ and $\delta_{u,i}^j$, or $M_{v,k}^j$ and $\delta_{v,k}^j$ with the understanding that $M_{u,i}^j (M_{v,k}^j)$ is the centre element of the support set of $A_i^j(B_k^j)$, and $\delta_{u,i}^j(\delta_{v,k}^j)$ is the half-width of the support set. Hence A_i^j and B_k^j may be expressed as

$$A_{u,i}^j = (M_{u,i}^j, \delta_{u,i}^j) \quad B_{v,k}^j = (M_{v,k}^j, \delta_{v,k}^j). \quad (9.5)$$

By using the above notation, the jth rule can be written as

IF $(M_{u,1}^j, \delta_{u,1}^j)$ AND $(M_{u,2}^j, \delta_{u,2}^j)$ AND ... AND $(M_{u,n}^j, \delta_{u,n}^j)$
THEN $(M_{v,1}^j, \delta_{v,1}^j)$ AND $(M_{v,2}^j, \delta_{v,2}^j)$ AND ... AND $(M_{v,m}^j, \delta_{v,m}^j)$.

In the rest of this section and the next subsection, we will focus on the IF part of the above rule, and leave the THEN part to be treated later on. Let input space $\Omega = (\bar{U}_1 \times \bar{U}_2 \times \ldots \times \bar{U}_n) \in R^n$ be a compact product space, and $M_u^j = (M_{u,1}^j, M_{u,2}^j, \ldots, M_{u,n}^j) \in \Omega$ and $\Delta_u^j = (\delta_{u,1}^j, \delta_{u,2}^j, \ldots, \delta_{u,n}^j)$ be two n-dimensional vectors. Then the condition part of the jth rule may be viewed as creating a subspace $\Omega^j \in \Omega$ or a hypercube whose centre and radius are M_u^j and Δ_u^j respectively. Thus the *condition* part of the jth rule can be simplified further to 'IF $M\Delta_u(j)$', where $M\Delta_u(j) = (M_u^j, \Delta_u^j)$. Similarly n current inputs $u_{0i} \in \bar{U}_i (i = 1, 2, \ldots, n)$, with u_{0i} being a singleton, can also be represented as an n-dimensional vector u_0 in Ω.

It is helpful to view the IF part of a rule and a measured input as patterns to be called a rule pattern and an input pattern respectively. Geometrically, a rule pattern can be visualized as consisting of a set of points (vectors) centred at M_u^j with a neighbourhood defined by Δ_u^j with constraints imposed by the corresponding membership grades. P rule patterns partition Ω into P subspaces which are typically overlapped to some degree along the boundaries due to the effect of fuzziness. On the other hand, a measured input is just a determined point situated in the same space as are the rule patterns.

The fuzzy control algorithm can be considered to be a process in which an appropriate control action is deduced from a current input and P rules according to some prespecified reasoning algorithms. We split the whole reasoning procedure into two phases: *pattern matching* and *weighted averaging*. The first operation deals with the IF part for all rules, whereas the second one involves an operation on the THEN part of the fired rules.

PATTERN MATCHING

From the pattern concept introduced above, we need to compute the matching degrees between the current input pattern, a point in Ω, and each rule pattern, a set of points in Ω. Because the two patterns are now formulated numerically in the same manner and are interpreted geometrically in the same space, it is straightforward to adopt some metrical concepts to measure the similarity of the two patterns. There are at least two approaches to performing this task, based on the notions of volume ratio or relative distance. For the sake of later use in this chapter, we present only the distance algorithm as follows.

Denote the current input by $u_0 = (u_{01}, u_{02}, \ldots, u_{0n})$. Then the matching degree denoted by $S^j \in [0, 1]$ between u_0 and the jth rule pattern $M\Delta_u(j)$ can be measured by the complement of the corresponding relative distance given by

$$S_j = 1 - D^j(u_0, M\Delta_u(j)) \tag{9.6}$$

where $D^j(u_0, M\Delta_u(j)) \in [0, 1]$ denotes relative distance from u_0 to $M\Delta_u(j)$. D^j can be specified in many ways and three computational definitions are given below.

Relative Euclidean distance:

$$D^j_E(u_0, M\Delta_u(j)) = \begin{cases} \dfrac{\|M^j_u - u_0\|}{\|\Delta^j_u\|} & \text{if } \|M^j_u - u_0\| \leq \|\Delta^j_u\| \\ 1 & \text{otherwise} \end{cases} \tag{9.7a}$$

where $\|\cdot\|$ denotes Euclidean norm.

Relative Hamming distance:

$$D^j_H(x_0, M\Delta_u(j)) = \begin{cases} \dfrac{\sum_{i=1}^{n} |M^j_{u,i} - u_0 i|}{\sum_{i=1}^{n} \delta^j_{u,i}} & \text{if } \sum_{i=1}^{n} |M^j_{u,i} - u_0 i| \leq \sum_{i=1}^{n} \delta^j_{u,i} \\ 1 & \text{otherwise} \end{cases} \tag{9.7b}$$

Relative maximum distance:

$$D^j{}_M(x_0, M\Delta_u(j)) = \begin{cases} \underset{1 \leq i \leq n}{\text{Max}} \left[\dfrac{|M^j_{u,i} - u_0 i|}{\delta^j_{u,i}} \right] & \text{if for all } i \, | M^j_{u,i} - u_0 i | \leq \delta^j_{u,i} \\ 1 & \text{otherwise} \end{cases} \quad (9.7c)$$

It is evident from (9.6) and (9.7) that if u_0 and $M\Delta_u(j)$ are fully matched, i.e. u_0 is exactly the same as the centre vector M^j_u, then $D^j = 0$, leading to the matching degree S^j being 1. On the other hand, if they are completely unmatched, i.e. u_0 is outside the boundary of $M\Delta_u(j)$ determined by the corresponding metric, then $D^j = 1$ and thus $S^j = 0$. Otherwise $0 < D^j < 1$ and $0 < S^j < 1$, indicating a partial matching.

WEIGHTED AVERAGING
Recall that under the unique definition of the membership function, each rule can be expressed as

IF $M\Delta_u(j)$ THEN $(M^j_{v,1}, \delta^j_{v,1})$ AND ... AND $(M^j_{v,m}, \delta^j_{v,m})$.

In what follows, we assume that $\delta^j_{v,k}$ are identical with respect to all k and j. Suppose that a current input pattern u_0 and a specific rule pattern j are given. If the matching degree $S^j = 1$, the deduced control values should be $v_k = M^j_{v,k}, k = 1, 2, \ldots, m$. This conclusion implies the utilization of the *maximum membership decision* scheme. However, it is also identical to the scheme referred to as centre of gravity (COG) if we notice that the membership functions are assumed to be symmetrical about their centres. If $S^j = 0$, on the other hand, the jth rule has no contribution to the final controller output. Otherwise, $0 < S^j < 1$ and there is more than one rule contributing to the control values.

Suppose that for a specific input u_0 and P rules, after the matching process is completed, there exist Q matching degrees satisfying $0 < S < 1$ and they are relabelled as $S^1, S^2, \ldots, S^Q$ with corresponding Q groups of centres of the THEN parts denoted by

$$\{M^1_{v,1}, M^1_{v,2}, \ldots, M^1_{v,m}\}.$$
$$\{M^2_{v,1}, M^2_{v,2}, \ldots, M^2_{v,m}\}$$
$$\vdots$$
$$\{M^Q_{v,1}, M^Q_{v,2}, \ldots, M^Q_{v,m}\}.$$

Self-organizing fuzzy-neural control for blood pressure management 271

Then the kth component of the deduced control action v_k is given by

$$v_k = \frac{\sum_{q=1}^{Q} S^q M_{v,k}^q}{\sum_{q=1}^{Q} S^q} = \sum_{q=1}^{q} \bar{S}^q M_{v,k}^q \qquad (9.8)$$

where

$$\bar{S}^q = \frac{S^q}{\sum_{q=1}^{Q} S^q}.$$

It can be seen that Equation 9.8 gives a weighted averaging value with respect to the fired rules' THEN parts. How large a percentage a specific rule contributes to the global value is determined by the corresponding matching degree. Because only the centres of the THEN parts of the fired rules are utilized and they are the only elements having the maximum membership grade 1 on the corresponding support sets, the algorithm can be understood as a modified maximum membership decision scheme in which the global centre is calculated by the COG algorithm. However, notice that compared with the traditional defuzzification COG algorithm where the centre is determined by all the elements in $\bar{V}_k$, here it is computed only by the local centres of Q fired rules. Because symmetrical membership functions with identical widths are assumed, the effect produced by omitting the width attached to the THEN part can be neglected, thereby suggesting that the algorithm (9.8) is justified, also the widths in the THEN parts can be removed from the original rules, and accordingly the rule form can be further simplified to

$$\text{IF } M\Delta_u(j) \text{ THEN } M_v^j \qquad (9.9)$$

where $M_v^j = [M_{v,1}^j, M_{v,2}^j, \ldots, M_{v,m}^j]$ is a centre value vector of the THEN part.

9.3 Representation and reasoning by CPN

9.3.1 CPN network

By combining a portion of the self-organizing map of Kohonen and the outstar structure of Grossberg, Hecht-Nielsen developed a new type of neural network named the counterpropagation network (CPN) (Hecht-Nielsen, 1987, 1988, 1990). Functionally, the CPN is designed to approximate a continuous function $f: A \in R^n \to R^m$, defined on a compact set A by means of a set of samples (μ^s, v^s) with μ^s vectors being randomly drawn from R^n in accordance with a fixed probability density function p. The trained CPN functions as a statistically optimal self-adapting look-up table. Possible applications of CPNs include pattern recognition, function approximation, statistical analysis, and data compression (see Hecht-Nielsen, 1988).

Figure 9.1 shows a schematic of the *forward-only* version of the CPN which will be used in this chapter. It consists of an input layer, a hidden Kohonen layer, and a Grossberg output layer with n, N and m units respectively. In what follows, the forward algorithm used during normal operation of the CPN is presented, whereas the backward algorithm used during training will be described in the next section. Denoting the input vector and output vectors at the Kohonen and Grossberg layers by $\mu = [\mu_1, \mu_2, \ldots, \mu_n]^T$, $\zeta = [\zeta_1, \zeta_2, \ldots, \zeta_N]^T$ and $\nu = [\nu_1, \nu_2, \ldots, \nu_m]^T$ respectively, the single winner forward algorithm of the CPN in regard to a particular input μ_0 is outlined as follows:

- Determine the winner unit J at the Kohonen layer competitively, according to the distances of weight vector $\omega^j(t)$ with respect to μ_0

$$D(\omega^J, \mu_0) = \underset{j=1,N}{\text{Min}} \; D(\omega^j, \mu_0) \tag{9.10}$$

where $\omega^j = [\omega^j_1, \omega^j_1, \ldots, \omega^j_n]$ is the weight vector connecting n input units to the jth unit at the Kohonen layer.

- Calculate the outputs $\zeta^j \in \{0, 1\}$ of the Kohonen layer by a winner-takes-all rule

$$\zeta^j = \begin{cases} 1 & \text{if } j = J \\ 0 & \text{otherwise.} \end{cases} \tag{9.11}$$

- Compute the outputs of the Grossberg layer by

$$\nu_k = \sum_{j=1}^{N} \zeta^j \pi^j_k \tag{9.12}$$

where $\pi^j = [\pi^j_1, \pi^j_2, \ldots, \pi^j_m]$ is the weight vector connecting the jth Kohonen unit to m Grossberg output units and $k = 1, 2, \ldots, m$.

To improve the mapping approximation accuracy, the trained CPN can also be operated in a multi-winner mode or an interpolation mode. The basic idea is that more than one Kohonen unit can win the competition with

Self-organizing fuzzy-neural control for blood pressure management

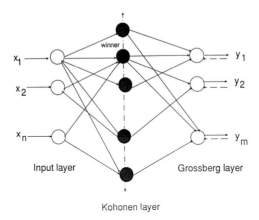

Figure 9.1 *The forward-only counterpropagation network.*

respect to the current input μ_0, and therefore the computed net output is a combination of look-up table entries associated with the winning Kohonen units. A problem arises as to how to split the unit output signal ($\zeta^j = 1$), which was previously assigned to a single winner, into several portions distributed to each winner. Hecht-Nielsen (1988) suggested that the win criterion can be based either on distance measurement between the current input and winning weights or on the basis of a fixed number of Kohonen units winning. As pointed out by Hecht-Nielsen (1990), this partitioning scheme used to split the ζ output signal is one of the major open research issues in connection with the CPN network.

9.3.2 Equivalence between SFCA and CPN

As mentioned in the first section, we are seeking structural mapping from the SFCA onto the CPN such that control knowledge represented formerly in rule form can be represented by the topology of the CPN and associated weights, and the reasoning algorithm can be carried out by operating the network directly. By carefully examining these two paradigms, we have found that there exist some striking similarities between the SFCA and the CPN which provide a basis for performing our objective.

The first aspect of similarity involves the issue of knowledge representation. More specifically, after training is terminated the CPN has been trained and arranged in such a way that N associations (ω^j, π^j) can function as a look-up table. In other words, the knowledge acquired via training is entirely represented by associated weights ω^j and π^j. Furthermore, as will be explored in the next section, the learned vectors ω^j are approximately equi-probable with respect to μ vectors drawn from A and each ω^j is in fact a representative of a set of vectors surrounding it. It becomes very clear that, by being analogous to the simplified rule form (9.9), each CPN association (ω^j, π^j) can be expressed as a rule:

$$\text{IF } \omega^j \text{ THEN } \pi^j \tag{9.13}$$

Equivalently, each Kohonen unit defines a rule by regarding the weight vectors connecting to and emanating from that unit as IF and THEN parts respectively. However, the difference between (9.9) and (9.13) lies in the specification of the width related to the IF part of the rule. While the width is explicitly present in (9.9), it is in fact implicitly embedded in (9.13) and becomes effective during the operation stage in a nearest-neighbour sense. Recall that M_u^j in rule (9.8) is a centre vector with maximum membership grade 1 and plays the same role as ω^j in (9.13). In this view, each rule in the form of (9.9) can be directly mapped into a Kohonen unit with M_u^j and M_v^j being corresponding weight vectors.

The similarity between these two systems can be made even clearer by exploring the algorithmic aspect in CPNs and the reasoning process in the SFCA. Both of them are intended to provide an approximate output ν or v by operating the existing knowledge (ω^j, π^j) or (M_u^j, M_v^j) with respect to the current input μ or u. Comparing (9.6), (9.7), and (9.8) in the SFCA with (9.10), (9.11) and (9.12) in a CPN, it can be concluded that the matching degree stage in the SFCA is functionally similar to the competition process in CPNs, and also the weighted average in the SFCA corresponds to the computation of the output at the Grossberg layer. An interesting and important analogy is the correspondence between matching degree S^j in the SFCA and the activation value ζ^j at the Kohonen layer in CPN. S^j usually takes a value in the range of $[0, 1]$, indicating a graded or soft matching and leading to an approximate output by averaging all the M_v^j with $S^j > 0$. In terms of a CPN, the SFCA allows several winners to be active and therefore naturally works in an interpolation mode. On the contrary, in the single winner mode the CPN works in a hard matching manner by setting one and only one output signal of the Kohonen unit to be 1, i.e. $\zeta^j \in 0, 1$. It is evident that the interpolation mode in CPN as suggested by Hecht-Nielsen bears some resemblance to the approximate reasoning process undertaken by the SFCA. A significant implication of this analogy is that the matching degree interpretation and associated algorithm in the SFCA provide an alternative and immediate solution to the split problem encountered in applying the interpolation mode for CPNs, a problem which was identified by Hecht-Nielsen and discussed at the end of the previous subsection.

9.4 Self-construction of the rule-base

So far the knowledge representation and reasoning problems have been solved by structural mapping and the associated forward algorithm, provided that the rule-base is available. It is noted that no training process is needed under this assumption because of the close correspondence which exists between the rule-base and the net structure. It would be apparently insignificant if we merely made a simple structural equivalence without taking full advantage of the adaptive property of neural networks. In other words, this localized knowledge representation paradigm would be more attactive and more useful only by removing the assumption of availability of the rule-base, thereby representing an extremely challenging problem which is referred to as knowledge acquisition and is essential for the creation of a knowledge-based system. To this end, the adaptive property of the network must be fully exploited to provide self-organizing and self-learning of the required rule-base directly from the controlled environment. In terms of CPN, this means that the number of units in the Kohonen layer must be self-organized and the associated weights with each unit must be self-learned. In the following, we first describe the standard training algorithm of the CPN, then present a modified scheme capable of carrying out the above task.

9.4.1 CPN training algorithm

Basically, the CPN training algorithm is a supervised training process by which the weights of the network are determined by exposing it to a set of paired training samples (μ^s, ν^s). The algorithm consists of two parts: a Kohonen scheme which is unsupervised in nature and is used to learn ω^j, and a Grossberg scheme which is truly supervised and is used to learn π^j.

More specifically, assuming that the number of Kohonen units is specified in advance and remains fixed during the training, the Kohonen algorithm can be described as follows. The training vector μ^s drawn randomly from A is presented to the CPN, and the input layer distributes to each of the units of the Kohonen layer through connecting weight vectors Ω^j. The competition then takes place among all the Kohonen units so as to determine which unit wins the current competition by determining which unit is closest to the current ν^s in the sense of the defined metric. Following the competition, the output of the winning unit J is set to 1, whereas outputs of all the other units are set to 0. The above two steps follow the same computing equations ((9.10) and (9.11)) as used during normal operation. The winner's weight vector ω^J is then updated by adding a time-varying scale difference $\mu^s - \omega^J$ such that the modified ω^J is closer to μ^s, whereas the weights of all the other units remain unchanged. More formally, the update law is given by

$$\omega^j(t) = \omega^j(t-1) + \alpha_t[\mu^s(t) - \omega^j(t-1)]\zeta^j \qquad (9.14)$$

where $\zeta \in 0, 1$ is determined by (9.10) and (9.11). $0 < \alpha_t < 1$ is a gain sequence decreasing monotonically with time in a linear or exponential manner. It is well known that if the coefficients α_t satisfy

$$\lim_{p \to \infty} \sum_{t=1}^{p} \alpha_t = +\infty \qquad (9.15)$$

$$\lim_{p \to \infty} \sum_{t=1}^{p} \alpha_t^2 < \infty \qquad (9.16)$$

then convergence can be guaranteed in the sense of mean-squared performance measure. In what follows, a harmonic series $\alpha_t = 1/t$ satisfying the aforementioned conditions will be used. The resultant weight vectors ω following the above training procedure can be considered to be approximately equi-probable with respect to μ vectors in a nearest-neighbour sense (Hecht-Nielsen, 1990) and to be N optimally quantized representatives of the input space A in some metric sense.

Once the Kohonen layer has stabilized, ω^j can be frozen and the Grossberg layer begins to learn the desired output ν for each frozen weight vector ω^j by adjusting the weights connecting the Kohonen units to the Grossberg units. More specifically, the update law at this layer is given by

$$\pi_k^j(t) = \pi_k^j(t-1) + \beta[-\pi_k^j(t-1) + \nu_k^s]\zeta^j \qquad (9.17)$$

where π_k^j is a weight from the jth Kohonen unit to the kth Grossberg (output) unit. β is a constant update rate within the range $[0, 1]$. ν_k^s is the kth component of the training sample ν^s.

Since each time only the winning Kohonen unit J produces the output $\zeta^J = 1$, (9.17) essentially modifies those weights connecting the Jth unit to the Grossberg units. By the assertion made in the last section, the weight vector π^J only is updated. It has been observed that the learned π^j in (9.17) are the exponential average of the ν^s vectors associated with the μ^s vectors which led the jth Kohonen unit to win, or in other words, those μ^s which are within the neighbourhood of ω^j.

9.4.2 Self-organizing of the IF part of the rule-base

There are several difficulties in applying the CPN training algorithm described above to our case where real-time adaptation is required. However, the major problems lie in the fact that: (a) the number N of the Kohonen units must be specified in advance; and (b) the correct or desired output at the Grossberg layer must be supplied. By assumption, the above required knowledge is unavailable and instead must be learned on-line as well as the learning of associated weight vectors. This section focuses on the problems relevant to the Kohonen layer or equivalently the IF part of the control rule, leaving the problems associated with the Grossberg layer or the THEN part to be handled in the next subsection.

Since the CPN network functionally plays the role of a controller, the distribution feature of the input data varies from case to case in an unknown manner depending largely on the characteristics of the controlled process, the form of command inputs and performance requirements. In this circumstance, it is very difficult to specify the number of the cluster centroids, or equivalently of the control rules, especially if a high dimensional input of the CPN is involved. Therefore, it is necessary to develop a modified Kohonen algorithm so as to learn not only the weight vectors ω as the original algorithm does, but also to learn the required number of the Kohonen units. Thus we need a truly self-organizing learning algorithm and a dynamically variable CPN structure in response to on-line incoming data.

Comparing the IF part of (9.9) in the SFCA with (9.13) in the CPN, there is a width vector Δ_u^j associated with the former. As discussed before, Δ_u^j can be visualized roughly as defining a neighbourhood for the jth rule centred at M_u^j. This viewpoint, together with the concept of relative distance (9.7), provides some insight into finding a solution for the problem. A vital idea is to associate with each existing Kohonen unit a valid radius and a local update gain such that each subregion represented by the weight vector ω, and restricted by the associated radius, is treated as a completely localized region although the overlap along the boundaries between the adjacent regions is allowed. By assigning each Kohonen unit a predefined width vector Δ_u^j, the winner J not only has a minimum distance among all the existing units in regard to the current input μ as determined by (9.10), but also must satisfy the condition of μ falling into the winner's neighbourhood as designated by Δ_u^j. Thus if these two conditions are met, then unit J is considered to be the winner and the associated weight vector is adjusted using (9.14) but with a local update gain. On the other hand, if these conditions are not satisfied with respect to all the units, it indicates that no existing unit is adequate to assign μ as its member and therefore a new unit should be created. It is clear that, starting from an empty state, the Kohonen layer can be dynamically self-organized in terms of the number of units and weight vectors ω associated with each unit, thereby establishing the IF part of the rule-base.

Incorporating the above ideas into the standard Kohonen algorithm, we develop a modified algorithm and present it as follows, where l, t and T denote the iteration number, the sampling instant and maximum sampling time respectively. In addition, α^j is the local gain controlling the speed of the adaptive process for ω^j, and is inversely proportional to the active frequency n^j of the jth unit up to the present time instant, $N^l(t)$ stands for the number of the Kohonen units at the lth iteration and at time t, and it is assumed that all δ_i^j are identical being denoted by δ.

MODIFIED KOHONEN ALGORITHM
(a) Initialization. $\omega_1^1(0) = u(0)$; $n_1^1(0) = 1$; $\alpha_1^1(0) = 1/n_1^1(0)$; $N_1(0) = 1$.
(b) At the lth iteration, do the following at each sampling time t.
    (b1) Find the unit J which has the minimum distance to the current μ by

$$D(\omega_l^J, \mu) = \|\omega_l^J(t) - \mu(t)\| = \min_{j=1,N} \|\omega_l^j(t) - \mu(t)\|. \qquad (9.18)$$

    (b2) Determine the winner using the following rule:

$$\begin{cases} \text{if } D(\omega_l^J, \mu) \leq \delta \to J \text{ is the winner} \\ \text{if } D(\omega_l^J, \mu) > \delta \to \text{create a new unit.} \end{cases} \qquad (9.19)$$

    (b3) Modify or initialize parameters;
        If J is the winner:

$$\begin{cases} n_l^J(t) = n_l^J(t-1) + 1; \; \alpha_l^J(t) = 1/n_l^J(t) \\ \omega_l^J(t) = \omega_l^J(t-1) + \alpha_l^J[\mu(t) - \omega_l^J(t-1)] \\ N_l(t) = N_l(t-1) \\ \zeta^J = 1. \end{cases} \qquad (9.20)$$

        If a new unit is created:

$$\begin{cases} N_l(t) = N_l(t-1) + 1 \\ \omega_l^{N_l}(t) = \mu(t) \\ n_l^{N_l}(t) = 1 \\ \zeta^{N_l} = 1 \end{cases} \qquad (9.21)$$

(c) After the lth iteration, remove all inactive units and reinitialize all active units:

$$\begin{cases} N_{l+1}(0) = N_l(T) - N_l^{\text{inactive}} \\ \omega_{l+1}^j(0) = \omega_l^j(T) \\ \alpha_{l+1}^j(0) = \alpha_l^j(T) \\ j = 1, 2, \ldots, N_{l+1}(0). \end{cases} \qquad (9.22)$$

Compared with the standard Kohonen algorithm, the proposed algorithm above possesses two notable features. The first one is that the input space is partitioned in a soft or fuzzy manner in the sense that each Kohonen unit occupies a hyper-region, part of which is shared by other existing neighbouring clusters. The second feature is that the partition of the input space is a dynamical process altering the structure of the CPN continuously along both temporal and spatial dimensions.

9.4.3 Self-learning the THEN part of the rule-base

As mentioned previously, the major difficulty in deriving the weight vectors π connecting the Kohonen layer to the Grossberg layer, or equivalently the THEN parts of the rules, stems from the unavailability of the teacher signals ν^j guiding the supervised training. More generally, lacking a teacher is a common obstacle facing any kind of neurocontroller and can be regarded as a bottleneck. Although considerable effort has been recently devoted to constructing the teacher signals explicitly or implicitly for neurocontrollers with various net topologies (e.g. Barto, 1990), it is far from being completely and satisfactorily solved. Here we propose a simple but efficient scheme capable of carrying out the task of training π. The approach comprises essentially two steps. First, the teacher signals are constructed explicitly at the beginning of each iteration by an iterative learning approach. Then the derived signals are supplied to the Grossberg layer of the CPN so as to adjust the π vectors using the standard algorithm (9.17).

Figure 9.2 shows a block diagram of the learning system consisting of a reference model and a learning mechanism. The reference model is designed to specify what the process responses y_p should be when both the model and the process are subject to the same command signal r. For the sake of simplicity, we again adopt the non-interacting model with second-order linear transfer functions.

Denoting the learning error by e_L, defined as the difference between the output y_d of the reference model and the output y_p of the process, the overall goal of the learning system is to force the learning error $e_L(t)$ asymptotically to zero or to a predefined tolerant region ε within a time interval of interest $[0, T]$ by repeatedly operating the system. More specifically, we require that $\|e_L, l_{L,l}(t)\| \to 0$ or $\|e_L, l_{L,l}(t)\| < \varepsilon$ uniformly in $t \in [0, T]$ as $l \to \infty$, where l denotes the iteration number, $\varepsilon > 0$ is a predefined error tolerance, and $\|\cdot\|$ stands for the norm. It is clear that whenever convergence occurs, the corresponding control action at that iteration is regarded as the desired control γ_d with which the corresponding response y_p of the controlled process will be close enough to y_d.

By taking the process time-delay into account, the learning law is given by

$$\gamma^{l+1}(t) = \gamma^l(t) + \mathbf{P}_L \cdot e_{L,l}(t + \lambda) + \mathbf{Q}_L \cdot c_{L,l}(t + \lambda) \tag{9.23}$$

where $\gamma^{l+1}, \gamma^l \in R^m$ are on-line learning teacher vector-valued functions at the $(l+1)$th and the lth iterations respectively, $e_{L,l}, c_{L,l} \in R^m$ are learning

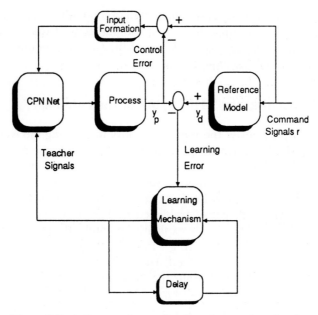

Figure 9.2 *A diagram for on-line learning teacher signals.*

error and change of learning error defined by $c_{L,l}(t) = e_{L,l}(t+1) - e_{L,l}(t)$, λ is an estimated time advance corresponding to the time delay of the process, and $\mathbf{P}_L, \mathbf{Q}_L \in R^{m \times m}$ are constant learning gain matrices.

A variety of special algorithms can be obtained with different selections of learning gain matrices. For example, the simplest version is when $\mathbf{P}_L$ is diagonal whereas $\mathbf{Q}_L = 0$. In this case, the rate of change of the error is not considered, nor are the loop interacting effects. The learning action in each loop is totally dependent on its own error. Learning gain matrices $\mathbf{P}_L$ and $\mathbf{Q}_L$ should be chosen carefully. As would happen in any other learning system, too big or too small gain values will typically lead to either divergence or too slow convergence speed. Thus a trade-off between speed and convergence should be made. In practice, this selection is not a very hard task because the learning system is relatively robust with respect to the values of the gains.

It is noted that the control update at the $(l+1)$th iteration is entirely based on the information derived at the lth iteration, i.e. the previous control action and the resulting performance measured by the error and its derivative. Accordingly, all the information at the lth iteration must be stored, and all the $\gamma(t) \in [0, T]$ at the $(l+1)$th iteration are adjusted simultaneously. Thus at the beginning of each iteration, γ is available at each time instant t and can be used to guide the weight vector adjustment at the Grossberg layer by

$$\pi_k^j(t) = \pi_k^j(t-1) + \beta[-\pi_k^j(t-1) + \gamma_k^l(t)]\zeta^j. \qquad (9.24)$$

Self-organizing fuzzy-neural control for blood pressure management

The above equation is the same as (9.17) except that here the desired signal ν^s is replaced by γ. Assume that, by appropriately choosing $\mathbf{P}_L$ and $\mathbf{Q}_L$, the desired output y_d can be approached asymptotically with a learned control sequence γ_d. The γ_d can then be embedded into π^j vectors by (9.24) with a suitably chosen β. Thus, with increasing iterations the THEN parts of the rules are gradually learned along with the learning process of γ.

9.5 Application to blood pressure control

We have applied the proposed approach to the problem of blood pressure control as described in Chapter 7. A set of simulations were performed, aimed at demonstrating the feasibility of the proposed scheme and examining its self-organizing and self-learning behaviours when applied to this multivariable control problem. More specifically, we investigated the adaptive ability and convergence property of the system during the learning mode and the generalizing property in the reasoning mode. Throughout this work, the EC-type controller defined in Section 9.2 was employed and the following values were used. The time interval of interest contains 100 sampling points with the sampling time being 30 s. Set-point changes for CO and MAP were set to be 20 ml s^{-1} and -10 mmHg changing from nominal values of 100 ml s^{-1} and 120 mmHg respectively. The maximum iteration number was 10. The other parameters used will be given accordingly.

9.5.1 Adaptive ability

By adaptive ability, here we mean the capability of the system to deal with various situations with respect to controller environments, in particular to variations of the process parameters and desired performance requirements, and to the noise measurements, while keeping the controller parameters fixed. In this case, learning gain matrices $\mathbf{P}_L = \text{diag}\{0.05, -0.05\}$ and $\mathbf{Q}_L = 0$, Grossberg update date $\beta = 0.5$, and Euclidean distance with the valid radius $\delta = 0.1$ were used. To measure the performance, a normalized squared sum of errors (NSSE) has been defined by

$$\text{NSSE}^l = \frac{\text{SSE}^l}{\text{SSE}_{\max}} \qquad (9.25)$$

where

$$\text{SSE}^l = \sum_{i=1}^{100}[(y_{d,CO}(i) - y^l_{p,CO}(i))^2 + (y_{d,MAP}(i) - y^l_{p,MAP}(i))^2] \qquad (9.26)$$

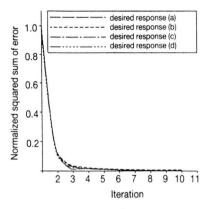

Figure 9.3 *Adaptive capability for different desired responses.*

is the squared sum of error at the lth iteration and SSE_{max} is the largest SSE^l chosen from all the SSE^l produced by using different parameters within the same group at all the iterations from $l = 1$ to $l = 10$.

Figure 9.3 shows the results of NSSE versus the iteration number when different performance requirements were demanded by specifying the parameters in the reference model as follows:

(a) $\xi_{CO} = 0.8$ $t_{s,CO} = 240$ s $\xi_{MAP} = 0.7$ $t_{s,MAP} = 240$ s
(b) $\xi_{CO} = 0.7$ $t_{s,CO} = 240$ s $\xi_{MAP} = 0.8$ $t_{s,MAP} = 240$ s
(c) $\xi_{CO} = 0.8$ $t_{s,CO} = 240$ s $\xi_{MAP} = 0.8$ $t_{s,MAP} = 240$ s
(d) $\xi_{CO} = 0.9$ $t_{s,CO} = 400$ s $\xi_{MAP} = 0.7$ $t_{s,MAP} = 240$ s.

It can be seen that the system is capable of handling the various desired responses using a set of fixed controller parameters. The NSSEs quickly approach small and stable values, indicating a fast learning process. It can be seen that a relatively large NSSE was observed for case (b). In fact, the actual process responses are quite acceptable even for this seemingly worst case, as indicated in Figure 9.4.

By altering the process parameters in the model given in Section 7.2.2, a set of NSSEs were obtained and are depicted in Figure 9.5, where three cases are displayed with parameter variations of 10%. Although slightly different convergence behaviour with different cases was observed, stable and small NSSEs were achieved after a few iterations in all cases.

To examine the learning ability in a noise-contaminated environment, we carried out a simulation where the outputs of the process were corrupted by random noise with a uniform distribution, and therefore both controller inputs and adaptive inputs were contaminated by noise. Figure 9.6 shows the outputs of the process after ten iterations with a noise amplitude of 10% at the set-points. It can be seen that the responses are satisfactory.

Self-organizing fuzzy-neural control for blood pressure management 283

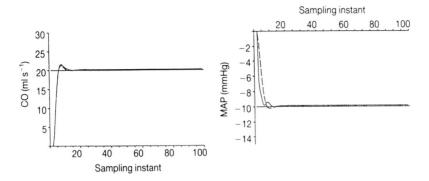

Figure 9.4 *Outputs of the process corresponding to case (b) of Figure 9.3.*

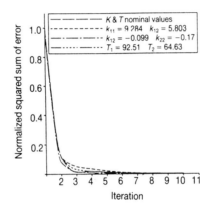

Figure 9.5 *Adaptive capability for different process parameters.*

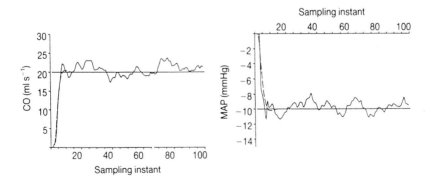

Figure 9.6 *Outputs of the process at the 10th iteration under noise measurements.*

9.5.2 Convergence property

By keeping the process parameters and the reference model fixed, the convergence properties of the system were investigated with respect to various controller parameters in terms of how these parameters influence the convergence process measured by the NSSE.

LEARNING MATRIX $\mathbf{P}_L$

The values of the learning matrix $\mathbf{P}_L$ have a great effect on the learning process. Bigger values will speed up the convergence process but at the risk of divergence. On the contrary, smaller values will slow down the learning process in a sometimes unacceptable manner. Figure 9.7 gives the results with $\mathbf{P}_L = \text{diag}\{0.05, -0.05\}$, $\text{diag}\{0.1, -0.1\}$, and $\text{diag}\{0.03, -0.03\}$ respectively. As would be expected, the results agree well with the above remarks.

GROSSBERG LEARNING RATE β

As mentioned before, β plays the role of controlling the update of π in an exponential manner. The bigger it is, the more important the current teacher signal γ is, and therefore the more quickly the previous learned π is forgotten. Figure 9.8 shows the results with $\beta = 0.5, 0.1$, and 0.9 respectively. It appears that too big or too small β values will generally result in a slower convergence process, indicating that values around 0.5 are good choices. However, the choice is not very sensitive.

VALID RADIUS δ

δ is mainly used to control the self-organizing process in the CPN. It has a direct effect on the number of Kohonen units or control rules. The smaller δ is, the more units the CPN creates, and therefore the more rules in the rule-base. By choosing $\delta = 0.01, 0.1$, and 1.0 respectively, we obtained respective rule-bases with rule numbers of 22, 14 and 8. However, as expected, the convergence is not very sensitive to this parameter as indicated in Figure 9.9.

DISTANCE METRICS

Finally, we examined the effect of the distance metrics used in the self-organizing process at the Kohonen layer. Because different distance metrics define different shapes of the neighbourhood of each rule, it is expected that they have some effect on the number of created rules and less effect on the control or learning performances. We carried out comparative studies by using three frequently used metrics: Euclidean, Hamming and maximum distances, D_E, D_H and D_M. Three almost identical convergence processes, as shown in Figure 9.10, verified our expectation. However, it is

Self-organizing fuzzy-neural control for blood pressure management 285

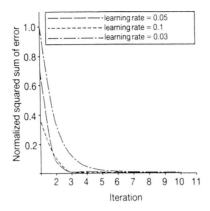

Figure 9.7 *Convergence property with learning rate* $\mathbf{P}_L$.

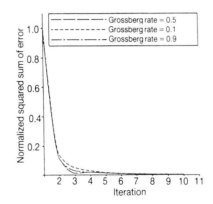

Figure 9.8 *Convergence property with Grossberg rate* β.

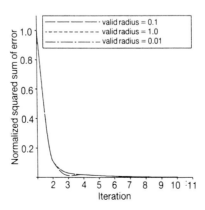

Figure 9.9 *Convergence property with valid radius* δ.

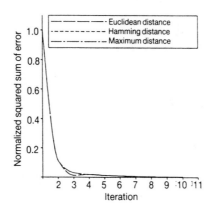

Figure 9.10 *Convergence property with distance metric* D.

interesting to note that the rule numbers produced by these metrics are 14, 16 and 13 respectively. These results can be explained by the fact that, with the same valid radius δ, the neighbourhood defined by D_M has the biggest volume, therefore the smallest rule number 13, the one defined by D_H has the smallest volume, therefore the highest rule number 16, leaving the defined volume and the produced rule number as D_E in the middle. Compared with the case of the valid radius, the different metrics have much less influence in controlling the rule number.

9.5.3 Approximate reasoning property

The proposed CPN-based controller can work in two modes: real-time control with or without learning. In the latter case, it is assumed that an appropriate CPN structure with corresponding weights has been obtained during the learning stage. With this learned CPN or rule-base, it is expected that the controller can perform similar tasks in an acceptable manner by replacing a winner-take-all competitive scheme with a soft matching cooperative strategy. This requires the CPN to have some generalizing or interpolative capability or, equivalently, robustness with respect to some new situations. Table 9.1 gives the performance indices ISE and ITAE obtained at the 10th iteration during the learning mode (the first row) and those obtained using the learned CPN (14 rules) with the approximate

Table 9.1 *Performance indices for learning and learned modes*

	ISE_{CO}	$ITAE_{CO}$	ISE_{MAP}	$ITAE_{MAP}$
Learning	16.08	126.70	3.16	54.82
Learned	15.82	70.80	3.10	34.93

Self-organizing fuzzy-neural control for blood pressure management 287

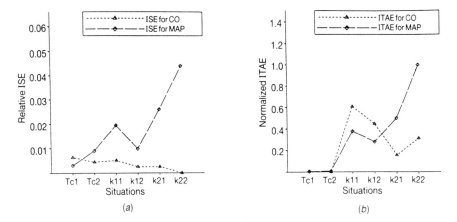

Figure 9.11 *Robustness of learned CPN controller (a) relative ISE; (b) normalized ITAE.*

scheme (the second row). The table indicates that the performances given by the latter are better than those given by the former. This may stem from the utilization of the interpolative reasoning. It is worth pointing out that for a safe use of the learned CPN, a bigger valid radius δ must be used to ensure the coverage of the whole possible input space by the learned rules. In our case, we assigned $\delta = 0.6$ instead of 0.1 which was used during the learning mode.

By using a learned CPN with 14 rules, we investigated the robustness property with variations of process gains, time constants and in a noise-contaminated environment. Figure 9.11 shows the results in terms of performance indices 'Relative ISE' (Figure 9.11(*a*)) and 'Normalized ITAE' (Figure 9.11(*b*)) versus the varying parameters, where

$$\text{Relative ISE} = \frac{|\text{ISE}^* - \text{ISE}|}{\text{ISE}^*} \tag{9.27}$$

$$\text{Normalized ITAE} = \frac{|\text{ITAE}^* - \text{ITAE}|}{\text{Max}|\text{ITAE}^* - \text{ITAE}|} \tag{9.28}$$

where ISE*(ITAE*) and ISE(ITAE) are the performance indices obtained with nominal and changed process parameter values (5% in this case) respectively. From Figure 9.11, we may conclude that (a) the system possesses good robustness as indicated by low Relative ISE values (Figure 9.11(*a*)); (b) the system is less sensitive to time constants than to process gains in the steady-state stage (Figure 9.11(*b*)); (c) in most cases, the *MAP* is more sensitive to the variation of parameters than *CO*.

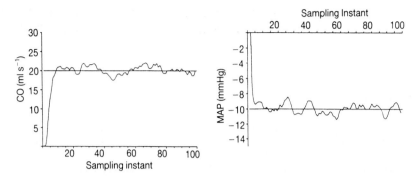

Figure 9.12 *Outputs of the process using learned CPN under noise measurements.*

Finally, Figure 9.12 shows the output responses when the measured process outputs were corrupted by random noise with an amplitude of 10% at the set-points. It can be seen that the system works satisfactorily in such a noise-contaminated environment.

9.6 Conclusion

We have introduced a unified framework for constructing automatically a control rule-base constrained by prespecified control performance requirements. The underlying principles of the approach rely on a combination of ideas from various fields. In particular, the SFCA provides a very efficient interpolative look-up table paradigm suitable for use with multivariable numerical environments, and CPNs offer some insight into the idea of how a fixed-structure network can be developed adaptively into a multidimensional look-up table. Also, the concepts of relative distance in the SFCA and the learning strategy in the learning control make it possible to extend the original CPN training algorithms at both Kohonen and Grossberg layers into a highly self-organized and completely unsupervised algorithm. The approach reported here out-performs the existing fuzzy control algorithms in many aspects. In particular, we claim that the approach is generic in the sense that, in principle, control rule-bases of arbitrary dimension can be constructed automatically while satisfying chosen desired, but physically achievable, performance requirements. The learning process involved is extremely fast due to the simple network topology and the efficiency of the learning algorithms. Another point is that very little prior knowledge about the controlled process is required in the implementation of the algorithm, but at the price of iterative operation, a price that must be paid regardless of whether using human or machine learning. Extensive simulations on a problem of multivariable blood pressure control have demonstrated the learning, adaptive, and approximate reasoning capabilities of the system. It has been found that the proposed approach is extremely efficient in terms of simple topological structure, fast learning speed, and good robustness properties.

References

Barto, A.G., 1990, 'Connectionist learning for control: an overview', in W.T. Miller et al. (Eds), *Neural Networks for Control*, pp. 5–58, Cambridge, MA: MIT Press.
Hecht-Nielsen, R., 1987, Counterpropagation network, *Applied Optics*, **26**, 4979–84.
Hecht-Nielsen, R., 1988, Applications of counterpropagation network, *Neural Networks*, **1**, 131–9.
Hecht-Nielsen, R., 1990, *Neurocomputing*, Reading, MA: Addison-Wesley Publishing Company.
Nie, J., 1987, 'Expert fuzzy control systems', MS thesis, Xidian University, Xi'an, China.
Nie, J., 1989, 'A class of new fuzzy control algorithms', in Proceedings of the IEEE International Conference on Control and Applications, Israel.

Chapter 10
Neural network control for unconsciousness anaesthesia

H. U. Rehman

10.1 Introduction

Sleep and anaesthesia are both states of unresponsiveness which vary in depth. Sleep is natural, healthy and has a circadian rhythm (a rhythm of approximately twenty-four-hour period) (Oswald, 1989). Anaesthesia is an artificial state maintained by the continuing presence of chemical (anaesthetic) agents in the brain. Using anaesthetic agents there are several complications and side effects, which may cause death under extreme conditions. However, the quality and safety of the procedures have improved significantly in various ways since the introduction of anaesthetic techniques. New anaesthetic agents have been introduced providing better anaesthetic techniques. Attention has also been paid to the control of the three basic components of anaesthesia i.e. narcosis (sleep), analgesia (pain relief) and muscle relaxation (Carrie and Simpson, 1988). These can be controlled by supplying a single anaesthetic agent at high dosage, but this can lead to undesirable side-effects. Better control can be achieved by supplying a precise dose of several drugs each aimed at a specific feature. This also allows the patient to be operated upon under lighter general anaesthesia than before, thus giving safer procedures. Since there is no direct method to measure the depth of anaesthesia, various techniques have been used to suggest safe amounts of anaesthetic drug, considering the conditions of an individual patient.

The effect of anaesthetic agents on the respiratory system, cardiovascular system, central nervous system and muscles (Vickers and Schnieden, 1984) may provide a monitoring system for the safe use of anaesthetic agents. Monitoring of electroencephalogram (EEG) signals, colour of skin, pupil size, patient movement and other clinical signs such as heart rate (HR), respiration rate (RR), systolic arterial pressure (SAP), mean arterial pressure (MAP), etc., are used by anaesthetists to determine the depth of anaesthesia (Linkens et al., 1986) and to decide the correct dosage of anaesthetic agent. However, quick action needs to be taken when rapid changes take place in clinical signs, which may be misleading and hence cause an incorrect dosage to be supplied. Furthermore, there is a considerable variation in the importance and interpretation applied to each clinical sign.

The advent of computers and their vast application has also led to their use during surgery in different ways such as monitoring, record keeping, checking HR, blood pressure, etc. Various studies have been carried out with computer-controlled depth of anaesthesia using both open-loop and closed-loop techniques (Titel et al., 1968; Chilcoat, 1980; O'Callaghan et al., 1983; Chilcoat et al., 1984). Those instruments that can measure automatically some of the changes in the patient's state during anaesthesia have been interfaced with computers to give on-line advice and control. The aim of these studies is not to replace the anaesthetist by computers but to help him to perform more demanding human tasks (Linkens and Hacisalihzade, 1990). In an ideal situation physicians are also part of the control loop, with computers playing an important role (Rampil and Smith, 1984) as represented in Figure 10.1.

For automatic control of anaesthetic depth various indicators have been considered as measurement variables. EEG signals have been observed and analysed by computers during anaesthesia. Changes in these signals have been correlated with the depth of anaesthesia and used to control the anaesthetic agent. One of the studies by Schwilden et al. (1989) describes an adaptive feedback controller using the drug propofol. Another recent study carried out by Chi et al. (1991) used computer analysis of the power spectrum of an EEG during drug infusion in humans. Considerable changes in the EEG were observed at the start, but a steady state was obtained,

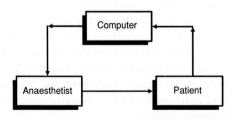

Figure 10.1 *Relationship of computer, anaesthetist and patient under closed-loop conditions.*

regardless of increasing dose, which suggests that the power spectrum of the EEG fails to respond to a dose increase after the initial changes.

The effects of different anaesthetics on EEG differ widely (Clark *et al.*, 1971), and a careful inspection is needed to reveal consistent changes that correlate well with the assessment of anaesthetic depth or the anaesthetic dose. Accurate monitoring and analysis of the changes in EEG are difficult during surgical operations since they require high skill and time. As the use of EEG signals as a measurement variable requires very sophisticated equipment, more studies are needed to explore fully the method and to devise easy analysis during surgery. Studies have also been carried out to infer anaesthetic drug concentration, using pharmacokinetic compartmental models (Mapleson *et al.*, 1980). Computer models based on various parameters have been developed to simulate the uptake and distribution of anaesthetic agents (Tatnall *et al.*, 1981). Suppan (1977) was the first to use systolic arterial pressure (*SAP*) in closed-loop control as an indicator of the adequacy of anaesthesia for the control of the administration of halothane (Asbury, 1991). Mean arterial pressure (*MAP*) has also been used by various workers for controlling the depth of anaesthesia (Schils *et al.*, 1983; Gray and Asbury, 1986).

A rule-based automatic controller for general anaesthesia with enflurane was developed by Robb *et al.* (1988) based on the initial study of Gray and Asbury (1986). *SAP* was used as an index of the anaesthetic depth, since it reaches its target very quickly and contains enough information to allow some form of control. The task of the computer program was to maintain the target value of *SAP*, which was 90% of the predicted *SAP* by age and sex, by controlling enflurane and morphine. It was found that during the operation the anaesthetic state produced by the controller was acceptable to the supervising anaesthetist (Robb *et al.*, 1991). The feasibility of single-input–single-output (*SAP*-vapour delivery) control was demonstrated, and the use of *MAP* was rejected as most of the anaesthetists did not use this in actual practice. The use of this system may be successful in normal operations but was not suggested seriously for complicated operations. A review of studies relating to the automatic control of anaesthetic depth has been carried out in detail by Rehman (1992).

Another study was performed by Linkens *et al.* (1986) to develop an expert system for the control of the depth of anaesthesia using different clinical signs. As most clinical signs are not numerically quantifiable, a small study was conducted by A. J. Asbury, in which colleague anaesthetists ranked ten clinical signs of different types. Table 10.1 shows the mean of raw rank and order of mean. The expert system considered the following clinical signs; *SAP*, HR, RR, sweating, patient movement, pupil size and pupil position. Certain assertions, questions, rules and goals were developed to provide knowledge representation for the system. Later, the system was called RESAC (realtime expert system for advice and control) (Linkens *et al.*, 1990), and it comprises a rule-based backward chaining inference engine

Table 10.1 *Ranking of clinical signs*

Clinical signs	Mean of raw rank	Order of mean ranks
Movement and response to surgery	7.40	1
Respiration rate	5.80	2
Heart rate	5.30	3
Low muscle tone	5.00	4
Lacrimation	4.90	5
Arterial pressure	4.84	6
Sweating	4.77	7
Pupil position	4.60	8
Pupil diameter	3.40	9
Capillary refill	2.50	10

with about 400 rules, and makes use of fuzzy logic and Bayesian reasoning (see Chapter 2). RESAC was tested in several clinical trials, and after each trial, improvements were made in the knowledge-base of the system (Greenhow, 1990). The quality of RESAC's advice was determined by anaesthetists stating whether the performance was very good, good, OK, poor, or very poor (Linkens *et al.*, 1990). RESAC gives the certainty of the anaesthetic state and suggests the drug dosage by giving output hypotheses of anaesthetic OK (AO), anaesthetic light (AL) and anaesthetic deep (AD). In the final clinical trial the dose suggested by RESAC was administered during all the operations and RESAC was rated as 'good' or 'very good' in five operations out of the seven (Greenhow, 1990). The size of the rule-base within RESAC appears to be at the threshold of realistic rule acquisition, editing, debugging and verification for a knowledge base. Neither rule-based nor frame-based artificial intelligence paradigms are easy to manage with this size of knowledge domain.

In the study presented in this chapter, an alternative attempt has been made to use the newly developed technique of artificial neural networks (ANNs), since ANNs offer a better possibility of rapid knowledge acquisition via their self-organizing learning properties. They have the ability to learn functionalities in those cases where it is possible to specify the inputs and outputs but difficult to define the non-linear relationships between them. They are also tolerant to noise in the input data. These attributes of ANNs are suitable for the realm of anaesthesia because the relationships between clinical signs are not clear. Using this technique there is no problem associated with the number of rules as the relationships are developed by the ANN itself.

10.2 Experimental procedures

For this study, patients' data such as *HR*, *SAP*, *RR*, percentage of anaesthetic agent, temperature, etc., were logged into a computer, during several surgical operations. These operations were carried out in two series, one for spontaneously breathing patients and the other for ventilated patients. Controllers and patient models (PMs) for the spontaneous and ventilated patients are discussed separately in this chapter.

As RESAC advice was rated by anaesthetists as giving excellent control, the surgical data were input to RESAC to get smooth data, and to compare the results obtained via ANN and regression with those of RESAC. It was observed in the initial stages of the study that ANN took less time and gave better results if the data were smooth rather than having large transitions (Rehman, 1992). The outputs of RESAC were certainty values from -500 to 500 for the three states of anaesthesia, i.e. AO, AL and AD, with suggested dosage ranging from 0 to 5%. These outputs were later used for developing drug controllers using ANNs and regression.

The ANN back-propagation (BP) learning algorithm (Rumelhart et al., 1986) has been used to train the programme. BP is the most popular learning algorithm for ANNs, suggested and used successfully by Rumelhart et al. (1986). This algorithm produces a multilayer network, for example, a network with three layers has an input layer, an output layer, and an intermediate layer, not connected directly to the input or the output, being the so-called hidden layer.

The network must first be trained. When an input is presented to an untrained network, a random output is produced. An error function is defined, that represents the difference between the network's current output and the actual output. To get the desired output, the value of the error function is continually reduced by adjusting the weights of the links between the units. This is done by propagating the error value for each actual output backwards, to the hidden layer. The adjustments for the weights in the hidden layer are calculated using the derivatives of the error functions that are used to adjust the weights for the output layer units. The procedure repeatedly adjusts the weights of the connections in the network so as to minimize the error function. As a result of the weight adjustment, internal hidden units come to represent important features of the task domain, and the regularities in the task are captured by the interaction of these units.

10.3 Controllers and models for spontaneously breathing patients

The development and results of two controllers, one using ANN techniques and the other using non-linear regression (NLR) are discussed later. The drug controllers have been connected to other programmes that model the patient. Two PMs have been developed via ANNs and linear regression analysis. The data files used for model identification were selected from those surgical operations in which only small amounts of morphine were used, since the use of morphine may affect clinical signs.

10.3.1 ANN controller

One of the initial requirements of the BP algorithm is reliable data on which the network is to be trained and tested. For training the BP programme the legal input values are from 0 to 1, thus the surgical data were normalized with a global normalization factor.

The initial trainings were carried out with inputs of age, weight, gender, *HR*, *SAP* and *RR*. After a series of training and testing sessions, results were compared to those of RESAC and found to be very promising. In subsequent trainings, time delays in the anaesthetic dose were introduced, as the effect of a previous dose remains for some time. Comparison of results with one time-delay and two time-delays in dose showed that the former gave a better result than the latter (Linkens and Rehman, 1992a). This agrees with the pharmacology of the anaesthetic agent (isoflurane was used in all operations) which suggests that the uptake and the elimination of isoflurane is quicker than other anaesthetic agents such as enflurane (Stoelting and Miller, 1989). Also, 'delta target' values (delta target = target–actual) for *HR*, *SAP* and *RR* set by anaesthetists for individual patients undergoing sugery were included as inputs for the training of the programme.

Successive trainings were carried out with ten inputs and four outputs, selecting different numbers of hidden units in the network. The minimum value of the total sum of squares (Rumelhart *et al.*, 1986) was obtained with three hidden units. Figure 10.2 shows the structure of network with inputs,

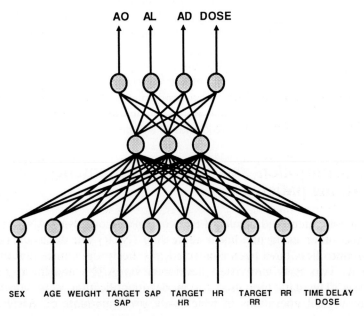

Figure 10.2 *Structure of network for training of ANN controller.*

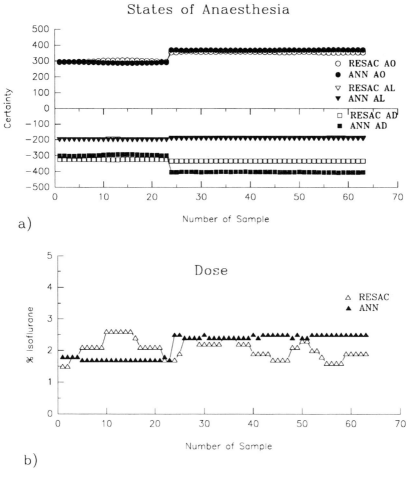

Figure 10.3 *Outputs from RESAC and ANNAD, (a) three states of anaesthesia i.e., anaesthetic OK (AO), anaesthetic light (AL) and anaesthetic deep (AD), and (b) percentage dosage. Sample period is approximately 1 minute.*

hidden units and outputs. For initializing the training network, random biases and weights were selected, also the learning rate and momentum term for upgrading the weights were gradually increased as the training proceeded. This gradual increase in learning rate and momentum term helps the system to converge more rapidly. After successful training and testing, a computer program called ANNAD (artificial neural networks for anaesthetic dose) was developed, using the weights from the above training runs. ANNAD suggests three states of anaesthesia and the dosage of anaesthetic agent, after receiving time-related inputs. In the experiments conducted so far the three states of anaesthesia and suggested dosage by ANNAD have been almost the same as that suggested by RESAC. Figure 10.3 shows the states of anaesthesia and suggested dose by RESAC and ANNAD for one particular patient.

An interesting feature of ANNAD was demonstrated when two different sets of target values of *HR*, *SAP* and *RR* were presented to it (Linkens and Rehman, 1992b). It was observed that the outputs from ANNAD for each set of target values were different thus indicating that ANNAD does indeed take account of target values.

10.3.2 Non-linear regression controller

An attempt was also made to develop a controller via regression analysis and to compare its performance with ANN controllers. A graphical computer package 'Sigmaplot' was used to find the best fit non-linear model. An approach of least-squares regression which minimizes the sum of squared residuals is used in that package. However, it has been reported that the least median of squares regression, which minimizes the median squared residual, is more robust and can describe the bulk of data provided half of the data are not outliers (Dallal and Rousseeuw, 1992). There are some limitations with NLR, such as the fact that the overall contribution and significance of each variable decreases with a large number of dependent variables. To find suitable dependent variables and their multiples, there are some tedious statistical tests (Kleinbaum *et al.*, 1988) which involve a great deal of computation and time.

The NLR for AO, AL, AD and dosage was obtained in terms of *SAP*, *HR*, *RR*, their multiples and their squares. The same data file as in the case of an ANN was used for finding the regression. The coefficients obtained from the above NLR analysis were then used in developing a controller for anaesthetic depth. The same data as in Figure 10.3 were tested on the above controller and the results were published by Rehman *et al.* (1992). The results from the test have shown that the three states of anaesthesia and percentage of dose calculated by NLR were almost the same as those from RESAC. Later when this controller was connected in closed-loop with the PM, it gave anomalous results. An improved NLR controller in which target values for *SAP*, *HR* and *RR* were included as inputs has also been developed. Four non-linear equations, i.e. three anaesthetic states and dosage, were obtained in terms of target *SAP*, *SAP*, target *HR*, *HR*, target *RR*, *RR*, *SAP* × *HR*, *SAP* × *RR* and *HR* × *RR*. Figure 10.4 shows the testing of data on this NLR controller. The performance of this controller in closed-loop is discussed in section 10.5.1.

10.3.3 ANN patient model (ANN-PM)

An ANN-PM was obtained using the BP algorithm on the data of a second patient collected during a similar surgical operation as for the controller

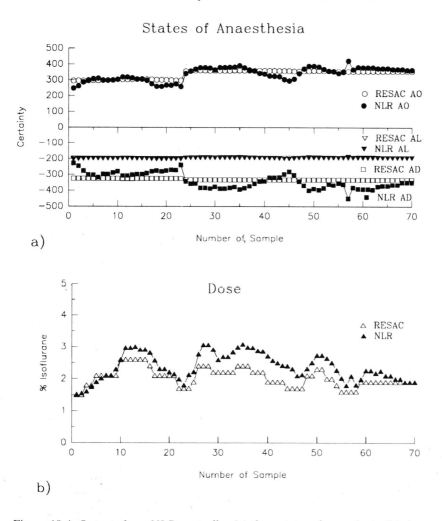

Figure 10.4 *Outputs from NLR controller (a) three states of anaesthesia (b) dose.*

design. The outputs were *SAP*, *HR* and *RR*. Three separate ANNs were obtained for each output with a different combination of inputs for the spontaneously breathing patient simulator (Linkens and Rehman, 1992b).

The inputs for calculating *SAP* were dose, *HR*, *RR*, and delayed versions of dose, *HR* and *SAP*. For *HR*, the inputs were the same except that *HR* was replaced by *SAP*, and finally for *RR* the inputs were dose, *HR*, *SAP*, with delayed versions of dose, *HR*, *SAP* and *RR*. The three networks for training are shown in Figure 10.5. Figure 10.6 shows typical outputs from this PM. All three clinical signs were driven by only one variable, i.e. dose. Changes in *SAP* and *HR* are visible from the figure, but there is little variation in *RR* caused by the change in given dose.

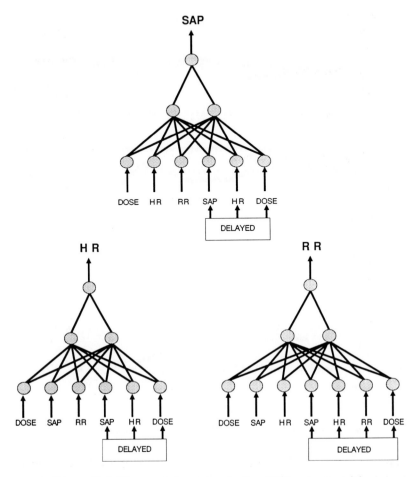

Figure 10.5 *Three training networks for ANN patient model.*

10.3.4 Patient model via linear regression (LR-PM)

Multivariate linear regression analysis has been used to develop another PM that calculates *SAP*, *HR* and *RR*, and simulates a patient under anaesthetic effect. The same data were used for regression as in the ANN-PM. The dependent variables were dose, time-delay dosage, time-delay *SAP*, time-delay *HR* and time-delay *RR*. The three outputs (*SAP*, *HR* and *RR*) obtained are shown in Figure 10.7, the inputs being the same as for Figure 10.6. It can be seen that the values of *SAP* and *HR* decreased at the beginning and increased when dose was decreased. A significant change can also be seen in *RR* when the dose was decreased. Altogether eight PMs were developed via regression and tested in closed-loop with the ANNAD.

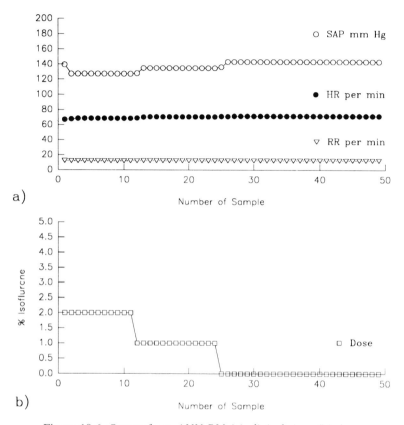

Figure 10.6 *Output from ANN-PM (a) clinical signs (b) dose.*

The aim was to check the performance of the PM and get a reliable model for validating the controllers. The PM discussed in this section gave the best results.

10.4 Controllers and models for ventilated patients

A controller and a PM for ventilated patients have been developed via an ANN. A linear regression PM has also been obtained. The controller was then studied in closed-loop with the two patient simulators obtained via an ANN and linear regression respectively.

10.4.1 ANN controller for ventilated patients

The same BP algorithm was used to train the ANN controller as in Section 10.3.1. After several attempts at training, success was achieved with three

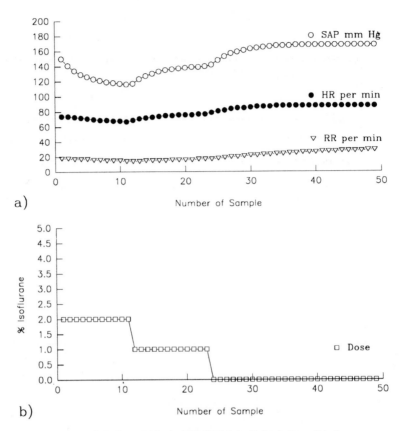

Figure 10.7 *Output from LR-PM (a) clinical signs (b) dose.*

hidden units. The inputs were gender, age, weight, target *SAP*, *SAP*, target *HR*, *HR* and delayed dose, while the outputs were AO, AL, AD and dosage. A fully connected network as shown in Figure 10.2 was used for training. The only difference was in the inputs, since *RR* and target *RR* are not relevant when a ventilator is used for breathing.

The training of the data for the controller is shown in Figure 10.8, while for testing, data from a second patient were selected. Figure 10.9 shows the testing of the data. It can be seen that the curves for the states of anaesthesia are not well-overlapping the RESAC curves, but the suggested dose is almost the same as for RESAC.

10.4.2 ANN ventilated patient model (ANN-VPM)

The configuration for training the BP programme for this model was different from the case of the spontaneous ANN-PM. The inputs were dose, time-delay dose, time-delay *SAP* and time-delay *HR*, while the outputs were

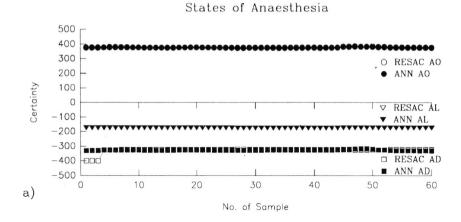

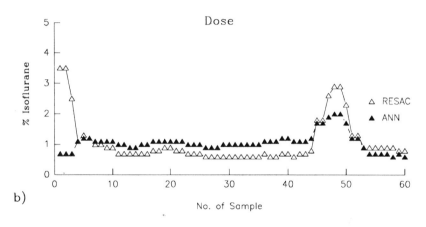

Figure 10.8 *Training of data for ventilated patient controller, (a) three states of anaesthesia and (b) percentage dosage.*

SAP and *HR*. The number of hidden units was three, the configuration of the network being shown in Figure 10.10. The data for testing were selected from another patient and results are shown in Figure 10.11. Another test was conducted by giving dosages from 2% to 1% and then to 0%. Figure 10.12 clearly shows the change in *SAP* and *HR* due to the drop in dosage.

10.4.3 Ventilated patient model via linear regression (LR-VPM)

Applying the technique of linear regression analysis, equations for *SAP* and *HR* were obtained for an LR-VPM. The same data were used for regression as in ANN-VPM. An equation for *SAP* was obtained in terms of dose, delay

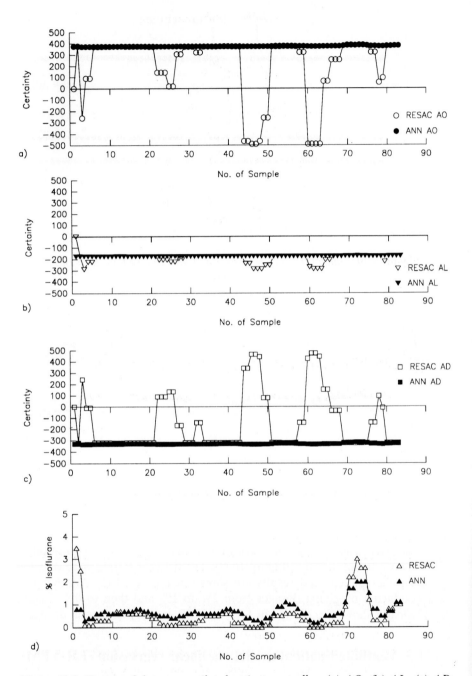

Figure 10.9 *Testing of data on ventilated patient controller, (a) AO, (b) AL, (c) AD and (d) percentage dosage.*

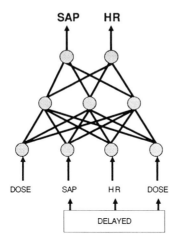

Figure 10.10 *Configuration of network for ANN ventilated patient model.*

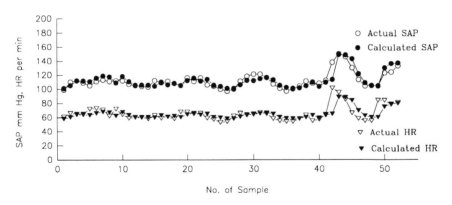

Figure 10.11 *Testing of data on ANN ventilated patient model.*

dose, delay *SAP*, *HR* and delay *HR*. For *HR* the independent variables were dose, delay dose, *SAP*, delay *SAP* and delay *HR*. After comparative studies, the constants in the regression equations were replaced by a proportion of the respective target values. As a result, the system converged to the required target values and a steady state was obtained. These proportions were adjusted so that they were almost the same as the constants in the regression equations.

The same testing data were chosen as in Figure 10.11, and the results for the test on the linear regression model are shown in Figure 10.13. The outputs of this LR-VPM are shown in Figure 10.14, when a hypothetical dose of 2% was given first and then dropped to 1% and finally to 0%, as in previous cases.

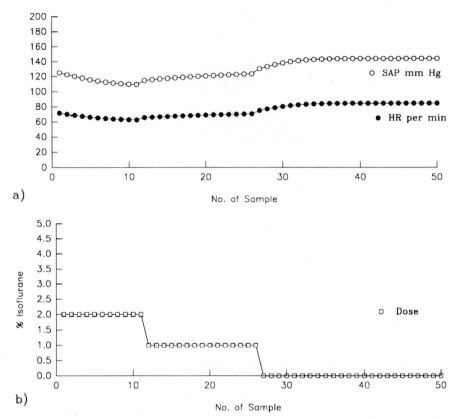

Figure 10.12 *Outputs from ANN ventilated patient model with hypothetical dose changes, (a) clinical signs and (b) dose.*

10.5 Closed-loop control

Closed-loop studies were performed by combining the controller and PM together, the patient simulator supplying clinical signs to the controller which in turn supplied the suggested doses which influenced the PM. Figure 10.15 represents the structure for closed-loop control of the controller and the PM for the spontaneous cases. The same structure was used for the ventilated series except there were no *RR* and target *RR* inputs to the controller from the PM. The tests of these two series are discussed in the following subsections.

10.5.1 Closed-loop control for spontaneous patients

The controller programme, ANNAD, was connected to ANN-PM and LR-PM respectively for closed-loop studies. The NLR controller was only

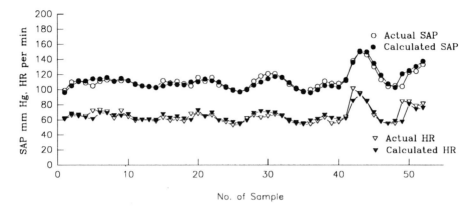

Figure 10.13 *Testing of data on ventilated patient model obtained via regression.*

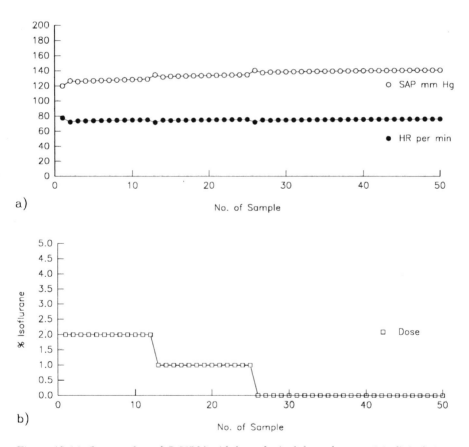

Figure 10.14 *Outputs from LR-VPM with hypothetical dose changes, (a) clinical signs and (b) dose.*

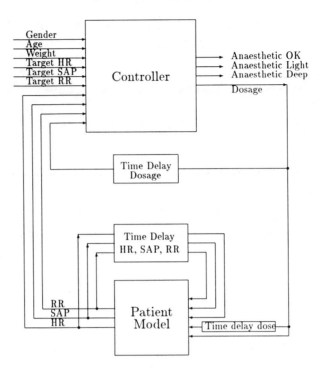

Figure 10.15 *Schematic of closed-loop control of drug controller and patient model.*

connected to the LR-PM. The same inputs were used for each combination of models, and the performance under closed-loop conditions for the three combinations is discussed.

Firstly, ANNAD was combined with ANN-PM in closed-loop. Figure 10.16 shows the three states of anaesthesia and suggested dose by ANNAD and clinical signs by ANN-PM. The overall system tended to equilibrium quickly and the values of *SAP*, *HR* and *RR* settled to their target values.

Secondly, ANNAD was connected to the LR-PM to check its compatibility. Figure 10.17 shows the three states of anaesthesia and the percentage of suggested dose together with the clinical signs supplied by the PM. The system tended to an equilibrium which depended upon target values and initial data of the patient. The transient response was very good, and slightly superior in terms of speed of convergence to the previous result.

Thirdly, the NLR controller was combined with the LR-PM, the structure of closed-loop being the same as in Figure 10.15, except that gender, age and weight were not inputs for the NLR controller. The results are shown in Figure 10.18. The values of the clinical signs changed significantly due to a high percentage of dose. In this case there were considerable oscillations in the transient response, showing inferior performance to the previous

Neural network control for unconsciousness anaesthesia

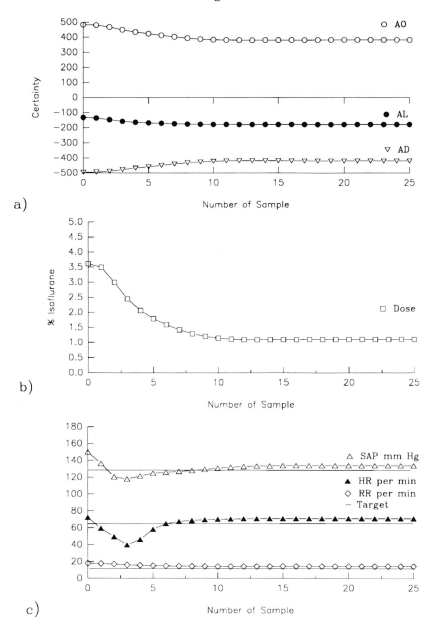

Figure 10.16 *Outputs from ANNAD and ANN-PM closed-loop control.* (a) *Three states of anaesthesia,* (b) *drug dose from ANNAD and* (c) HR, SAP *and* RR *from ANN-PM.*

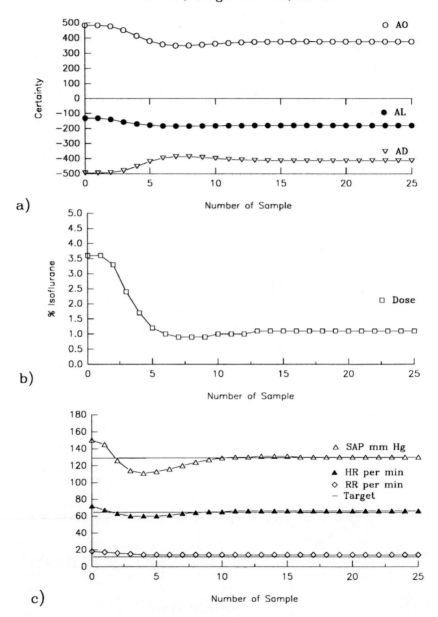

Figure 10.17 *Outputs from ANNAD and LR-PM closed-loop control. (a) Three states of anaesthesia, (b) Drug dose from ANNAD and (c) HR, SAP and RR from LR-PM.*

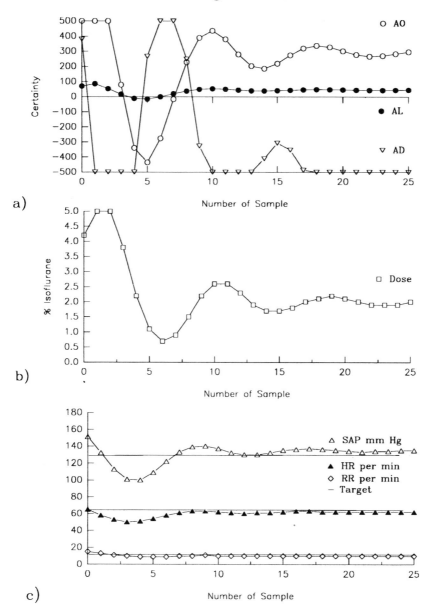

Figure 10.18 *Outputs from NLR and LR-PM closed-loop control (a) Three states of anaesthesia, (b) drug dose from NLR controller and (c) HR, SAP and RR from LR-PM.*

Table 10.2 RMSE *for* SAP, HR *and* RR

No. of Tests	SAP RMSE	HR RMSE	RR RMSE
1	9.7	8.6	5.6
2	77.2	29.1	1.0
3	60.6	14.3	2.3
4	41.6	11.5	7.2
5	42.7	9.5	6.5
6	10.4	22.4	4.7
7	39.3	13.6	3.1
8	42.7	26.0	3.2
9	72.9	73.0	3.0
10	24.6	12.2	3.1
11	49.4	7.2	8.2
12	54.3	18.2	6.5
13	18.3	16.6	2.2
14	49.0	18.9	3.2
15	17.7	3.6	4.1
16	46.6	1.8	6.5
17	29.5	10.9	3.3
18	36.3	6.6	4.6
19	74.1	71.1	1.1
20	31.7	1.0	2.9

configurations. However the performance of this combination is far better than the one discussed by Rehman *et al.* (1992).

Furthermore, the robustness of the system to parameter changes in LR-PM was also calculated by a Monte Carlo method. The coefficients of the dependent variables were randomly increased or decreased by 10% for calculating *SAP*, *HR* and *RR* within the second closed-loop system (ANNAD and LR-PM). Twenty such sets were performed each for 50 data samples. The target values for *SAP*, *HR* and *RR* were 124, 70 and 16 respectively. Root mean square errors (RMSE) were calculated for *SAP*, *HR* and *RR* compared with base-line data. The values RMSE for *SAP*, *HR* and *RR* are given in Table 10.2. The average RMSE for *SAP*, *HR* and *RR* was ±41, ±18 and ±4 respectively. The percentage error due to the parameter sensitivity was ±33% for *SAP*, ±27% for *HR* and ±25% for *RR*. Figures 10.19 and 10.20 are for tests 9 and 15 which show the results of ±10% change in the regression equations of *SAP*, *HR* and *RR*. The control of test 9 is an example of control for extremely unfavourable values whereas test 15 gave the best average results. The response of ANNAD respecting three clinical signs is also evident from Figures 10.19 and 10.20, which are predicting different dosages and states of anaesthesia.

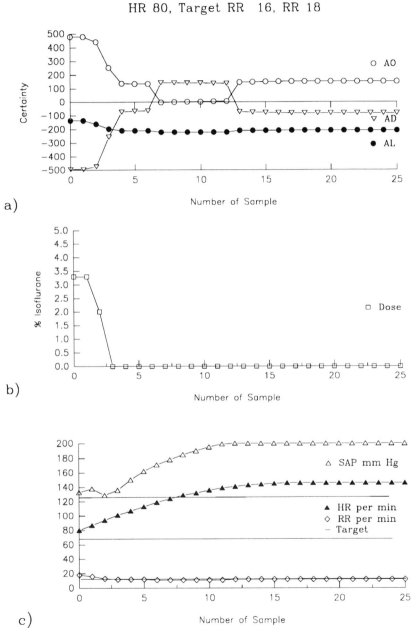

Figure 10.19 *Outputs from ANNAD and LR-PM closed-loop control for test 9 for ±10% sensitivity of LR-PM.*

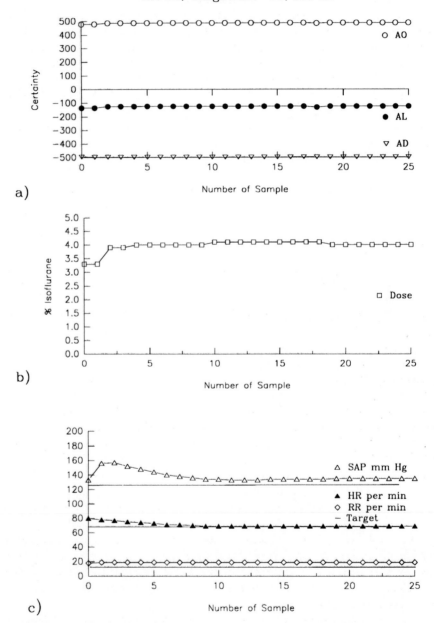

Figure 10.20 *Outputs from ANNAD and LR-PM closed-loop control for test 15 with ±10% sensitivity of LR-PM.*

10.5.2 Closed-loop control for ventilated patients

Closed-loop studies of the ANN-controller for ventilated patients coupled to the patient simulators were carried out. The results of the tests from each closed-loop are given in Figures 10.21 and 10.22. The first closed-loop structure of this series of experiments was a combination of an ANN controller and ANN-VPM, while the second closed-loop format was a combination of an ANN controller and LR-VPM. Figure 10.21 shows the results of the test when the ANN controller was connected to the ANN patient simulator. After a few samples the system tended to a steady-state equilibrium condition. The corresponding results of closed-loop control of the ANN controller with a regression patient simulator are shown in Figure 10.22. The system again tended to the set targets and settled to steady-state conditions.

In both tests of this series, the values of *SAP* and *HR* were slightly less than the desired targets. This was not always true for other tests conducted (results are not included).

10.6 Conclusions

The results demonstrate the ability of an ANN controller to replicate advice from RESAC, and also to produce good control performance obtainable when this is coupled to patient simulators.

A series of tests was carried out with each closed-loop configuration by providing data from various patients with different age, weight and sex. Also, the starting values of clinical signs and the target values during surgery, were varied. The results from all these experiments showed that for the spontaneous series the best combination is when ANNAD is connected to the LR-PM. This combination is more robust and can also work with very high target values or high clinical signs. The low sensitivity to changes in the LR-PM case also demonstrates the superiority of this combination. Although the regression controller gave inferior performance it was presented with less information than the ANN controller, thus not providing an entirely equivalent comparison.

The results from the closed-loop study of ventilated patients show almost as good performance. There were no large significant changes in the three states of anaesthesia for the test data used in this research. However, when significant changes occurred within the closed-loop simulations, AO, AL and AD varied accordingly.

The controllers have not yet been tested during surgical operations on patients. Having established good performance from an off-line simulation protocol, the next phase would be to perform clinical trials. In actual clinical trials controllers would be interfaced to work with a Dinamap blood

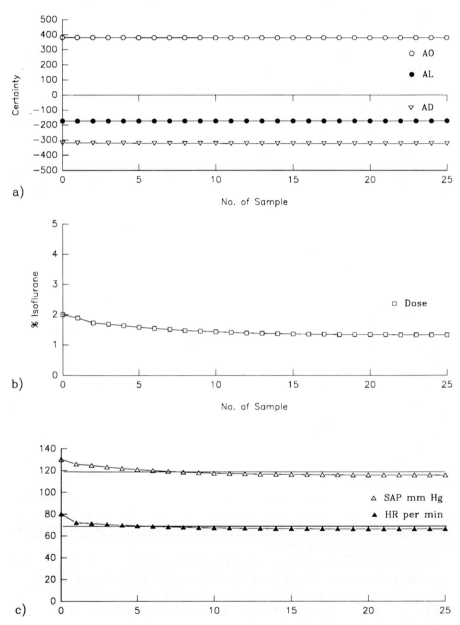

Figure 10.21 *Outputs from ANN ventilated patient controller and ANN-VPM closed-loop controller. (a) Three states of anaesthesia, (b) drug dose from ANN controller and (c) HR, SAP and RR from ANN-VPM.*

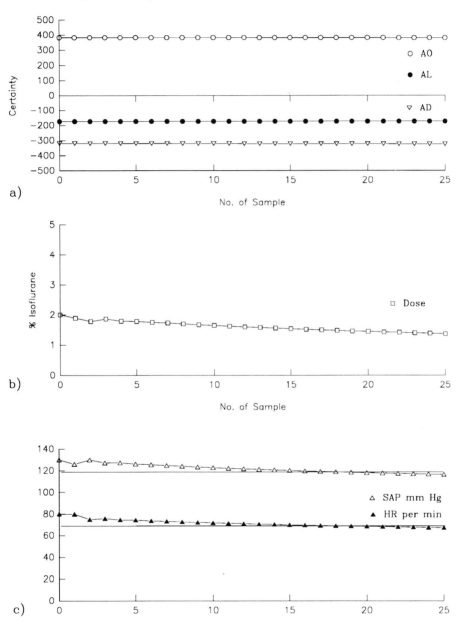

Figure 10.22 *Outputs from ANN ventilated patient controller and LR-VPM closed-loop control. (a) Three states of anaesthesia, (b) drug dose from ANN controller and (c) HR, SAP and RR from LR-VPM.*

pressure monitor and other instrumentation to supply the necessary on-line information directly. Other information, such as patient age, weight, sex, etc., would be entered interactively by an anaesthetist into the computerized system.

The overall results obtained are a foundation for further studies providing a methodology and demonstration of the ability of ANN to control depth of anaesthesia in patients in the operating theatre. The controllers and PM developed can be used in various studies for off-line simulations of this innovative technique. Further work is under progress to calculate the robustness of the control strategies to the sensitivity of the ANN-PM for both series and LR-VPM.

References

Asbury, A.J., 1991, Comments on the letter of Prof. J.M. Couto da Silva, *British Journal of Anaesthesia*, **67**, 506.
Carrie, L.E.S. and Simpson, P.J., 1988, *Understanding Anaesthesia*, 2nd Edn, pp. 1–6, London: Heinemann.
Chi, O.Z., Sommer, W. and Jasaitis, D., 1991, Power spectral analysis of EEG during sufentanil infusion in humans, *Canadian Journal of Anaesthesia*, **38**, 275–80.
Chilcoat, R.T., 1980, A review of the control of depth of anaesthesia, *Transactions of the Institute of Measurement and Control*, **2**, 38–45.
Chilcoat, R.T., Lunn, J.N. and Mapleson, W.W., 1984, Computer assistance in the control of depth of anaesthesia, *British Journal of Anaesthesia*, **56**, 1417–31.
Clark, D.L., Hosick, E.C. and Rosner, B.S., 1971, Neurophysiologic effects of different anesthetics in unconscious man, *Applied Physiology*, **31**, 884.
Dallal, G.E. and Rousseeuw, P.J., 1992, LMSMVE: A program for least median of squares regression and robust distances, *Computers and Biomedical Research*, **25**, 384–91.
Gray, W.M. and Asbury, A.J., 1986, 'Measurement and control of depth of anaesthesia in surgical patients', presentation at the 3rd IMEKO Conference on Measurement in Clinical Medicine, Edinburgh, pp. 167–72.
Greenhow, S.G., 1990, 'A knowledge based system for the control of depth of anaesthesia', PhD thesis, University of Sheffield, UK.
Kleinbaum, D.G., Kupper, L.L. and Muller, K.E., 1988, *Applied Regression Analysis and Other Multivariable Methods*, USA: PWS-KENT.
Linkens, D.A., Greenhow, S.G. and Asbury, A.J., 1986, An expert system for the control of depth of anaesthesia, *Biomedical Measurement Information and Control*, **1**, 223–8.
Linkens, D.A., Greenhow, S.G. and Asbury, A.J., 1990, 'Clinical trials with the anaesthetic expert advisor RESAC', presentation at Expert Systems in Medicine, 6th Annual Meeting, London, pp. 11–18.
Linkens, D.A. and Hacisalihzade, S.S., 1990, Computer control systems and pharmacological drug administration: a survey, *Journal of Medical Engineering and Technology*, **14**, 41–54.
Linkens, D.A. and Rehman, H.U., 1992a, 'Neural networks controller for depth of anaesthesia', presentation at the Colloquium on Applications of Neural Networks to Modelling and Control, Liverpool, UK.

Linkens, D.A. and Rehman, H.U., 1992b, 'Nonlinear control for anaesthetic depth using neural networks and regression', in Proceedings of the 1992 IEEE International Symposium on Intelligent Control, Glasgow, UK.

Mapleson, W.W., Lunn, J.N., Blewett, M.C., Khatib, M.T. and Willis, B.A., 1980, Computer assistance in the control of depth of anaesthesia, *British Journal of Anaesthesia*, **52**, 234P.

O'Callaghan, A.C., Hawes, D.W., Ross, J.A.S., White, D.C. and Wloch, R.T., 1983, Update of isoflurane during clinical anaesthesia: servo-control of liquid anaesthetic injection into a closed-circuit breathing system, *British Journal of Anaesthesia*, **55**, 1061–4.

Oswald, I., 1989, 'The physiology and pharmacology of sleep', in Nimmo, W.S. and Smith, G. (Eds), *Anaesthesia*, Vol. 1, pp. 3–9, Oxford: Blackwell.

Rampil, I.J. and Smith, N.T., 1984, Computers in anesthesiology, Saidman, L.J. and Smith, N.T. (Eds), *Monitoring in Anesthesia*, pp. 441–96, London: Butterworth.

Rehman, H.U., 1992, 'Nonlinear control for anaesthetic depth using neural networks and regression', PhD thesis, University of Sheffield, UK.

Rehman, H.U., Linkens, D.A. and Asbury, A.J., 1993, Neural networks and nonlinear modelling and control of depth of anaesthesia for spontaneously breathing and ventilated patients, *Computer Methods and Programmes in Biomedicine*, **40**, 227–47.

Robb, H.M., Asbury, A.J., Gray, W.M. and Linkens, D.A., 1988, Towards automatic control of general anaesthesia with enflurane, *British Journal of Anaesthesia*, **61**, 109P–110P.

Robb, H.M., Asbury, A.J., Gray, W.M. and Linkens, D.A., 1991, Towards a standardized anaesthetic state using enflurane and morphine, *British Journal of Anaesthesia*, **66**, 358–64.

Rumelhart, D.E., Hinton, G.E. and Williams, R.J., 1986, 'Learning internal representations by error propagation', in Rumelhart, R.E., McClelland, J.L. and The PDP Research Group, MIT (Eds), *Parallel Distributed Processing: Explorations in the Microstructure of Cognition*, Vol. 1, pp. 318–362, Cambridge, MA: MIT Press.

Schils, G.F., Sasse, F.J. and Rideout, V.C., 1983, Automated control of halothane administration—computer model and animal studies, *Anesthesiology*, **59**, A169.

Schwilden, H., Stoeckel, H. and Schuttler, J., 1989, Closed-loop feedback control of propofol anaesthesia by quantitative EEG analysis in humans, *British Journal of Anaesthesia*, **62**, 290–6.

Stoelting, R.K. and Miller, R.D., 1989, *Basics of Anesthesia*, Churchill–Livingstone.

Suppan, P., 1977, Feed-back monitoring in anaesthesia, IV: the indirect measurement of arterial pressure and its use for the control of halothane administration, *British Journal of Anaesthesia*, **49**, 141–50.

Tatnall, M.L., Morris, P. and West, P.G., 1981, Controlled anaesthesia: an approach using patient characteristics identified during uptake, *British Journal of Anaesthesia*, **53**, 1019–26.

Titel, J.H., Lowe, H.J., Elam, J.O. and Grosholz, J.R., 1968, Quantitative closed-circuit halothane anesthesia, *Anesthesia and Analgesia*, **47**, 560–9.

Vickers, M.D. and Schnieden, H., 1984, *Drugs in Anaesthesia Practice*, London: Butterworth.

Chapter 11
Genetic algorithms in the control of anaesthesia

H. Okola Nyongesa

11.1 Learning in control

In classical deterministic control theory, the design of an optimal controller for a process should always be preceded by complete knowledge of the characteristics of the process. The mathematical description of the process must be known, and all inputs and disturbances to the process are assumed to be deterministic functions of time. Any deviations from the assumed characteristics results, usually, in a deterioration in the performance of the controller. Such systems are called, *deterministic*. Later developments introduced *stochastic* control theory, to take into account the uncertainties that may be present. Thus, if all or part of the *a priori* information about the process can be described statistically, for example, in terms of probability distribution or density functions, then stochastic design techniques are used. However, if the *a priori* information is partially or completely unknown, in general, an optimal design cannot be obtained by the classical methods.

In order to design an optimal controller for a completely or partially unknown process it is, usually, necessary to gather further information about the process or to adapt to the process. In conventional adaptive control theory, on-line modelling techniques can be used to derive a model structure for the process, after which a design of a controller can be obtained based on this model. An alternative approach is to regard the control problem as a learning task, and hence, derive the parameters of a controller through learning methods. Psychologists define learning as any systematic change in a system's behaviour or performance with respect to a specified goal. The name learning in systems engineering, thus, has been used to define problems which are approached in a behavioural manner. This comprises a wide spectrum of problems from control of systems with uncertainties in their dynamics, to advanced decision-making, pattern recognition and classification problems. Learning control systems, therefore, characterize a class of systems that is much more sophisticated than conventional control systems.

Learning control represents attempts to imitate human behavioural decision-making, in defining control strategies. A learning control system is one which acquires the information necessary to control a process with unknown dynamics, by interacting with it. Learning may be performed *off-line*, in which case, the controller is said to be trainable or is 'supervised', or, *on-line*, in which case it is 'unsupervised'. Another term that is commonly used in this field is *self-organizing* control. When the learning system must actually operate in the unknown environment, then non-supervised or on-line learning schemes are the only alternative. Self-organization is a control systems theory especially developed, to treat systems with completely or partially unknown dynamics, operating in a deterministic or stochastic environment. It is characterized by the additional features of explicit or implicit identification and, on-line modelling of the unknown system. The identification and modelling provides information that is used to adjust the controller for near-optimal performance. In this respect, performance-adaptive self-organizing controllers are systems designed to drive completely or partially unknown processes using on-line 'unsupervised' learning. Such systems act to improve the performance of the controlled process, rather than identifying its structure. They function on the principle that the selection of a control action is based upon the achievement or improvement of a sub-goal, such as a per-sample performance criterion.

One of the earliest models of learning to be applied to control problems were learning automata introduced by Tsetlin (1961), to model the behaviour of biological systems. A learning automaton is a stochastic finite state machine which receives reinforcement from an interacting environment. More recently, new approaches to learning control have emerged from the use of learning techniques modelled on analogies with natural biological systems. These artificial biological systems include: the appropriately named, neural networks (NN) (Miller *et al.*, 1990), immune networks (IN) (Bersini and Varela, 1990) and genetic algorithms (GA) (Holland, 1975; Goldberg, 1989). Neural networks are an implementation of an algorithm that attempts to imitate the function of a 'biological brain'. They are composed of several nodal units called *neurons*. Neurons are usually organized in layers of which there are usually three types; one input layer, one output layer and one or more hidden layers. The output of a neuron is a non-linear function of the weighted sum of its inputs. Neurons can be used to model non-linear input–output relationships by repeated procedures through the network, until their outputs match given target values. Immune networks are very recent, and hence, there have been few studies on them. They were devised from an analogy with the immune systems of biological systems. They are characterized by differential equations that govern the quantitative changes of different types of *lymphocytes* in a fixed-size population of lymphocytes, and an algorithm for removal of certain lymphocyte types and their replacement by new types (produced in bone marrow). Each lymphocyte type represents a point in the search space. Genetic algorithms, on the other hand, are modelled on the concepts of natural evolution, and utilize such nature-imitation processes as, reproduction, crossover, mutation and deletion. All these artificial life systems are characterized by an ability to reconfigure and adapt themselves to changing environments. Immune networks and genetic algorithms, however, are evidently quite similar in nature and their adaptability relies on a constant generation of innovative solutions beyond the capabilities of the connectionist neural networks. Whereas there have been numerous reported studies on the application of neural networks in control, the study of immune networks and genetic algorithms is very recent and is only beginning to emerge. In this chapter, we shall describe the application of genetic algorithm techniques to the control of multi-variable anaesthesia processes.

11.2 Identification of the multi-variable anaesthesia model

Anaesthesia is a temporary physiological state induced by the presence of chemical (anaesthetic) agents in the body. The anaesthetic agents affect respiratory, cardiovascular, muscular and central nervous system functions. Multi-variable general anaesthesia involves the control of three functions: muscle relaxation (or paralysis), unconsciousness (also called the depth of anaesthesia) and pain (or analgesia). Paralysis is necessary, during surgical operations, to stop involuntary muscle twitches, especially during surgical operations on small and delicate organs, such as the eye or the brain. Unconsciousness is necessary to reduce body activity and remove awareness, so that the patient may have no memory of the operation. During the period of unconsciousness, although the sensation of pain is still present, the patients' reaction to it is altered so that they can tolerate levels of pain that they would otherwise not. Each of the above effects, in general, requires the use of a different drug of which there are several types available.

The anaesthesia environment is a complex and dynamic system where a large amount of data is constantly generated and displayed. Throughout the surgical procedure, the anaesthetist has to maintain the patient's vital functions stable and within normal ranges, and also keep a record of all procedures and actions taken. Maintaining a patient's functions involves monitoring several key clinical signs from the patient. The monitoring task can, thus, impose a high work load on the anaesthetist, especially during complicated operations, since multiple patient signs, measured signals and alarms must be continually checked and correlated. A computerized system working in association with anaesthetists, therefore, could enhance their performance and, the patients' safety (Ahmed *et al.*, 1990).

Identification information has been obtained in previous studies by Weatherley *et al.* (1983) for atracurium and, by Millard *et al.* (1986, 1988) for isoflurane. Drug characteristics are defined by their *pharmacokinetics* and their *pharmacodynamics*. The pharmacokinetics relate the time-profile of the drug and its metabolites in the body fluids and tissue (Godfrey, 1982). The pharmacodynamics describe the pharmacological effect of the drug. The pharmacokinetics of a drug administered via an intravascular (or intravenous) route (direct injection into the blood system) are characterized by the two phases of distribution and elimination, while those administered through extravascular routes, such as oral administration, have an additional absorption phase. Plasma concentration of the muscle relaxant drug, atracurium, after a bolus intravenous injection in the normal dose range—(0.3–0.6) mg kg^{-1}—has been observed to decline in two exponential phases (Weatherley *et al.*, 1983), which correspond to distribution and elimination of the drug. Furthermore, the distribution of the drug is represented by a 'two-compartment' model comprising: distribution in a central compartment, which is made up of the systemic blood and well-perfused tissues; and distribution in a peripheral compartment corresponding to the less well perfused tissues. Then, there is a third compartment, the effect compartment, representing drug concentration at the points where its effects are felt. Therefore, the pharmacokinetics of the drug can be represented by a 'three-compartment' model comprising the central, peripheral and effect compartments. These characteristics were also observed in an identification by Khelfa *et al.* (1988), using measurement data obtained during a surgical operation.

From the rate constants obtained in the experimental identification studies, the drug kinetics are represented by a third-order transfer

$$\frac{1.0\, e^{-s}(1 + 10.64s)}{(1 + 3.08s)(1 + 4.81s)(1 + 34.42s)}. \qquad (11.1)$$

In addition, the relationship between the dynamic effect of the drug and the concentration in the 'effect compartment' is modelled by a Hill equation:

$$E = \frac{1}{1 + (X_{50}/X_E)^\alpha} \qquad (11.2)$$

where E, is the effect of the drug, X_E is the drug concentration in the effect compartment, $\alpha = 2.98$ and $X_{50} = 0.404$.

The mode chosen for closed-loop control of the depth of anaesthesia is the cardiovascular system, that is by controlling the mean arterial blood pressure. This has been studied by, among others, (Smith et al., 1984; Gray and Asbury, 1986; Robb et al., 1988, 1991, 1993). Fukui et al. (1982) and Millard et al. (1986, 1988) have studied the control of arterial pressure in anaesthesia, although their concern was not control of the depth of anaesthesia. Automatic control via systolic or mean arterial pressure was shown by Smith et al. (1984) and Monk et al. (1989) to be as good as, and in some cases superior to, manual control by an anesthetist.

Millard et al. (1988) conducted an identification study of the pharmacokinetics and pharmacodynamics of the anaesthetic drug isoflurane on mean arterial pressure (MAP). This study used on-line identification, where step and bolus responses were determined. Off-line identification techniques, such as PRBS excitation, would be preferable, in order to obtain a more accurate model. However, it is not in general possible to apply this method during routine surgical operations, partly for ethical considerations, but also due to limitations on time and space during surgery. Off-line methods, on the other hand, have been applied in some situations, for example in the identification of muscle relaxant characteristics in dogs (Linkens et al., 1982).

In the study by Millard et al. (1988), step changes in the concentration of the inspired anaesthetic agent were applied when the patient was in a stable anaesthetic state. The results obtained showed that there is a transport delay which was observed to vary between 15–30 s. In addition, if the changes in the inhaled drug concentration are small (0–5%), the response showed linear characteristics, otherwise the response is non-linear and time-varying. The dominant time constant was of the order of 1–2 minutes. Thus, the model can be approximated by first-order linear characteristics. The gain was estimated to be 15 mmHg drop in mean arterial pressure for a 1% change in drug concentration. Therefore, the model relating the mean arterial pressure change to isoflurane drug concentration can be expressed as:

$$\frac{\Delta MAP(s)}{U(s)} = \frac{K e^{-\tau s}}{1 + Ts} \quad (11.3)$$

where $\tau = 25$ s, $K = -15$ mmHg/%, $T = 2$ min.

The simultaneous control of muscle relaxation and depth of anaesthesia is a multi-variable process, and a significant effect of the drug isoflurane on muscle relaxation has been observed (Linkens et al., 1991). An effect of the muscle relaxant drug atracurium on the heart rate and arterial pressure was also observed. These latter effects, however, are small, transient changes lasting no more than a few seconds and were not registered in all patients. Interaction of atracurium on mean arterial pressure can for this reason be ignored. Linkens *et al.* (1991) studied the effect of isoflurane on muscle relaxation, and showed it to be representable by the transfer function:

$$\frac{K_3 e^{-\tau_3 s}}{(1+T_6 s)(1+T_7 s)} \tag{11.4}$$

where $\tau_3 = 1$ min, $K_3 = 0.27$ %/%, $T_6 = 2.83$ min, $T_7 = 1.25$ min.

The above transfer functions represent the multi-variable anaesthesia model that will be used in the simulations in this chapter.

11.3 An overview of genetic algorithms

Genetic algorithms (GAs) are exploratory search and optimization procedures that were devised on the principles of natural evolution and population genetics. The basic concepts of genetic algorithms were developed by J. Holland (1973, 1975), and subsequently in several research studies. Goldberg (1989) and Davis (1990) provide comprehensive overviews and introductions to GAs.

Much of the terminology in GAs was coined by Holland and was borrowed from the field of natural population genetics. We shall begin by introducing some of the more commonly used concepts in GAs.

- A genetic structure is a coded fixed-length string of bits drawn from an alphabet, the binary alphabet being the most commonly used.
- Each position (or locus) in the string code is called a *gene*.
- The possible values of each gene are called *alleles*.
- A complete string coding is called a *genotype*. Another term used for the string is *chromosome*.
- The functional behaviour or property of a genotype is called its *phenotype*.
- A collection of genotypes is called a *population*.
- Each genotype has associated with it a *fitness* which determines its survival in the population.
- A population of strings is also called a *gene pool*.
- The process of applying genetic operators to develop better solutions is called *evolution*.

There are several differences between the functioning of GAs and the more traditional optimization techniques, especially those based on gradient methods. These differences include:

- GAs work on a coding of the parameters to be optimized, rather than the parameters themselves.
- GAs search a space using a population of trials, representing possible solutions to the problem. The initial population, usually consists of randomly generated individuals.
- GAs use an objective function assessment, to guide the search of the problem space.
- GAs use probabilistic rules to make decisions.

Typically, the GA starts with little or no knowledge of the correct solution, and depends entirely on responses from an interacting environment and its evolution operators to arrive at good solutions. By dealing with several independent points the GA samples the search space in parallel and is, hence, less susceptible to getting stuck on sub-optimal solutions. As has been stated above, the genetic algorithm processes imitate natural evolution, and include such operations as: reproduction, crossover and mutation. A simple GA has four parameters: population size, reproduction, crossover and mutation. The GA proceeds by evaluating each individual in the population, and then applying the genetic operators to generate new trials. Reproduction is a process in which a new generation of population is formed by randomly selecting strings from an existing population according to their fitness. This process results in individuals with higher fitness values obtaining more copies in the next generation, whilst low fitness individuals may have none. It is, for this reason, referred to as a *survival of the fittest* test. Crossover is the most dominant operator in a GA, responsible for producing new trial solutions. Under this operation, two strings are selected to produce new *offspring* by exchanging portions of their structures (see Figure 11.1). The offspring may then replace weaker individuals in the population. Mutation is a local operator, which is applied with a very low probability of occurrence typically, 0.001 per bit, or less. Its operation is to alter the value of a random position on a gene string. When used in this way, together with reproduction and crossover operators, mutation acts as an insurance against total loss of any bit value in a particular position, throughout the population, by its ability to introduce a value which may not have existed due to limited population size or was lost through application of the other operators. The processes of evaluation, reproduction, crossover and mutation are iterated until there is a convergence to an acceptable solution.

$Parent_1$ = 010 ! 10011
$Parent_2$ = 001 ! 01001
$Offspring_1$ = 010 01001
$Offspring_2$ = 001 10011

Figure 11.1 *A single-point crossover operator.*

11.4 Genetic algorithms in control

Genetic algorithms are blind search techniques that usually operate without knowledge of the task domain, utilizing only the fitness of evaluated individuals. Furthermore, the initial individuals are randomly generated binary bit-strings. Their direct application to control of a process could, therefore, potentially have dire consequences. However, GAs can offer substantial advantages or improvements to conventional controllers, if appropriately applied. The first, and most obvious, way to apply GAs is to use them directly to generate process control signals. The genetic coding in such a case would, for example, represent ⟨Stimulus⟩:⟨Response⟩ or ⟨Condition⟩:⟨Action⟩ production rules. This approach requires a suitable partitioning of the input space, so that there is one production rule for each partition, from which a control action can be derived. The use of this approach, however, requires substantial training, and hence the process must be capable of tolerating erroneous inputs. It has, for example, been successful in non-critical bench-mark experiments, such as cart-pole balancing (Odetayo and McGregor, 1989). The basis for fitness assignment in this case is related to the time a trial structure will hold the pole in a balanced position. The disadvantages with this approach include:

- it is dependent on the availability of *a priori* knowledge about the task environment, in order to suitably partition the input space;
- the number of different observable states defined by environment sensors can be quite large, which in turn implies that a large number of production rules may be required to achieve reasonable control;
- there is also the possibility that the actions of the GA could inflict drastic consequences on the process.

The use of a GA to directly control a process is, in general, limited because of restrictions on the nature of inputs and how poor a level of performance can be tolerated in practice.

The second method through which a GA could be used in process control is to apply the GA techniques to optimize the parameters of a conventional controller. In this case, the GA codings represent the parameters of an implementable controller, such as a PID regulator. The optimization process then consists of testing hypothetical controllers, represented by genetic codes, on a model of the process and obtaining a measure of the controller's global performance, which is then directly related to the fitness of the genetic code. Improved, plausible controllers are generated using GA reproduction and recombination operators. The resultant controller is, however, only as good as the conventional one and will suffer the same limitations. Furthermore, this method is only applicable if an accurate model of the process is available and is, in general, an off-line technique. On the other hand, the technique introduces objective criteria in optimizing the parameters of a conventional controller, and the learning phase can incorporate anticipated disturbances, such that the resultant controller will be robust with respect to these disturbances.

A third possibility is a hybrid genetic algorithm–conventional controller combination in which a conventional controller functions in its usual manner. However, the GA is operated on a supervisory level, modifying the actions of the conventional controller in order to improve the global performance. The fitness function in this case is a global observer of the controller's performance, and hence the approach affects long-term improvements. This approach has two apparent advantages:

- a GA can be coupled to an existing control system;
- the implementation ensures that the performance of the hybrid system is at least as good as the conventional controller, and where improvement is not achievable the GA can be disassociated, or at least does not modify the actions of the conventional controller.

The fourth possibility extends the hybridization method by integrating the GA within a conventional controller. This is an on-line application of GAs. This means that, instead of merely providing corrections to the actions of a conventional controller, the total control action is from the outset influenced by the GA. This approach affords the full learning capability of GAs and is more realistic than the direct method, especially when the GA-based system is incorporated in a robust controller that can moderate its behaviour, for example a fuzzy logic controller. However, its application is associated with a number of constraints:

- because the GA takes part in real-time control the individuals in a population are evaluated over a period of only one sample;
- the fitness function must provide a per-sample performance measure;
- there may be no model on which to evaluate the individuals;
- there are time constraints on the amount of processing in each sample interval.

One more possible way of implementing GAs in control is the dual controller-identifier mode, common to indirect adaptive control methods. In the identifier part, a genetic coding represents a model of the process. The fitness or viability of these trial models is based on their ability to predict future states, using given input–output data. The usual cost functions, for example least squares, can be used. In the controller part, GA chromosomes represent actual control strategies, such as the parameters of a PID controller or fuzzy control rules. To derive the control strategies, a model of the process obtained from the identifying part is used. The application of this approach, however, is hindered by the fact that GAs, in general, require a considerable amount of time to converge to a suitable solution, and hence its real-time use is limited.

In our research we have been interested in the application of GAs to on-line process control, particularly, when little *a priori* information is available about the process. In that respect, the hybridization method through which a GA is incorporated within a conventional fuzzy controller has been studied. We shall, next, briefly review the elements of a simple fuzzy controller.

11.5 Fuzzy logic control

Unlike traditional logic types, fuzzy logic aims to model the imprecise modes of human reasoning and decision making, which are essential to our ability to make rational decisions in situations of uncertainty and imprecision. This ability is dependent on the fact that human reasoning can utilize imprecise propositions and also infer imprecise consequences. Fuzzy logic was proposed by L.A. Zadeh (1965) to provide an approximate yet effective means of describing the behaviour of systems which are too complex or too ill-defined to be amenable to precise mathematical analysis. There are two reasons why classical logic systems cannot cope with inexact or incomplete information. First, they do not provide any means of representing imprecise propositions; and secondly, they do not possess a mechanism that would make an inference from such imprecise propositions (Zadeh, 1988). Fuzzy logic overcomes both these difficulties by the use of 'linguistic variables' and 'fuzzy' relations.

The fundamental concept of fuzzy logic that plays the major role in fuzzy expert systems and fuzzy controllers is the so-called linguistic variable (Zadeh, 1973). A linguistic variable is a variable whose values are expressions or words taken from a natural or constituted language. As an example, in an application to regulate temperature, 'Temperature' is a linguistic variable if the values it may take can be assigned as, 'Cold', 'Cool', 'Warm' and 'Hot'. It is immediately noticeable from this example that the values of the linguistic variable do not have a precise or 'crisp' meaning. Thus, the value of a linguistic variable represents a possibility distribution which shows the possibility of a particular deterministic value in a specified space taking that linguistic description. Thus, for example, there is a possibility that temperatures of 20 °C and 25 °C could be described as 'Cold'. Furthermore, there is a higher possibility that 20 °C is 'Cold' than that 25 °C

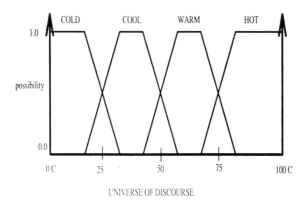

Figure 11.2 *Fuzzy linguistic variables.*

is also 'Cold'. This is commonly referred to as the linguistic value's membership function. Figure 11.2 shows the possibility distribution or membership functions of the four linguistic values of temperature mentioned above, where the specified span or universe of temperatures is between 0 and 100 °C.

11.6 Fuzzy controller applications

The development of fuzzy logic controllers owes a great deal to the work of Mamdani and coworkers (Assilian and Mamdani, 1977; King and Mamdani, 1977; Mamdani, 1974), who in an effort to devise a non-mathematical controller for a pilot-scale steam engine put to use the concepts of fuzzy reasoning, proposed by Zadeh (1965, 1973). It has long been recognized that, through practice, human beings can control many complex processes without explicit knowledge of their internal structures. The fuzzy controller attempts to elicit the subjective nature of human reasoning in order to deal with processes whose dynamics are unknown. This is obviously of considerable advantage in the control of complex and imprecise systems, as exist in many industrial and biomedical applications. The ability to cope with processes for which no mathematical model is obtainable has remained the most attractive aspect of fuzzy control. Fuzzy controllers offer clear advantages over conventional control techniques (Cellier and Alvarez, 1992).

- They can be designed with very little knowledge of the process they are supposed to control, consequently, the same controllers can be applied to different processes.

- Fuzzy controllers are less sensitive to parameter variations than conventional approaches, and hence can cope with time-varying processes.
- Because of the simplicity with which they can be designed, fuzzy controllers are also, in most cases, cheaper to implement.

Conceptually, fuzzy logic controllers are rule-based expert systems, consisting of sets rules of the form:

IF (Process_state$_1$ = Fuzzy_value$_1$) AND (Process_state$_2$ = Fuzzy_value$_2$) AND . . .
THEN (Control_action = Fuzzy_value$_M$);

where the process states are approximate or fuzzy values of some process variables. In most cases these approximate values are real process measurements that have been fuzzified. In our studies, only three process variables were used in fuzzy relations; E, the process error; CE, the change in process error; and U, an incremental change in the control signal.

Figure 11.3 shows a general configuration of a simple fuzzy logic controller. This consists of four main components: input interface, knowledge-base, inference logic and an output interface. The input interface computes values of the input state variables and performs scaling and 'fuzzification' to convert to fuzzy values in the universe of discourse. The knowledge-base is comprised of a data-base and a rule-base. The elements of a fuzzy data-base are:

(1) a universe of discourse;
(2) the fuzzy partitions (or linguistic term set);
(3) membership functions of the fuzzy variables.

Fuzzy control rules are generally specified using linguistic terms, and the fuzzy partition defines the number of elements in the term set, that is the number of distinct fuzzy sets. We have, in common with many other studies, adopted an eight-term linguistic set:

NB: negative big
NM: negative medium
NS: negative small
NZ: negative zero
PZ: positive zero
PS: positive small
PM: positive medium
PB: positive big.

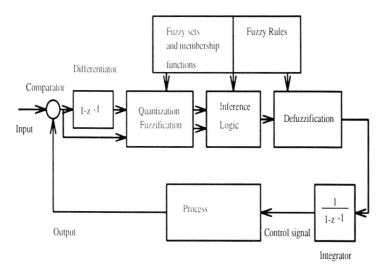

Figure 11.3 *Configuration of a simple fuzzy logic controller.*

Table 11.1 *Typical fuzzy rule-base*

E/CE	NB	NM	NS	NZ	PZ	PS	PM	PB
PB								
PM		PS					PB	
PS		PZ					PS	
PZ		NM			PZ		PM	
NZ				NZ				
NS		NS					NZ	
NM		NB					NS	
NB								

A fuzzy rule-base consists of a set of IF . . . THEN conditional statements that defines its control strategy. A typical rule-base is shown in Table 11.1. The table is interpreted as a list of rules of the form:

R_1: IF *E* is PM and *CE* is NM THEN *U* is PB;

R_2: IF *E* is PM and *CE* is PM THEN *U* is PS;

⋮

We can observe that several rules have not been included in the list. This is a typical occurrence, and is due to the fact that it is possible to infer an output from one rule for different input fuzzy subsets.

The inference logic is the decision-making component which utilizes fuzzy implication and rules of inference to derive a consequent output. This is based on the 'sup-min' compositional rules of inference proposed by Zadeh (1973). A fuzzy rule, stated as;

$$R_i: \text{IF } x \text{ is } X_i \text{ and } y \text{ is } Y_i \text{ THEN } z \text{ is } Z_i$$

is a fuzzy implication defined by a membership given by;

$$\mu_{R_i} = [\mu_{X_i} \wedge \mu_{Y_i}] \rightarrow \mu_{Z_i} \tag{11.5}$$

where x, y and z are linguistic variables representing the process state variables and control variable, and X_i, Y_i and Z_i are linguistic values of the variables, respectively. The relation is given by the Cartesian product of $X \times Y \times Z$. With given values of inputs, x and y, the consequent z is found using the compositional rule of inference as:

$$\begin{aligned}\mu_z &= (\mu_x, \mu_y) \circ \mu_R \\ &= \mu_x \circ (\mu_y \circ \mu_R) \\ &= \max[\min\{\mu_x, \max(\min(\mu_y, \mu_{R_i}))\}].\end{aligned}$$

In many control applications, a deterministic or 'crisp', rather than fuzzy, control action is required. The output interface performs defuzzification of the inferred output fuzzy sets to produce a non-fuzzy deterministic control action, and also performs scaling to values suitable for application to the controlled process. In general, one or more output fuzzy subsets are obtained from the application of each rule in the rule-base. Different defuzzification methods can be used to obtain a composite deterministic action. Among these are (Lee, 1990):

(a) the maximum criterion, which gives the point, from one rule, having the highest membership value;
(b) the mean of centres method which gives the weighted mean of the points with maximum membership values in each rule;
(c) the centre of area method which gives the centre of gravity of the distribution of output fuzzy subsets.

Although fuzzy logic controllers (or fuzzy expert systems) have been successfully applied in the control of many physical processes, the derivation of the linguistic rules has remained an intractable problem. There is no generalized method for the formulation of the fuzzy control rules and the choice of their membership functions. Hence, there is frequently a need to readjust the rules and membership functions.

Several studies have addressed techniques for automated derivation of fuzzy rules and their membership functions. The self-organizing technique introduced by Procyk and Mamdani (1979), was the first such implementation of an adaptive fuzzy technique. Adaptation in this case, was related to adjustment of the structure of the controller. Since then, several applications of this method have been reported (Daley and Gill, 1986, 1987; Hasnain, 1989; Abbod, 1992). Recently, however, there have been attempts to formulate other adaptive fuzzy techniques. In a similar manner to conventional adaptive control, fuzzy adaptive control can be put into two categories: direct fuzzy adaptive and indirect fuzzy adaptive systems.

FUZZY DIRECT ADAPTIVE SYSTEMS

Fuzzy direct adaptive systems use a fuzzy controller whose parameters can be altered on-line. The membership functions and control rules are defined in the usual way. However, either of them or both are allowed to change in response to some performance criteria. To relate this to conventional systems theory, the membership functions can be compared to the parameters of the controller, while the rules are comparable to its structure. The method of Procyk and Mamdani falls under this category. The criteria for controller adjustment in the study was a performance index, and hence, the self-organizing fuzzy controller is a performance-adaptive, rather than a parameter-adaptive controller. Another approach that is attracting interest is the technique of fuzzy self-tuning. In this approach the membership functions of the controller are adjusted, usually on the basis of an error performance index. This technique has been studied by Batur and Kasparian (1989), using an expert system supervisor to make the adjustments to membership functions. Chunyu *et al.* (1989) implemented fuzzy tuning by direct modification of a control look-up table. Look-up tables are usually derived from fuzzy control rules.

FUZZY INDIRECT ADAPTIVE SYSTEMS

In fuzzy indirect adaptive control the parameters of the process are estimated and a model of the process is derived, usually as fuzzy relations. This model is then used to derive the actual fuzzy controller parameters, as if this model were the actual process. For example in a study by Moore and Harris (1992) an intermediate process model derived from observed data is used to provide an on-line controller design. Fuzzy modelling techniques have also been reported by Linkens and Shieh (1992) and Cellier and Alvarez (1992).

In our research, we have considered a learning approach to the problem of deriving fuzzy controller structure and parameters. In this chapter, we shall present two different techniques, one off-line, and the other on-line, for automated acquisition and modification of fuzzy rules and their membership functions. Both these methods use GAs.

11.7 Fuzzy control design

Many studies have shown fuzzy logic control to be an appropriate method for the control of complex continuous, unidentified or partially identified processes (Mamdani, 1974; Assilian and Mamdani, 1977; King and Mamdani, 1977), many of which cannot easily be modelled in a mathematical way. This is because, unlike a conventional process controller such as a PID controller, no mathematical model is required in order to design a fuzzy controller and in many cases they can be implemented more easily as well. However, the simplicity with which they can be implemented also presents a bottleneck in their design. Fuzzy controllers rely on heuristic knowledge that is subject to the designer's interpretation and choice. There is to-date no generalized method for the formulation of fuzzy control strategies, and their design remains an *ad hoc* trial and error exercise.

The first step in a fuzzy design procedure is to obtain an understanding of the process' dynamics. This is necessary because it is usually not possible to design any controller without assuming certain characteristics about its environment. However, in the case of fuzzy controllers this is a less rigorous model of the process which may be expressed merely in terms of the gain sensitivity, the system delays and an estimate of the order of the system. The second stage of the design process is to define the boundaries of the fuzzy universe of discourse and the number of partitions within it. Most studies have used universes that range from ± 6 to ± 10, and partitions of between three and nine fuzzy sets (Daley and Gill, 1986; Linkens and Abbod, 1992; Procyk and Mamdani, 1979). In addition, the universes may be discrete or continuous functions. Modification of a fuzzy universe of discourse and its partitions alters the control surface and thus can be used as a means of tuning the controller. It has been argued by Daley and Gill (1986), that an even number of partitions should be used to provide control adjustment on either side of the set-point, to achieve a zero mean steady-state error. On the other hand, Cox (1992), has recently suggested that an odd number of partitions should, in general, be used. Neither of these views are strongly supported by other research studies. The GA technique uses binary coded strings which naturally define even numbers of coded parameters. Consequently, the number of partitions used in this study was chosen to be eight and the size of the fuzzy universe to be the range of ± 10.

After specifying the fuzzy universe and the partitions within, the membership functions of the fuzzy sets can then be defined. The shapes of membership functions used in most studies are continuous triangular, or Gaussian functions, although they have been discretely defined in other studies (Procyk and Mamdani, 1979; Daley and Gill, 1986; Abbod, 1992). Gaussian functions are considered suitable when the controller rule-base has very few rules (Peters *et al.*, 1992), since the function has non-zero membership grades all over the fuzzy universe. However, when the number of rules is large, Gaussian functions result in the 'firing' of several rules, some of which may be antagonistic. In this case, it is necessary to limit the number of rules which fire by defining a membership cut-off level, α-cut (Foster et al., 1992). Membership functions used in our studies were continuous triangular functions. They are simpler to use since it is only necessary to specify where the peaks of fuzzy sets are located in the universe, and how wide the fuzzy sets are. It is generally agreed that a certain amount of overlap of the fuzzy sets is desirable to provide continuous and smooth transitions on the control surface (Mizumoto, 1988). However, since the fuzzy controller is non-linear the amount of overlap and positioning of the fuzzy sets is very dependent on the process under consideration, and hence subject to tuning and modification in order to obtain the required performance.

The third stage in the design process is to decide a fuzzification and defuzzification strategy, to convert real measurements and data to the fuzzy domain and vice versa. Fuzzification and defuzzification can be viewed, in a simplified way, as choosing scaling factors for each of the predicates of a fuzzy relation. This step is critical in the design process because the scaling factors have a very profound effect on the other parameters of the fuzzy controller (Linkens and Abbod, 1992). In fact, it is usually easier to find a good set of sensible rules and membership functions to apply as a starting point in an iterative design scheme, than to find appropriate scale factors. In the fourth and final stage, the control rules are derived. This is the set of 'IF ... THEN' linguistic relations that form the expert knowledge of the controller. The usual method of obtaining these rules is a heuristic trial-and-error approach based on analysing process behaviour, and consequent iterative modification to obtain acceptable performance.

Among the problems to be resolved in fuzzy design are the determination of the linguistic state space, definition of the membership grades of each linguistic term and the derivation of the control rules. The traditional methods through which this sort of information has been gathered include interviews with experienced process operators, process knowledge experts, or other sources of domain knowledge and theory. This approach is laborious, time consuming and in most cases specific to each application. Other shortcomings that result from this approach include:

- process operators usually cannot easily translate their knowledge and experience into an algorithmic or rule-based form, necessary to convert to an automatic control strategy;
- the expert knowledge is not always available;
- multi-variable fuzzy control remains very difficult in terms of eliciting the rule-base.

Some of the problems encountered in fuzzy design can be solved by application of machine learning techniques. First, it is desirable to simplify and automate the specification of linguistic rules, their membership functions, and the scaling factors. Secondly, it is also desirable that modification of control rules or their membership functions be possible in order to cope with previously unknown or changing process dynamics. This would also have the advantage that knowledge-bases could be applied more generally, only requiring adjustments to either the rules, membership functions or scaling factors in order to be suited to a different control problem. The choice of a learning method depends on the nature of the task domain and the available information. Two types of learning methods have hitherto been used to generate rules dependent on the available information. If sufficient input–output data can be obtained then inductive learning methods are usually used (Michalski, 1983; Cellier and Alvarez, 1992). On the other hand, if extensive domain theory or expert sources of system behaviour exist then explanation-based methods are applied (Mitchell *et al.*, 1985). There are, however, situations in which none of the above information is available. An alternative method of developing rules in such cases involves testing hypothetical trials on a model of the task, or indeed the actual task itself, if it can sometimes tolerate erroneous trials. Better trials can then be evolved based on assessment of previous trials. Thus, two learning approaches can be envisaged, off-line learning, when a simulation model is available, and on-line learning, when no suitable model can be obtained. In both cases, a GA is a suitable technique to apply to automate and introduce objective criteria in defining fuzzy controller parameters. The incorporation of genetic learning into a fuzzy design process adds an 'intelligent' dimension to the fuzzy controller: the ability to create and modify its rules. GAs enable the possibility of adjusting membership functions down to the level of individual rules. This is unlike the usual knowledge-based systems in which the arguments of rules are constants or variables that have been peviously bounded, and which retain these bounds whenever the rules are used. In a GA, the rules can be allowed to develop new bounds for their individual predicates, such that the same variable may have different bounds in another rule at the same time, or in the same rule at a different time. The main considerations to be addressed include, the coding of the rule structures, their evaluation, and the evolution processes that generate improved structures.

11.8 A genetic algorithm for fuzzy control design

One of the attractions for researchers in using GAs as search and optimization techniques was that working as *blind* algorithms they could be used to find near-optimal solutions to different types of problem, without knowledge of their specific task domain, by simply manipulating bit string codes. GAs were in most of these cases applied to function optimization over real $\mathcal{R}^n$ object spaces. However, it was soon noted that the choice of a number of control parameters and even the representation itself could severely affect the performance of the GA when applied to other types of problems. Running a successful GA involves having to find settings for a number of control parameters. These control parameters include population size, the nature and rates of the recombination operators; crossover, mutation, and reproduction. A number of studies have investigated the selection of these parameters, and there have been attempts to overcome the representation difficulties by taking advantage of any available *a priori* knowledge about the task problem, and the design of specialized coding and genetic operators (Caruana and Schaffer, 1988; Schraudolph and Belew, 1992; Grefenstette, 1986). Indeed, it has been demonstrated in many studies that a specially adapted GA will out-perform other GAs on the specific problem. Specialized genetic plans are derived by controlling the rates of the tripartite processes; reproduction, crossover and mutation. Hence, it is desirable to adapt some of the more common GA techniques with a view to deriving a genetic plan suited for fuzzy learning. By 'genetic plan' is meant the processes through which successive populations are generated using evaluation, selection, mating and deletion. In the following we discuss the factors which will influence a GA for fuzzy design.

11.8.1. Coding the genetic algorithm

The type of coding used in this research is the classical *concatenated binary mapping*. This coding joins together segment codes of all parameters into one composite string. The genetic structure of a fuzzy rule is made up of the codings of the fuzzy sets of the linguistic predicates of the rule. Furthermore, a linguistic variable is definable by its membership function which, in the case of the chosen triangular shape, is determined by the position of its peak and the spread of its non-zero grades. Therefore, each fuzzy set in a rule has three parameters that are coded: its linguistic value (or name), the peak and the width of the set.

The coding of a fuzzy rule was contained within the basic data structure of the computer hardware used, which is 32 bits. This simplified the manipulation of the codes. Eight linguistic values, namely, {NB, NM, NS, NZ, PZ, PS, PM, PB}, were specified and hence the rule-base consisted of a maximum of 64 rules. By representing the total coding for the rule-base in the usual form of a two-dimensional table, the coding for the rule premises, *E* and *CE*, can be made implicit by the positions of rules in the table. Therefore, coding is only required for the peaks and the widths of the fuzzy sets and the linguistic value of the rule consequences. For each fuzzy rule, three bits were used to code the linguistic value of the rule consequence. In

Table 11.2 *Typical coding format of a fuzzy rule*

Bits	Parameter
Bit 1	Tag-rule used or not
Bit 2–5	Width of E
Bit 6–10	Peak of E
Bit 11–14	Width of CE
Bit 15–19	Peak of CE
Bit 20–23	Width of U
Bit 24–28	Peak of U
Bit 29–31	Linguistic value of U

addition, to determine whether a rule was applicable in a rule-base or not, a one-bit tag was used, which leaves 29 bits, out of the 32, for coding the peaks and widths of the three fuzzy sets, E, CE and U. Nine bits were thus allocated to each fuzzy set. Since a fuzzy controller's performance is less sensitive to small differences in the widths of fuzzy sets than to differences in the peak positions, more bits were allocated to the coding of the peaks. The coding format used is shown in Table 11.2. The code segments are subscripted l, w, p standing for linguistic value, width of fuzzy set and position of the peak, respectively. This coding was replicated for each rule in the rule-base. A typical representation of a rule within the data structure is shown in Figure 11.4. A complete control strategy for the multi-variable anaesthesia process consisted of three separate, decomposed rule-bases; one rule-base for the control of a single-variable MAP process and two rule-bases for the multi-variable muscle relaxation process. Each rule-base is also associated with another coding for scale factors. Hence, the three rule-bases were coded in a concatenation of 3×65 rule codes. A non-decomposed strategy, using the traditional approach, would have to deal with a possible 8^4 (4096) rules.

The coding of each attribute represents a value between predetermined minimum and maximum constraints, given by:

$$\lambda_i = \lambda_{\min} + \frac{\lambda_{\max} - \lambda_{\min}}{2^l - 1} \mathcal{R}(\chi) \tag{11.6}$$

where $\lambda_{\min}$ is the minimum parameter constraint, $\lambda_{\max}$ is the maximum parameter constraint, λ_i is the parameter value of the code, χ is the binary code, l is the length of the parameter code, and $\mathcal{R}$ stands for the real number equivalent of the code segment which is given by,

$$\left(\sum_{j=1}^{l} a_j 2^{j-1} \right) \tag{11.7}$$

where a_j are the code bits, numbered from the least significant.

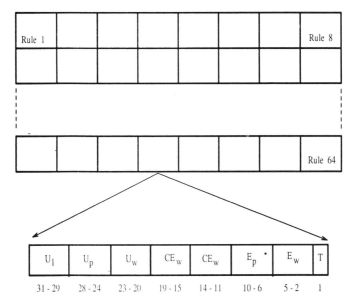

Figure 11.4 *Typical coding of fuzzy rule-base.*

11.8.2 Evaluation of trials

Each genotype in the population is a hypothetical knowledge-base for a fuzzy logic controller, containing a complete set of linguistic rules, their membership functions and a fuzzification/defuzzification strategy. The process of evaluating these knowledge-bases consists of submitting each to a simulation model, and returning an assessment value according to a given cost function. As an example, a test knowledge-base is made to control the model of the process for a pre-determined number of samples, and sums up errors over the response trajectory. The sum of errors is then directly related to the trial's objective fitness. The fitness of a trial is a measure of the overall worth of a solution which takes into account factors of an objective criterion, in this case, the performance of a controller implementable with the trial knowledge-base. The basic control objective is simply stated as its ability to follow a set-point with minimal error. The objective can thus be expressed in terms of minimization of controller performance indices in common use. These include: integral of absolute errors (IAE), integral of square errors (ISE) and integral of time multiplied by absolute errors (ITAE). Each of these indices has its own merits. For example, ITAE penalizes errors at large values of time and leads to reduction in steady-state errors at the expense of transient errors, while ISE is a criterion more suited to mathematical analysis. In our case it was found necessary to incorporate a penalty of excessive control effort into the evaluation cost function. The

GA, being a blind technique, is only able to optimize the characteristics explicit in the cost function. Thus, an index integral of absolute errors and control effort (IAECE), was derived:

$$J_1 = \Sigma(|(y(k) - r(k))| + |(u(k) - u(k-1))|) \qquad (11.8)$$

where $y(k)$ is the process output, $r(k)$ the reference input, and $u(k)$ the control signal, at sampling instant k, respectively.

11.8.3 Evolution process

In learning applications, as opposed to function optimization, one may not necessarily be interested in finding optimal solutions to problems. This is because, in most cases, the global optimal solution will not even be known. Hence, the GA can be used as a learning heuristic that finds good knowledge structures quickly which may, or may not, be global optima as well (DeJong, 1992). In order to improve the performance of a GA there is a need to maintain a balance between exploration and exploitation of the search space. Exploration is related to the number of new trials carried out while exploitation is related to the number of good candidates retained in a population to produce future offspring. An appropriate selection of the various genetic operators forms a suitable genetic or evolution plan.

A genetic plan can be defined as quintuple $\{P,R,C,M,F\}$, where P is the population size, R, C and M are the reproduction, crossover and mutation operators, respectively, and F is the fitness re-scaling technique. The choice of an appropriate population size is a fundamental decision to be taken in all GA implementations. If the population size is too small the GA will usually converge too quickly, and in many cases to a poor solution due to insufficient information in the population. Too large a population, on the other hand, will take a very long time to evaluate, and in addition result in slow progression towards its final solution. Furthermore, when the evaluation of a trial structure is computationally expensive, there is a need to impose a limitation on the size of population that the GA can reasonably support. This means obtaining a balance between the requirement for a large information capacity in the population and the need to produce a solution within a limited amount of time.

The most common evolution techniques are: generational replacement, generational gap and steady-state. By evolution, we mean the processes of producing new genetic trials that may be different from their parents. Generational replacement replaces the entire population with new offspring, while the generational gap method replaces a proportion of the population, called the generation gap. The steady-state method, on the other hand, introduces only one or two new offspring into the population. In addition, we studied another evolution technique, called selective breeding. As suggested by the name, this technique was meant to select deterministically which new offspring can become members of a new generation. Selective breeding could control which individuals enter or die from the population and, hence, reduce sampling errors. The scheme uses a replacement method in which the worst members of the population are replaced by offspring only if the offspring are better.

Traditionally, the number of crossover points used in a genetic algorithm, which determines the number of segments of the parent codes that are exchanged, has been set to 1. However, there have been experimental studies which have suggested the use of more crossovers and higher rates of mutation (Syswerda, 1989; Muhlenbein, 1992). Crossover and mutation in context-sensitive structures, do require careful application to avoid generating obviously unsuitable trials. It is also prudent to consider the use of knowledge-based genetic operators. For example, exchanging the linguistic values of different fuzzy rules could mean that the new offspring acquire membership functions that are obviously not suitable for them. Similarly, since the linguistic codes identify the premises of rules, mutation and crossover within these codes will create new premises that are merely duplicates of other rules. Hence, crossover was restricted to rules with the same goals, while mutation resulted in new fuzzy sets in the same 'neighbourhood'.

11.9 A real-time genetic algorithm for fuzzy control

Despite the blind nature of genetic search techniques, there are circumstances when the GA could be applied on-line and in real-time. Such circumstances include the following (Renders and Haus, 1992).

(a) A process model is available and the time interval between samples is long enough to allow processing of the GA to convergence. Convergence of the GA or the attainment of optimal solutions are, usually, not preconditions in this sort of problem, and it may be possible that a rapidly converging evolution scheme can be devised which produces a 'good enough' solution within a very short time. Another way this approach could feasibly be implemented is on massively parallel computer systems using, for example, one chromosome per processor (Manderick and Spiessens, 1989), which reduces the time taken to evaluate each trial.

(b) A GA is used for on-line adaptation of a 'well designed' controller. A typical example is when an off-line learning method has been used to derive the rules and membership functions of a fuzzy controller and, subsequently, an on-line GA is used to alter the rules and/or membership functions. The purpose of this sort of application would

(c) A GA is used with little or no knowledge about the process. The feasibility of this application, however, is limited by the fact that GAs are blind search processes that could inflict drastic consequences on a controlled environment. However, GAs can be applied to advantage within an expert environment that can moderate the direct actions of a GA. In the rare circumstances when the process can endure sometimes erroneous inputs, direct application of the GA may be feasible. Such processes are, admittedly, very unusual in practice.

In function optimization problems, a cost function is available which is used to evaluate the trial solution. Similarly, in off-line control applications where a model of the process is available, evaluation involves having a hypothetical controller represented by a genetic code, controlling the model of the process for a specified time and then obtaining a measure of the global performance. In applying the GA to the on-line control of an unmodelled dynamic process there are a number of constraints which arise.

(1) There is no objective function assessment available by which to rate the fitness of each individual, and hence the system may have to rely sometimes on a noisy performance feedback, from an unknown environment;
(2) The GA must provide an appropriate control action at each sample instant. What this means is that it is neither possible nor desirable to have a specific individual control the process for a length of time.
(3) There is a limitation on the amount of computation that can be done between sampling instants. This hinders the possibility of developing a model, on-line on which to evaluate the chromosomes.

In this latter case, a preferable course of action is an incremental GA, in which only one chromosome from a population is evaluated in each time interval (Fogarty, 1989). The other chromosomes in the population are then evaluated in successive time intervals. Another alternative approach is to evaluate only one chromosome from the population in each generation, and the evaluation of the rest of the population is then estimated based on this one evaluation. In our studies the method of estimating fitness was used.

An incremental genetic algorithm (IGA) overcomes some difficulties experienced with evaluating a population of different trials in real-time. Firstly, it is not possible to evaluate every individual from the same initial conditions of the process, since the process is always moved to a new state in each sample interval. This means that any fitness assignment function would have to take into account the characteristics of the response trajectory. Such a function would be very difficult to formulate. How, for example, would we rate a chromosome that adequately holds the process output at the equilibrium level, against one that drove the output to that state in the first place? The IGA, implemented in this research, thus begins with a population in which all individuals are assigned equal fitness. Notice that, in the usual GA, the fitness of an individual is a result of an objective cost function assessment. In each time-interval, an individual is selected from the population on the basis of its fitness and its suggested action is applied to the process environment. In order to estimate the fitness of the rest of the population, credit assignment, which is a reward–punishment algorithm, is subsequently applied to the whole population when a performance feedback is received from the environment. All individuals in the population are matched against the evaluated chromosome, which is assumed responsible for the current performance feedback from the interacting environment, and the amount of reward or punishment given to each then depends on the degree of this matching. The selection criteria, through which individuals are chosen to be applied to the environment or to be recombined, also involves a matching process to determine how selected individuals are related to current environmental conditions. This ensures that only the most suitable chromosomes are selected, otherwise, the learning process could severely disrupt the on-line controller behaviour. Hence, selection is a sort of bidding process where the amount each individual bids in order to be selected is related to its fitness and the degree to which it matches the environment's states. Winning individuals are chosen, probabilistically, on the basis of the highest bids. Similarly, the GA reproduction and recombination operators select individuals which are closely matched to the environment states, and newly formed offspring only replace those parents similar to them. On the other hand, this ensures that the population does not become dominated by a few specialized individuals who happen to have high fitness at that moment, thereby forgetting previously rehearsed situations or situations that are yet to be encountered.

The majority of studies and applications of GAs have been on search, function optimization and sequential learning tasks. This is not very surprising. Search and optimization problems are usually well defined with objective functions, constraints and decision variables, and hence provide a tame environment for any optimization technique. By contrast, machine learning problems have ill-defined goals, subjective evaluation criteria and numerous decision options. While the application of GAs in search and optimization has both tested and improved their use, it should be noted that the objective of pioneering GA research was to gain an abstraction of the adaptive learning mechanisms exhibited by natural systems and, consequently, to design artificial autonomous learning and decision-making systems. This type of learning system is, generally, referred to as a genetic-based machine learning (GBML) system, an example of which is a classifier system

(Goldberg, 1989; Holland, 1986). Classifier systems (CSs) are general purpose machine-learning systems that use GAs to learn simple rules which guide their performance in an arbitrary environment. Classifiers are in Condition/Action form. The conditions part specifies what kinds of messages activate the rule, and the action specifies what message is sent out when the condition part is satisfied. They can be programmed, initially, to implement whatever expert knowledge is available to the designer; learning then permits the system to expand and improve its performance (Booker et al., 1989). CSs have many similarities with rule-based expert systems, and in particular fuzzy systems, but with the following differences.

(a) CSs maintain several competing rules, called classifiers.
(b) Several classifiers can be active at the same time. There is no conflict between active classifiers because their only function is to post their actions onto a global list of messages. This concurrency avoids difficult conflict-resolution problems which arise in one-rule-at-a-time systems.
(c) The relative ratings of competing classifiers is evaluated during the learning process through competition and credit assignment.

The main elements of a CS are: a rule-message component, a GA and a credit assignment algorithm. There are, in addition, input and output interfaces that are used for interacting with external environments. A rule or classifier is a finite length string over an alphabet, consisting of an arbitrary number of conditions and one action. A message on the other hand is a string of the same length as the condition part of a classifier, and whose purpose is to test the matching of classifier conditions. Conditions, in general, are defined over the alphabet $\{0, 1, \#\}$ while messages and actions are defined over $\{0, 1\}$, where $\#$ in a condition matches both 0 and 1, and hence, can be used to generalize rules. A condition is, thus, a subset of all possible messages, and a classifier is satisfied when the tested message belongs to that subset. A satisifed classifier gets the chance to compete for reproduction or to affect its action. The actions of classifiers can also be passed on as messages that are matched against other classifiers. This is common in cases where long chains of rules are processed before there is any performance feedback from the environment, such as in game play systems. Credit assignment is the process of apportioning reward or punishment to classifiers that were activated during previous cycles, and which are responsible for the present performance measure. To effect this, each classifier in a population has associated with it a strength or fitness, which is adjusted by the credit assignment algorithm. In many classifier systems, this is achieved with the so-called *bucket brigade* algorithm (Goldberg, 1989; Riolo, 1988a, 1988b), which is a model of a competitive service economy in which classifiers compete for selection by making bids.

The amount bid by a classifier is proportional to its fitness and the degree to which it matches the input messages. The amount a classifier bids is subtracted from its fitness if it wins the bidding process. On the other hand, classifiers that send internal messages that are later matched by a winning classifier share out its bid. In a simpler case of credit assignment, where there are no sequences of messages posted by classifiers, and reward is received directly from the environment at each sample instant, those classifiers responsible for the environment pay-off have their fitness increased, or decreased, at each crediting instance. The fitness of a classifier is important in determining the competitiveness of a classifier when it bids, first, for a chance to effect its action, and secondly, to participate in the reproduction and recombination processes. These selection stages determine the short-term and long-term behaviour of the classifier system, respectively.

11.10 A fuzzy classifier system (FCS)

A fuzzy classifier system (FCS) is a classifier system which combines fuzzy reasoning and genetic learning techniques. This approach as stated earlier on, would ensure that the actions of the GA can be moderated by the fuzzy expert system. In general, classifiers in a fuzzy classifier system represent the usual fuzzy conditional statements. Each classifier is a binary string that encodes the rules and membership functions of fuzzy relations. However, unlike the usual fuzzy expert systems where there are only single rules for each set of input conditions, FCSs contain populations of similar and competing rules. A GA operates on the populations to develop better rules, using fitness values obtained with a credit assignment algorithm. Figure 11.5 shows a typical configuration of a fuzzy classifier system.

The task of acquiring fuzzy control rules is the main function of the FCS. The FCS functions by partitioning the input space, as does the usual fuzzy system. However, the number and forms of the partitioning are very much dependent on the process under consideration, and hence are a matter for learning algorithms. Thus, for every instance of environment messages, the FCS checks to find if there exist rules that can adequately handle the current conditions. If no adequate rule exists, then one or more can be created by generating populations of representative, plausible classifiers. It is easy to see that in this sort of situation it is not possible to maintain a single or fixed-size population of classifiers without having *a priori* information about the number of different partitions of the input space. FCS, therefore, maintains separate sub-populations for each category of input message that is encountered. These separate sub-populations, however, also simplify processing within the FCS since it becomes easier, for example, to determine which sub-populations are relevant to a particular set of environment messages. Hence, only those sub-populations that are relevant

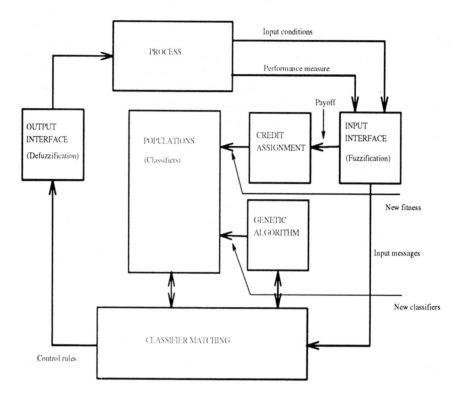

Figure 11.5 *Configurations of a fuzzy classifier system.*

to particular conditions are processed, instead of dealing with a very large population. Furthermore, any sub-population which becomes irrelevant to new environment states can be left undisturbed to preserve the learned information contained within it.

The determination of whether or not to create a new population of classifiers is based on matching the environment messages to the existing rules. If the degree of match to all existing populations falls below a pre-determined level, it means that the current rules are not adequate and, hence, a new population of classifiers ought to be created. Creation of a new population of rules involves determining the possible linguistic classes of the input messages, which then form part of the classifier conditions. Consequently, all categories of linguistic classes that are matched above another pre-determined level are used as a basis for the new populations of plausible rules. For example, new rule populations are created if the degree of matching to all existing populations dropped to below 0.5. When this happens, all linguistic classes which matched the input messages to a degree greater than 0.25 are used as the basis for new rule populations.

In these studies, initial populations in the FCS were seeded with simple heuristic rules, which were obtained by partitioning the fuzzy input space into a few regions of predictable behaviour. For example, it is predictable that if the output response is rapidly moving away from the desired set-point, then a large reversal control action ought to be applied. Similarly, if the response happens to be stable at the set-point then no further action needs to be taken. These rules are considered to represent minimal expert knowledge for control of a process. They are very general in nature, and do not relate to any *a priori* information about the process.

11.10.1 Performance assessment in FCS

A performance-adaptive learning controller, in order to improve its performance needs information as to how well it is performing at each instant. Performance assessment is the process through which the classifiers in FCS can be evaluated. Two types of performance measure are, in general, available. On one hand, a global criterion, such as integral of square errors (ISE), measures the overall performance of the controller over a complete response trajectory: in most cases a global criterion, can only be used as an off-line learning performance measure. A local criterion, on the other hand, measures the performance of the controller over a neighbourhood of only a few process states, and can be available at each sample interval. This type of criterion would be preferable when using an IGA, because it links credit assignment to individual actions. Unfortunately, local performance measures that can provide more information than binary (i.e. 'good' or 'bad') indications are difficult to formulate.

The primary objective of a controller is to achieve rapid transient response with minimal overshoots and small steady-state errors. At the same time, in an on-line application we only need to improve the system's behaviour over the interval Δt leading to the next decision point. A performance measure (e.g. IAE, ISE and ITAE) can be expressed in terms of minimization of a general integral function:

$$I = \sum_{k=0}^{n} \int_{t_k}^{t_k + \Delta t} \mathcal{F} \, dt \tag{11.9}$$

where $\mathcal{F}$ is usually an error function, Δt is the sample interval and n the number of samples. It can be shown that minimization of the sum of the integral functions is equivalent to minimization of the integral functions. This means that the performance objective can then be defined in terms of achieving the greatest possible descent towards the equilibrium state of the error function in each time interval. Furthermore, in order to avoid undesirable overshoots, it is necessary to predict future errors so that corrective action is taken in advance. Thus, the form of the integrand $\mathcal{F}$

which was used is given by $\mathscr{F} = |e_p|$, where e_p is a predicted error function. Accordingly, minimization of the integral function requires that:

$$\frac{d^N}{dt^N}|e_p| < 0 \qquad (11.10)$$

where N is the order of the highest derivative of the predicted error function.

A binary performance measure, P_0, which is based only on the polarity of the error signals, can be derived from the above expression as:

$$P_0 = \text{NOT}\left(\text{sign}\frac{d^N}{dt^N}|e_p|\right) \qquad (11.11)$$

where P_0 equal to logical 1 is an acceptable performance and P_0 equal to logical 0 is an unacceptable performance. In this case, positive sign of error signals (above the set-point) is logical 1, and positive sign of error-change (increasing error rate) is also logical 1. If the order of the highest derivatives is approximated to be 2, an equivalent Boolean formulation to Equation (11.11) is given by:

$$P_0 = \text{sign}(e_p)\overline{\text{sign}(\dot{e}_p)}\,\text{sign}(\ddot{e}_p) + \overline{\text{sign}(e_p)}\,\text{sign}(\dot{e}_p)\overline{\text{sign}(\ddot{e}_p)}. \qquad (11.12)$$

A simple expression for the predicted error function is given by:

$$e_p = e + T\dot{e} \qquad (11.13)$$

where T (>1.0) is the number of intervals predicted ahead.

11.10.2 Credit assignment in FCSs

There are two functions to be performed by a GA in a fuzzy classifier system: firstly, the rating of competing rules and, secondly, the discovery of new rules. Each rule has an associated *fitness* that is a measure of the rule's usefulness in achieving a system goal. The rating of a rule's usefulness is carried out through credit assignment, a reward–penalty algorithm that uses the external performance feedback from the interacting environment to assign new fitnesses to competing rules. Hence, classifiers which result in a 'positive' feedback are rewarded by increasing their strengths, while those leading to 'negative' feedback are punished by decreasing their strengths. The amount of reward (or punishment) also depends on the degree to which each classifier matches the environment states.

The success of fuzzy control in complex processes is partly due to the fact that control actions can be inferred from several parallel rules. Similarly in the FCS several classifiers are chosen, in this case one from each matched sub-population, which are used to compose the actual control action to the process environment. Selected classifiers are decoded into representative fuzzy sets and, subsequently, the 'mean-of-centres' or the 'centre-of-areas' defuzzification method can be used to obtain a deterministic output. Therefore, during credit assignment classifiers are rewarded or punished depending on their degree of matching the environment conditions and also their relation to the actual control action taken. The credit assignment process proceeds as outlined below.

- IF the Performance assessment is Good, AND the Control action was an Increment, THEN Reward those classifiers whose fuzzy actions are Greater or equal to the control action taken, and punish those whose actions are less.
- IF the Performance assessment is Good, AND the Control action was a Decrement, THEN Reward those classifiers whose fuzzy actions are Less than or equal to the control action taken, and punish those whose actions are greater.
- IF the Performance assessment is Bad, AND the Control action was an Increment, THEN Reward those classifiers whose fuzzy actions are Less than the control action taken, and punish those whose actions are greater or equal.
- IF the Performance assessment is Bad, AND the Control action was a Decrement, THEN Reward those classifiers whose fuzzy actions are Greater than the control action taken, and punish those whose actions are less or equal.

To achieve stability and convergence in fitness levels, that is to prevent run-away increments or decrements in fitness, reward and punishment are effected by classifiers receiving bonuses and also paying taxes, as defined in the bucket brigade algorithm. A rewarded classifier receives more bonus than the tax it pays, and conversely, a punished classifier pays more tax than the bonus it receives. Furthermore, the tax paid is proportional to an individual's fitness. Hence, if τ is a tax-rate and $\mathscr{B}$ the amount of bonus received, a classifier's fitness is adjusted according to the equation:

$$\mathscr{S}_{(nt+1)} = (1-\tau)\mathscr{S}_{nt} + \mathscr{B}. \tag{11.14}$$

However, the actual amount of reward or punishment received, as previously mentioned, is proportional to a degree of matching. Terminal fitness is reached when the bonus an individual receives is equal to the tax paid out, and is given by,

$$\mathscr{S}_{\infty} = \frac{\mathscr{B}}{\tau}. \tag{11.15}$$

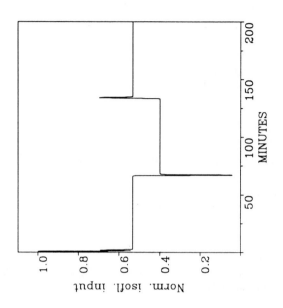
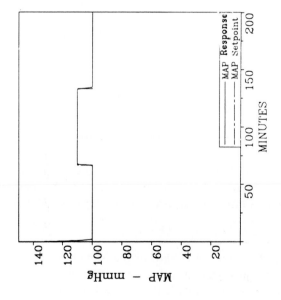

(a): MAP response

Genetic algorithms in the control of anaesthesia 353

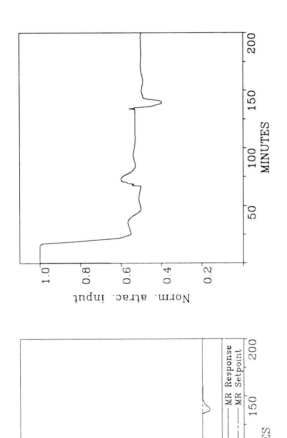

(b): MR response, showing
interactions from MAP

Figure 11.6 *Off-line fuzzy controller design.*

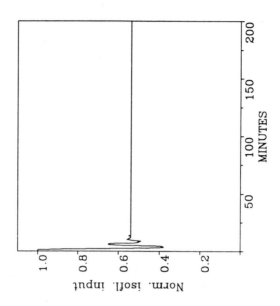

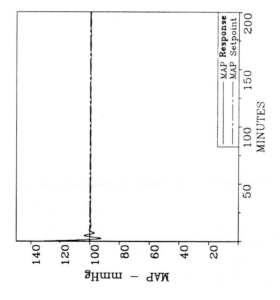

(a): MAP response

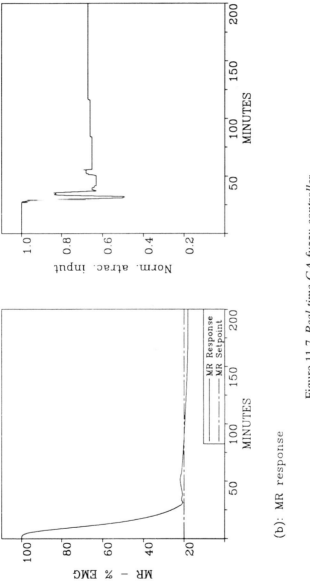

(b): MR response

Figure 11.7 *Real-time GA-fuzzy controller.*

11.11 Learning simulation results

In this section, we shall present the results from the implementation of the GAs to the problem of fuzzy control design when a model is available, and also the use of a fuzzy classifier system for on-line control and acquisition of fuzzy control rules. The simulation studies were carried out using the multi-variable anaesthesia process, presented in Section 11.2. In the on-line method, this model was only used to represent the dynamics of the controlled process and hence was not available to the classifier system. The experiments were conducted on an ATARI ATW 800 platform, which uses T800 transputers, and simulation programs were written in the 'C' programming language.

Figure 11.6 shows the results of simulated control using rules learned in the off-line optimization. These results show a good transient and steady-state performance by the resultant controller. However, the limitation of this method was that it could only respond satisfactorily to conditions for which the controller was trained. In order to cope with different initial conditions and changes in set-points, the controller had to be trained using several initial conditions.

Figure 11.7 shows the results of real-time control using the fuzzy classifier system. The FCS was initialized with a certain amount of expert knowledge. This is because, when no form of initial knowledge is available and there is no model on which to evaluate the initial random classifiers, it is not possible to operate the genetic-based classifier system in real-time. An application which does not start with any knowledge would have to be preceded by a long period of on-line training that may be intolerable in certain circumstances. However, the requisite initial knowledge is very general in nature, and does not relate to any particular process. It is observed that the FCS achieves satisfactory control of the process, which, however, is characterized by a steady-state error. This is partly due to convergence of the populations on non-optimal rules, and also due to the fact that the performance measure used is binary and does not incorporate any mechanism for detecting and compensating the steady-state errors.

11.12 Summary and conclusion

Our research is centred on the use of genetic algorithms for fuzzy logic control of anaesthesia. In this chapter we have outlined an implementation of fuzzy controller design, using a model obtained in previous identification studies. This was a training procedure that optimizes the parameters of the controller in order to respond appropriately to the given training conditions. The limitation of such off-line methods is that the system only learns to respond to conditions for which it was trained and will suffer substantial deterioration if it encounters new conditions. In real-world applications, however, the inputs and conditions to which the system may be subjected cannot be predicted in advance. To cope with this, we have investigated a new approach to real-time learning, using a rule-acquiring system called a fuzzy classifier system. This is a system which is able to generate fuzzy control rules without explicit knowledge of the dynamics of the process. It uses a genetic algorithm to improve and tune the rules that are created.

It has been demonstrated in the two types of implementation considered that acceptable performance of the learning controller is achievable without the burden of following a detailed control design strategy. The contribution of this particular study has been to demonstrate the integration of expert knowledge-based systems, such as fuzzy controllers, into genetic-based classifier systems to produce a hybrid, rule-acquisition, fuzzy control system. This scheme was implemented for the control of a practical problem of moderate complexity, being the control of a multi-variable anaesthesia process. While we consider the experimental results with fuzzy classifiers to be preliminary, there is a clear indication that utility of fuzzy expert systems can be improved by learning techniques.

References

Abbod, M.F., 1992, 'Supervisory intelligent control for industrial and medical systems', PhD dissertation, Department of Automatic Control and Systems Engineering, University of Sheffield.

Ahmed, F., Nevo, I. and Guez, A., 1990, 'Anaesthesiologist adaptive associate', presentation at the Annual International Conference of the IEEE Engineering in Medicine and Biology Society, Vol. 12, No. 3.

Assilian, S. and Mamdani, E.H., 1977, An experiment in linguistic synthesis with a fuzzy logic controller, *International Journal of Man Machine Studies*, 7, 1–13.

Batur, C. and Kasparian, V., 1989, 'A real-time fuzzy self-tuning control', in Proceedings 1989 American Control Conference, pp. 1810–5.

Bersini, H. and Varela, F.J., 1990, 'Hints for adaptive problem solving gleaned from immune networks', in Schwefel, H.-P. and Manner, R. (Eds), Proceedings of the First Workshop on Parallel Problem Solving from Nature, Dortmund, West Germany, pp. 343–53, Berlin: Springer.

Bersini, H. and Varela, F.J., 1991, 'The immune recruitment mechanism: a selective evolution strategy', in Belew, R. and Booker, L. (Eds) Proceedings of the Fourth International Conference on Genetic Algorithms, pp. 520–6, Cambridge, MA: Morgan Kauffman.

Booker, L.B., Goldberg, D.E. and Holland, J.H., 1989, Classifier systems and genetic algorithms, *Artificial Intelligence*, **40**, 235–82.

Caruana, R.A. and Schaffer, J.D., 1988, 'Representation and hidden bias: Gray vs. binary coding for genetic algorithms', in Proceedings 5th International Conference on Machine Learning, pp. 153–61, Cambridge, MA: Morgan-Kauffman.

Cellier, E.F. and Alvarez, F.M., 1992, 'Systematic design of fuzzy controllers using inductive reasoning', in Proceedings of the 1992 IEEE International Symposium Intelligent Control, Glasgow; pp. 198–203.

Chunyu, H.T., Toguchi, K., Shenoi, S. and Fan, L.T., 1989, 'A technique for design and implementation of fuzzy logic controllers', in *Proceedings of the 1989 American Control Conference*, pp. 2754–5.

Cox, E., 1992, Fuzzy fundamentals, *IEEE Spectrum*, **29**, 58–61.

Daley, S. and Gill, K.S., 1986, A design study of a self organizing fuzzy logic controller, *Proceedings of the Institution of Mechanical Engineers*, **200**, 59–69.

Daley, S. and Gill, K.S., 1987, Attitude Control of a spacecraft using a self organizing fuzzy logic controller, *Proceedings of the Institution of Mechanical Engineers*, **201**, 97–106.

Davis, L., 1990, *A Handbook of Genetic Algorithms*, New York: Van Nostrand–Reinhold.

De Jong, K.A., 1992, 'Are genetic algorithms function optimizers?', in *Proceedings of the Second Workshop on Parallel Problem Solving from Nature*, Brussels, Belgium, pp. 2–13, Berlin: Springer.

Fogarty, T.C., 1989, 'An incremental genetic algorithm for real time optimization', in *Proceedings of the 1989 IEEE Conference on Systems, Man, and Cybernetics*, pp. 321–6.

Foster, G.T., Kambhampati, C., Warwick, K., 1992, 'Quasi-decoupled fuzzy logic controller', in *Proceedings of the IEEE International Symposium Intelligent Control, 1992 Glasgow*, pp. 366–71.

Fukui, Y., Smith, N.T. and Fleming, R.A., 1982, Digital and sampled data control of arterial blood pressure during halothane anaesthesia, *Anaesthetics and Analgesia*, **61**, 1010–5.

Godfrey, K.R., 1982, Pharmacokinetics, *Transactions Institute of Measurement and Control*, **4**, 213–23.

Goldberg, D.E., 1989, *Genetic Algorithms in Search, Optimization and Machine Learning*, New York: Addison-Wesley.

Gray, W.M. and Asbury, A.J., 1986, 'Measurement and control of the depth of anaesthesia in surgical patients', presentation at the 3rd IMEKO Conference on Measurement in Clinical Medicine, Edinburgh, 1986, pp. 167–72.

Grefenstette, J.J., 1986, Optimization of control parameters for genetic algorithms, *IEEE Transactions Systems, Man, and Cybernetics*, **SMC-16**, 122–8.

Hasnain, S.B., 1989, 'Self organizing control systems and their transputer implementation', PhD dissertation, University of Sheffield.

Holland, J.H., 1973, Genetic algorithms and the optimal allocation of trials, *SIAM Journal of Computing*, **2**, 89–104.

Holland, J.H., 1975, *Adaptation in Natural and Artificial Systems*, New York: Addison-Wesley.

Holland, J.H., 1986, 'Escaping brittleness: the possibilities of general purpose learning algorithms applied to parallel rule based systems', in Michalski, R.S., Carbonelli, J.G. and Mitchell, T.M. (Eds), *Machine Learning: An Artificial Intelligence Approach*, Vol. II, pp. 593–623.

Karr, C.L., 1991, Genetic algorithms for fuzzy controllers, *AI Expert*, **6**, 26–33.

Karr, C.L., Freeman, L.M. and Meredith, D.L., 1989, 'Improved fuzzy process control of spacecraft autonomous rendezvous using a genetic algorithm', in *SPIE Intelligent Control and Adaptive Systems*, Vol. 1196, pp. 274–88, Bellingham, WA: SPIE.

Khelfa, M., Linkens, D.A. and Asbury, A.J., 1988, Non-linear identification of muscle relaxant drug dynamics, *Biomedical Measurement Information Control*, **2**, 130–6.

King, P.J. and Mamdani, E.H., 1977, The application of fuzzy control systems to industrial processes, *Automatica*, **13**, 235–42.

Lee, C.C., 1990, Fuzzy logic in control systems: fuzzy logic controllers, *IEEE Transactions Systems, Man, and Cybernetics*, **SMC-20**, 404–35.

Linkens, D.A. and Abbod, M.F., 1992, Self organizing fuzzy logic control and the selection of its scaling factors, *Transactions of the Institute of Measurement and Control*, **14**, 114–25.

Linkens, D.A. and Shieh, J., 1992, 'Self-organizing fuzzy modelling for non-linear system control', presentation at the 1992 IEEE International Symposium Intelligent Control, Glasgow, pp. 210–15.

Linkens, D.A., Asbury, A.J., Rimmer, S.J. and Menad, M., 1982, Identification and control of muscle relaxant anaesthesia, *Proceedings of the IEE*, **129**, 136–41.

Linkens, D.A., Mahfouf, M. and Asbury, A.J., 1991, 'Multi-variable generalized predictive control for anaesthesia', in Proceedings First European Control Conference, Grenoble, France, July, pp. 1681–3.

Mamdani, E.H., 1974, Applications of fuzzy algorithms for control of a simple dynamic process, *Proceedings of the IEE*, **121**, 1585–8.

Manderick, B. and Spiessens, P., 1989, 'Fine grained parallel genetic algorithms', in Schaffer, J. (Ed.), Proceedings of the Third International Conference on Genetic Algorithms, pp. 428–33, Cambridge, MA: Morgan Kauffman.

Michalski, R.S., 1983, A theory and methodology of inductive reasoning, *Artificial Intelligence*, **20**, 111–61.

Millard, R.K. et al., 1986, 'Self-tuning control of blood pressure during surgery', presentation at the 3rd IMEKO Conference on Measurement in Clinical Medicine, Edinburgh, 1986, pp. 173–8.

Millard, R.K. et al., 1988, Controlled hypotension during ENT surgery using self-tuners, *Biomedical Measurement and Information Control*, **2**, 59–72.

Miller, W.T., Suton, R.S. and Werborg, P.J., 1990, *Neural Networks for Control*, Cambridge, MA: MIT Press.

Mitchell, T.M., Mahadevan, S. and Steinberg, L., 1985, 'LEAP: a learning apprentice for VLSI design', in Proceedings of the 9th International Joint Conference on Artificial Intelligence, pp. 573–80, Cambridge, MA: Morgan Kauffman.

Mizumoto, M., 1988, Fuzzy control under various reasoning methods, *Information Science*, **45**(2), 129–51.

Monk, C.R., Millard, P., Hutton, J. and Prys-Roberts, C., 1989, Automatic arterial pressure regulation using isoflurane: comparison with manual control, *British Journal of Anaesthesia*, **63**, 22–30.

Moore, C.G. and Harris, C.J., 1992, Indirect adaptive fuzzy control, *International Journal of Control*, **56**, 441–68.

Muhlenbein, H., 1992, 'How genetic algorithms really work I: mutation and hill-climbing', in Grefenstette, J. (Ed.) Proceedings Second International Conference on Genetic Algorithms, pp. 15–25, Hillsdale, NJ: Lawrence Erlbaum.

Odetayo, M. and McGregor, D.R., 1989, 'Genetic algorithms for inducing control rules for a dynamic system', in Schaffer, J. (Ed.) Proceedings Third International Conference Genetic Algorithms, pp. 177–82, Cambridge, MA: Morgan Kauffman.

Peters, I., Beck, K. and Campasano, R., 1992, 'Fuzzy logic with dynamic rule-set', in Proceedings IEEE Symposium Intelligent Control, 1992, Glasgow, pp. 216–9.

Procyk, T.J. and Mamdani, E.H., 1979, A linguistic self organizing process controller, *Automatica*, **15**, 15–30.

Renders, J.M. and Haus, R., 1992, 'Biological learning metaphors for adaptive process control: a genetic strategy', in Proceedings of the 1992 IEEE International Symposium Intelligent Control, Glasgow, UK, pp. 469–75.

Riolo, R.L., 1988a, 'Bucket brigade performance I: long sequence of classifiers', in Proceedings of the 5th International Conference Machine Learning, pp. 184–95, Cambridge, MA: Morgan Kauffman.

Riolo, R.L., 1988b, 'Bucket brigade performance II: default hierarchies', in *Proceedings of the 5th International Conference Machine Learning*, pp. 196–201, Cambridge, MA: Morgan Kauffman.

Robb, H.M., Asbury, A.J., Gray, W.M. and Linkens, D.A., 1988, 'Towards automatic control of general anaesthesia', in *Medical Informatics: Computers in Clinical Medicine*, pp. 121–6, Conference of the British Medical Informatics Society, Nottingham.

Robb, H.M., Asbury, A.J., Gray, W.M. and Linkens, D.A., 1991, Towards a standardized anaesthetic state using enflurane and morphine, *British Journal of Anaesthesia*, **66**, 358–64.

Robb, H.M., Asbury, A.J., Gray, W.M. and Linkens, D.A., 1993, Towards a standardized anaesthetic state using isoflurane and morphine, *British Journal of Anaesthesia*, **71**, 366–9.

Schrauldolph, N.N. and Belew, R.K., 1992, Dynamic parameters encoding for genetic algorithms, *Machine Learning*, Vol. 9, pp. 9–21, Dordrecht: Kluwer.

Smith, N.T., Quinn, M.L., Flick, J., Fleming, R. and Coles, J.R., 1984, Automatic control in anaesthesia: a comparison in performance between the anaesthetist and the machine, *Anaesthesia and Analgesics*, **63**, 715–22.

Syswerda, G., 1989, 'Uniform crossover in genetic algorithms', in Schaffer, J. (Ed.) Proceedings of the Third International Conference on Genetic Algorithms, pp. 2–9, Cambridge, MA: Morgan Kauffman.

Tsetlin, M.L., 1961, On behaviour of finite automata in random media, *Automatic Remote Control*, **22**, 1210–19 (translation from Russian).

Weatherley, B.C., Williams, S.G. and Neill, E.A.M., 1983, Pharmacokinetics, pharmacodynamics and dose-response relationships of atracurium administered i.v., *British Journal of Anaesthesia*, **55**, 39S–45S.

Zadeh, L.A., 1965, Fuzzy sets, *Information and Control*, **9**, 338–53.

Zadeh, L.A., 1973, An outline of a new approach to the analysis of complex systems and decision processes, *IEEE Transactions System, Man, and Cybernetics*, **SMC-3**, 29–44.

Zadeh, L.A., 1988, Fuzzy logic, *IEEE Computer Magazine*, April, 83–92.

Chapter 12
Multifaceted knowledge representation and acquisition applied to the modelling of the cardiovascular system

E. Tanyi

The artificial intelligence (AI) phenomenon has extended computer programming well beyond the scope of numerical computation. The pursuit of this vision has resulted in an explosion of research activities in numerous directions. One such research theme is the notion of knowledge-based systems—computer programs which codify and process knowledge in specified domains. The importance of the knowledge-based theme is underscored by its endorsement by such gigantic AI projects as the European-based Alvey and the Japanese Fifth Generation projects. One variant of knowledge-based systems is, specifically, concerned with the emulation of the problem-solving strategies of the human expert in a given domain of application. These are Expert Systems, and they too have stimulated considerable research interest (Feigenbaum, 1979; Forsyth, 1984).

Knowledge-based systems can only truly fulfil their potential if they address two fundamental problems—knowledge representation (Hayes-Roth, 1984) and knowledge acquisition (Tanyi et al., 1990a). Knowledge representation refers to the concepts and structures which enable knowledge to be described (Linkens et al., 1988). Such concepts and structures should be sufficiently robust and versatile to capture the wide range of knowledge types encountered in most domains.

Knowledge acquisition refers to the addition of new knowledge to the system. It is essential that the facilities for knowledge acquisition be simple enough to be used by novices. The knowledge acquisition requirement is analogous to the notion of 'user-friendliness' in conventional programming.

An attempt by AI researchers to resolve the knowledge representation bottleneck has resulted in such paradigms as frames, object-orientation and rules. The frame paradigm organizes knowledge into a hierarchy of interrelated protypal classes (Tanyi and Linkens, 1987) which share information. The object-oriented paradigm extends the frame concept by allowing an object class to contain both a set of attributes and the numerical procedures required to compute some of these attributes. The rule-based paradigm models knowledge as a collection of antecedent–consequent pairs which can be 'chained' by an inference mechanism to reach a conclusion on a given hypothesis. The rule-based paradigm is suitable for heuristic knowledge. One firmly established result is that no single paradigm can adequately capture a wide range of knowledge types. For this reason, most knowledge representation software tools are hybrid systems incorporating two or more paradigms. This reality is reflected in commercial knowledge representation toolkits such as Knowledge Craft and KEE.

Two approaches are open to the knowledge-base designer. One is to use a general-purpose toolkit, and the other is to use customized software, specifically designed for the intended application. The commercial toolkit approach has several disadvantages when applied to modelling. The most severe disadvantage is the poor adaptability of such toolkits to the specific requirements of modelling. This is further compounded by the poor knowledge acquisition facilities, excessive cost and lack of portability which are characteristic of most toolkits.

The better approach is to construct a customized tool for modelling (Linkens, 1990). This was the motivation for the development of a knowledge acquisition module (KAM) (Tanyi *et al.*, 1991). KAM is a hybrid tool which supports frames, object-orientation, Petri nets and linguistic models. KAM implements these paradigms in the form of a pseudo-natural language, FKRL—a frame-based knowledge representation language. KAM is written in Prolog and it runs on an IBM PC or compatible machine.

12.1 Knowledge representation for systems modelling

Before showing how KAM is used, it is necessary to outline the knowledge representation paradigms which form its conceptual foundation. The choice of paradigms is closely linked to the types of model for which representation is sought.

12.1.1 Types of model

Three types of model are commonly used to describe systems—continuous-time, discrete and linguistic models. The combination of two or more model types facilitates the multi-faceted description of a system (Zeigler, 1984). Continuous-time models are differential equations which express the physical laws governing the behaviour of a system. Such laws might express mass, energy, or force balance. A discrete model describes the events which characterize a system and the logical conditions governing the passage from one event to another. A linguistic model is a natural-language description of a system. These are the three types of model for which KAM was designed.

12.1.1.1 Continuous-time models

A central feature of continuous-time models is that a single equation can describe a class of elements. This makes it possible to model a wide range of systems from a repository of elemental models. The frame paradigm is best suited to the construction of the model repository. A second feature of such models is that they often include parameters which are computed from prescribed formulae. For instance, the volume of any cylindrical conduit is defined by

$$V = 3.14 \times L \times D \times D/4$$

Where V, D and L are the volume, diameter and length respectively. The object-oriented paradigm of message-passing is best suited to the procedure-handling which facilitates the computation of such parameters.

12.1.1.2 Discrete models

Unlike continuous-time models, there is no standard AI paradigm for describing discrete models. One very convenient tool is the Petri net formalism (Willson and Krogh, 1990) proposed by the contemporary German mathematician Karl Adam Petri. A description of this formalism is presented in Section 12.1.4.

12.1.1.3 Linguistic models

For a linguistic model to be useful it must satisfy a number of requirements:

(i) emphasize the key entities and concepts which describe a system,
(ii) provide a top-down description which contains more abstract concepts at the top level and more detailed descriptions at the lower levels,

(iii) facilitate efficient retrieval of the description of any entity of the system, so that the model serves as an electronic text book,
(iv) allow time-dependent operations to be described.

There is no standard AI paradigm which satisfies these requirements. For this reason, an abstract data structure called a PROCESS was formulated to facilitate linguistic modelling.

The four paradigms mentioned in this section form the conceptual foundation of KAM.

12.1.2 The frame paradigm

A frame (Minsky, 1977) is a template for creating objects of a given class. Such a template description specifies the attributes of the object as well as its default values. In AI terminology, attributes are called SLOTS while attribute values are called SLOTVALUES.

In addition to describing objects and object classes, the frame concept allows relationships between objects or object classes to be defined. Two types of relationship are possible—class–subclass and object–class relationships. A class–subclass relationship links two classes of objects and is denoted by the 'IS A' semantic link. The object–class relationship assigns an object membership of a class and is denoted by the 'INSTANCE OF' semantic link.

These relationships between objects and object classes bind several frames into a hierarchical structure, with the more abstract entities at the top and more specific objects at the lower reaches. Such hierarchy forms the basis of information-sharing. This mechanism of information-sharing is called INHERITANCE.

As an illustration of the frame concept consider the frames shown in Figure 12.1.

Figure 12.1 shows four frames. The unidirectional valve is a subclass of the valve frame, while the aortic and tricuspid valves are members (instances) of the class of unidirectional valves. The hierarchy between the four frames is shown in Figure 12.2.

Each frame in the hierarchy can acquire (inherit) the attributes of those higher frames to which it is linked.

For the purpose of modelling it is useful to define a generic frame called COMPONENT which represents the class of elemental models. Various subclasses of this frame can be constructed for as many component types as required. A component frame is defined as:

```
frame      : COMPONENT
variables  :
equations  :
```

```
frame              : valve
IS A               : flow-element
inlet pressure     : P1
outlet pressure    : P2
flow               : Q
resistance         : R
equation           : Q = R(P1 − P2)

frame              : unidirectional valve
IS A               : valve
equation           : Q = 0 if P2 > P1; Q = R(P1 − P2) if P1 > P2

frame              : aortic valve
INSTANCE OF        : unidirectional valve

frame              : mitral valve
INSTANCE OF        : unidirectional valve
```

Figure 12.1 *Illustration of the template structure of frames.*

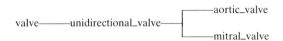

Figure 12.2 *Hierarchical relationship between the valve frames.*

Components are the basic building blocks of systems. However, due to the complexity of most systems, it is useful to introduce the notion of a subsystem—a collection of components. A system is, thus, defined as a collection of subsystems. This definition implies a different type of hierarchy which contains the system at the highest level, subsystems at an intermediate level and components at the lowest level. Such system hierarchy is different from the class hierarchy in Figure 12.2.

The system and sub-system frames are defined as:

```
frame        : system
subsystems   :
equations    :
variables    :

frame        : subsystem
components   :
equations    :
variables    :
```

The attribute 'components' is a list of objects of the class component. Similarly 'subsystems' is a list of subsystem frames.

12.1.3 The object-oriented paradigm

The central feature of the object-oriented paradigm is the so-called 'message-passing', which is the mechanism by which a procedure defined within an object can be used by related objects. This involves exchange of data between the host object and its relatives. It is this exchange of data which is referred to as message-passing. In AI jargon, the procedures attached to an object are called METHODS. Three methods are particularly useful in KAM. These are called the 'parameter-computation', 'equation-initializer' and 'simulator'. The parameter-computation is used for the calculation of any attribute of an object expressed as a formula. The equation-initializer converts a generic equation into a more specific form. The simulator converts the equations of a system into code for the ESL simulation language. ESL—ESA Simulation Language—was designed to meet the requirements of the European Space Agency (ISIM Simulation, 1988). In KAM, methods are attached to frames.

In order to appreciate the functionality of these three methods, consider the following frames:

```
frame       : artery
diameter    : D
length      : L
pressure    : P
flow        : Q
volume      : V = 3.14 × D × D × L/4
equation    : Q = V dP/dt

frame       : artery1
instance of : artery
diameter    : 2
length      : 10
pressure    : P1
flow        : Q1.
```

If it is desired to obtain the volume of artery1, it is calculated from the formula provided in the artery frame to which artery1 is related. This invokes the parameter-computation which takes data from artery1 ($D = 2$ and $L = 10$) to return the result, $V = 31.4$. Similarly, if it is desired to generate an equation for artery1, the generic equation defined in the artery frame is initialized by replacing the variables Q, V and P by their specific values $Q1$, 31.4 and $P1$ to obtain the equation:

$$Q1 = 31.4 \, dP1/dt.$$

It is in this initialized form that an equation can be simulated. The

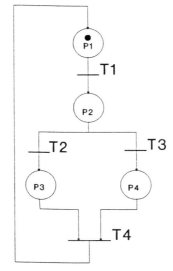

Figure 12.3 *An example of a Petri net.*

conversion of the initialized equation to ESL code is performed by the simulator.

12.1.4 The Petri net formalism

A Petri net (Rene, 1991) is a graphical model describing the relationship between the events which characterize a system and the conditions which define the transition from one event to another. The formalism provides a convenient way of describing sequential operations. For example, the flow of blood through the human cardiovascular system can be modelled as a Petri net in which the events represent the opening and closing of various heart valves and the transitions depend on the pressure levels at the inlet and outlet of each valve.

In Petri net jargon, events are called PLACES. Petri nets are constructed according to a convention in which places are represented by circles and transitions by horizontal bars. Some authors use rectangles to represent places. An example of a Petri net is shown in Figure 12.3.

The Petri net has four places P1, P2, P3, P4 and four transitions T1, T2, T3 and T4. The place containing a dot represents the initially active state of the system.

The knowledge representation problem is to define constructs for places and transitions. In a KAM, places are represented by a NODE construct while transitions are represented by a TRANSITION construct. The node construct consists of an identifier for the node, the input nodes, and the input transitions connected to the node. The transition construct consists of an identifier and the input nodes connected to the transition.

In addition to the description of the structure of a Petri net, it is necessary to analyse the net to obtain behavioural information. One useful analytical technique is the REACHABILITY TREE which shows all possible ways in which a net can evolve from an initial configuration of active states. The reachability tree usually reveals any hidden features of a system such as concurrency of events.

12.1.5 The process construct

The process construct is defined as:

> PROCESS = IDENTIFIER SUBPROCESSES DESCRIPTION

where

> IDENTIFIER is a text string identifying the process;
> SUBPROCESSES are a list of entities and concepts in terms of which the process is described;
> DESCRIPTION is a natural language description of the process.

An example of a process is:

> Process blood_circulation with subprocesses=[heart, blood-vessels, vascular-systems, blood_pressure]
> {The flow of blood through the human body is controlled by two pumps the left and right ventricles of the heart. The left ventricle supplies oxygenated blood from the lungs to the body while the right ventricle returns deoxygenated blood to the lungs}.

The process identifier is 'blood-circulation'. The subprocesses are 'heart', 'blood_vessels', 'vascular_systems' and 'blood_pressure'. A more detailed description of the process can be provided by further describing the subprocesses.

The process construct satisfies three of the four requirements for linguistic modelling specified in Section 12.1.1.3. These include emphasis of key concepts (subprocesses), top-down (hierarchical) description and incorporation of time. The description part of a process can contain time-based events. A fourth requirement—efficient retrieval of textual descriptions—is achieved by implementing a 'hypertext' type facility which allows the description of a selected subprocess to be displayed on the screen.

KAM contains a structure which extracts timed events from a process description and displays them on a graph with time on the horizontal axis and the duration of events on the vertical axis. Such a graph is called an

EVENT DIAGRAM. A twin construct called a SEQUENCE DIAGRAM displays a sequence of events in the form of a flow chart.

12.1.6 Glossary of knowledge representation concepts

The concepts and paradigms described in Sections 12.1.2–12.1.5 can be summarized as follows:

FRAME	:	A template for creating objects of a given class
COMPONENT	:	A generic elemental model
SUBSYSTEM	:	A collection of components
SYSTEM	:	A collection of subsystems
CLASS HIERARCHY	:	Levels of abstraction in a group of related objects
SYSTEM HIERARCHY	:	Decomposition of a system into subsystems and components
INHERITANCE	:	The mechanism by which related frames share information
MESSAGE-PASSING	:	The mechanism by which numerical procedures are shared by related objects
METHODS	:	Numerical procedures attached to an object
NODE	:	An event in a discrete model
TRANSITION	:	A condition in a discrete model
PETRI NET	:	The collection of nodes and transitions in a discrete model
REACHABILITY TREE	:	The set of all possible sequences which can result from a Petri net
PROCESS	:	A linguistic description of a system
PROCESS HIERARCHY	:	Levels of detail in a linguistic model
EVENT DIAGRAM	:	A graphical display of timed events
SEQUENCE DIAGRAM	:	A flow chart describing a sequence of operations.

12.2 The knowledge acquisition module (KAM)

The concepts and paradigms outlined in Section 12.1.6 are the blueprint from which KAM was designed. The various paradigms were implemented in the form of a pseudo-natural language, FKRL—a frame-based knowledge representation language. In this section, the syntax of FKRL is outlined together with the knowledge acquisition facilities of KAM.

frame valve is a flow-element with inlet_pressure, $P1$; outlet_pressure, $P2$; flow, Q; resistance, R; equation = $[Q = R(P1 - P2)]$.

frame artery is a flow_element with diameter, D; length, L; volume, $V = 3.14 \times D \times D \times L/4$.

frame artery1 instance of artery with $L = 20$; $D = 2$.

node n1 with input node n8 and input transition T1.

transition T1 if $(P1 - P2) > 20$ then activate n1.

process blood-circulation with subprocesses =[structure, function, blood_vessels, vascular_systems]
{The flow of blood through the human body is controlled by two pumps—the left and right ventricles of the heart. The left ventricle supplies oxygenated blood from the lungs to the body while the right ventricle returns de-oxygenated blood from the body to the lungs}.

Figure 12.4 *Illustration of the Syntax of FKRL.*

12.2.1 The syntax of FKRL

The syntax of FKRL is illustrated by the knowledge-base profile shown in Figure 12.4. The knowledge-base consists of six items—three frames, a node, a transition and a process.

The syntax of a frame consists of three parts—the name of the frame, the relationship between the frame and some other frame, and a list of attributes, separated by semicolons. The name of the frame is preceded by the keyword 'frame'. Its relationship to another frame is either the 'IS A' link or the 'INSTANCE OF' link depending on whether it is a subclass or a member of a class. The relationship part of the frame is optional and need not be specified if the frame has no relative or if it is the highest frame in the hierarchy. Attributes which serve as variables are assigned a symbol which is separated from the attribute by a comma. An example of this is the flow attribute of the valve frame which is assigned the symbol, Q. The equality sign is used to assign values to attributes. There are three kinds of attribute values—constants, lists and formulae. The attribute, $L = 2$, is an example of a constant. Lists are enclosed in square brackets. Equations are always represented by a list. A formula is similar to an equation except that it is not enclosed in square brackets. All formulae are evaluated through message-passing. The KAM's inference engine is designed to recognize formulae and to convert them to Prolog procedures.

The syntax of a node, transition and process is also indicated.

12.2.2 The KAM user-interface

The KAM user-interface consists of the box-menu shown in Figure 12.5.

The EDIT option enables a knowledge-base to be entered into the KAM. The COMPILE option checks the syntax of the knowledge-base. Any errors

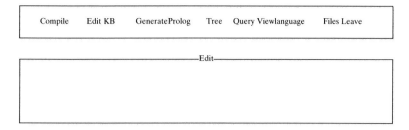

Figure 12.5 *The KAM box-menu.*

detected are interactively corrected. An error-free knowledge-base is converted to Prolog code via the GENERATEPROLOG option (Tanyi *et al.*, 1990b). The FILE option enables knowledge-base files to be transferred to and from disk. The TREE option is used to sketch knowledge-base hierarchies, including class, system and process hierarchies. A reachability tree can also be displayed via the TREE option. The QUERY option enables information to be retrieved from the knowledge base through pseudo-natural language queries. Sample queries include:

SHOW FRAMES
SHOW ARTERY
SHOW EQUATIONS OF ARTERY
FIND AN ARTERY WITH DIAMETER = 2

The first query gives a list of all frames in the knowledge base. The second shows the template structure of a prototypal artery. The third retrieves the equations of a prototypal artery, while the fourth searches the knowledge-base for any artery having a diameter of 2 units.

12.2.3 Knowledge acquisition with KAM

The knowledge acquisition procedure is a three-stage cycle which includes design, compilation and processing of the knowledge base. In the design phase, the types of models (viewpoints) for the intended application are specified. The elements of each model are then expressed in terms of appropriate KAM constructs which are then converted to FKRL code.

The compilation phase involves entry of the FKRL knowledge-base into KAM, verification of the FKRL syntax via the COMPILE option and conversion of FKRL to Prolog code via the GENERATEPROLOG option. It is in its Prolog form that the knowledge-base can be processed by the inheritance mechanism.

The processing phase involves two main operations—verification of the knowledge-base hierarchy via the TREE option and retrieval of information via the QUERY option. Verification of the knowledge-base hierarchy is a useful way of checking the conceptual validity of the knowledge-base (Tanyi et al., 1992).

12.3 Application of KAM to the modelling of the cardiovascular system

The knowledge acquisition procedure outlined in Section 12.2.3 is best illustrated by a typical case study—the modelling of the human cardiovascular system.

12.3.1 Design of the knowledge-base

The system can be modelled using all of the viewpoints supported by KAM—mathematical, discrete and linguistic.

12.3.1.1 The mathematical viewpoint

The mathematical description of the system is based on the well-documented PHYSBE model (McCleod, 1966) of which the block diagram is shown in Figure 12.6.

The model is an interconnection of various flow volumes representing elements of the circulatory system and the heart chambers. Each flow volume is described by lumped-parameter equations relating blood flow to pressure, resistance and compliance. The chambers of the heart are interlinked by four valves—the tricuspid, pulmonary, mitral and aortic valves.

A single heart beat causes a variation in the compliance of the left and right ventricles. This temporal variation in compliance is the driving function for the system.

THE VALVES
The four valves in the system are all uni-directional. This characteristic is modelled by assigning each valve a near infinite resistance when the outlet pressure exceeds the inlet pressure, and a small nominal resistance in the forward-flow condition. The template structure of a generic valve is:

```
frame             : valve
IS A              : component
inflow_resistance :
resistance        : R
inlet_pressure    : P_iv
```

Multifaceted knowledge representation and acquisition 373

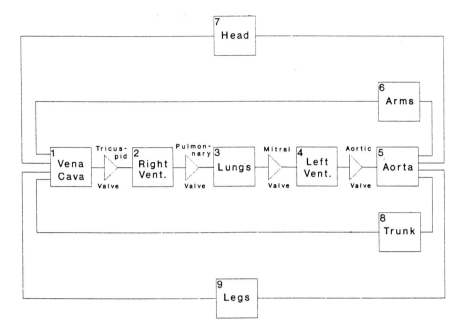

Figure 12.6 *Block diagram of the PHYSBE model.*

outlet_pressure : P_{ov}
equation : If $P_{ov} > P_{iv}$ then $R = 10 \text{ EXP}(20)$
  else $R = R_v$

The four valves are all instances of the valve class as indicated in the knowledge-base in Figure 12.7.

FLOW VOLUMES
Three types of flow volume are identifiable from Figure 12.6—resistive, passive and flow-junction. The outlet of a resistive volume is connected to a valve, and this affects the outlet pressure. The outlet of a passive volume is connected to another flow volume. A flow-junction is a volume in which either the inlet or outlet is connected to two or more volumes. Resistive and passive volumes have standard equations. The equations of a flow-junction, however, cannot be specified *a priori* since these depend on the number and types of elements connected to its inlet and outlet. From Figure 12.6, it can be observed that there are three instances of resistive volume—right ventricle, lungs and left ventricle. There are four instances of passive volume—arms, head, trunk and legs. The aorta and vena cava are instances of a flow-junction.

```
frame cardio_vascular is a system with views=[continuous_time,discrete,linguistic].
frame physbe instance of cardio_vascular with view=continuous_time;
equations;subsystems= [inflow,outflow].
frame inflow instance of system with subsystems =[vena_cava,tricuspid_valve,right_ventricle,
pulmonary_valve,lungs].
frame outflow instance of system with subsystems =[mitral_valve,left_ventricle,aortic_valve,aorta,
legs,arms,trunk,head].
frame flow_volume is a component with inlet_resistance,Ri;outlet_resistance,Ro;
inlet_pressure,Pi;outlet_pressure,Po;pressure,P;compliance,C;inlet_flow,Qi;
outlet_flow,Qo;volume,V.
frame flow_junction is a flow_volume with inlet_components;outlet_components;equations.
frame passive_volume is a flow_volume with equations =
           [Qi=(Pi-P)/Ri, Qo=(P_Po)/Ro, dV/dt=Qi-Qo].
frame resistive_volume is a flow_volume with outlet_valve_resistance,Rv;
outlet_volume_pressure,Pv;equations=
   [Po=(P*Rv+Pv*Ro)/(Rv+Ro),Qi=(Pi-P)/Ri,Qo=(P-Po)/Ro,dV/dt=Qi-Qo].
frame valve is a component with inflow_resistance,Rv;resistance,R;
inlet_pressure,Piv;outlet_pressure,Pov;equation=[R=Rv].
frame venacava instance of flow_junction with Pi=Pi1;Po=Po1;P=P1;Ri=R1;Ro=Ro1;V=V1;
equations=[Pi1=(P1/Ri1+P6/Ro6+P7/Ro7+P8/Ro8+P9/Ro9)/(1/Ri1+1/Ro6+1/Ro7+1/Ro8+1/Ro9),
       Po1=P1*Ri2+P2*Ro1/Ri2+Ro1,dV1/dt=pi1-P1/Ri1-P1-Po1/Ro1+Fe1].
frame aorta instance of flow_junction with Pi=Pi5;Po=Po5;P=P5;Ri=Ri5;Ro=Ro5;V=V5;
equations=[Po5=(P5/Ro5+P6/Ri6+P7/Ri7+P8/Ri8+P9/Ri9)/(1/Ro5+1/Ri6+1/Ri7+1/Ri8+1/Ri9),
       dV5/dt=((pi5-P5)/Ri5)-((P5-Po5)/Ro5)+Fe5].

frame rightventricle instance of resistive_volume with
Pi=Po1;Ro=Ro2;Ri=Ri2;RV=Ro2;Pv=P3;Po=Po2;P=P2;V=V2.
frame leftventricle instance of resistive_volume with
Pi=Po3;Ro=Ro4;Ri=Ri4;RV=Ro4;Pv=P5;Po=Po4;P=P4;V=V4.
frame lungs instance of resistive_volume with
Pi=Po2;Ro=Ro3;Ri=Ri3;Rv=Ri4;Pv=P4;Po=Po3;P=P3;V=V3.
frame head instance of passive_volume with Ro=Ro7;Ri=Ri7;Pi=Pi7;Po=Po7;P=P7;V=V7.
frame arms instance of passive_volume with Ro=Ro6;Ri=Ri6;Pi=Pi6;Po=Po6;P=P6;V=V6.
frame legs instance of passive_volume with Ro=Ro9;Ri=Ri9;Pi=Pi9;Po=Po9;P=P9;V=V9.
frame trunk instance of passive_volume with Ro=Ro8;Ri=Ri8;Pi=Pi8;Po=Po8;P=P8;V=V8.
frame tricuspid_valve instance of valve with R=Ri2;Pi=1;Po=2;Rv=Riv2.
frame pulmonary_valve instance of valve with R=Ro2;Pi=P2;Po=P3;Rv=Rov2.
frame mitral_valve instance of valve with R=Ri4;Pi=P3;Po=P4;Rv=Riv4.
frame aortic_valve instance of valve with R=Ro4;Pi=P4;Po=P5;Rv=Rov4.

node Xo with inputnodes TVc, PVo, MVc, Avo and inputtransition Ti.
node TVo with inputnode Xo and inputtransition Tc.
node PVc with inputnode Xo and inputtransition Tc.
node MVo with inputnode Xo and inputtransition Tc.
node AVc with inputnode Xo and inputtransition Tc.
node TVc with inputnodes TVo, PVc, MVo, Avc and inputtransition Tr.
node PVo with inputnodes TVo, PVc, MVo, Avc and inputtransition Tr.
node MVc with inputnodes TVo, PVc, MVo, Avc and inputtransition Tr.
node AVo with inputnodes TVo, PVc, MVo, Avc and inputtransition Tr.
transition Tc if Pi2>P2 then activate TVo.
transition Tr if Pi4>P4 then activate TVc.
transition Ti if P4=Pi4 then activate Xo.
```

Figure 12.7(*a*) *The knowledge-base of the cardiovascular system describing the continuous-time and discrete models.*

```
process blood_circulation with subprocesses=[heart,blood_vessels,blood_pressure]
    { The cardio_vascular system is a closed circuit linking
      the heart, blood vessels and capillaries}.
process heart with subprocesses = [structure, function]
    { The heart is a pump which supplies the blood vessels through its rythmic contractions}.
process structure { The muscle tissue of the heart consists of three hollow muscles,
                    the superior vena cava and inferior vena cava}.
process function with subprocesses = [compression_relaxation, heart_sounds, electro_cardiograph]
    { The compression of the muscle tissue of the heart reduces the volume of the
      heart chambers resulting in a pressure drop inside the chambers. This causes the
      blood to flow in the direction in which the pressure is low. The compression stroke
      lasts about 0.4 second followed by a relaxation stroke of about 0.6 second. During
      the compression_relaxation cycle the heart emits sounds. It also generates an electric
      potential which is called an electro-cardiograph  }.
process blood_pressure with subprocesses =[greater_circulation, lesser_circulation, pressure_regulation].
process greater_circulation with subprocesses=[arterial_pressure,venous_pressure,capillary_pressure]
    { The left ventricle pushes the blood under high pressure through the arteries
      to the capillaries. The arterial, venous and capillary pressures are maintained at different levels}.
process lesser_circulation { The right ventricle pumps the blood through the capillaries
                             of the lungs via the arteries of the pulmonary circuit}.
process blood_vessels with subprocesses=[arteries,veins,capillaries].
```

Figure 12.7(b) *The linguistic knowledge-base of the cardiovascular system.*

The template structure of the various classes of flow volume are:

frame	: flow-volume
IS A	: component
inlet_resistance	: R_i
outlet_resistance	: R_o
inlet_pressure	: P_i
outlet_pressure	: P_o
pressure	: P
compliance	: C
inlet_flow	: Q_i
outlet_flow	: Q_o
volume	: V
frame	: resistive_volume
IS A	: flow_volume
outlet_valve_resistance	: R_v
outlet_volume_pressure	: P_v
equations	: $[\, P_o = (P*R_v + P_v*R_o)/(R_v + R_o),$
	$\quad Q_i = (P_i - P)/R_i,$
	$\quad Q_o = (P - P_o)/R_o,$
	$\quad dV/dt = Q_i - Q_o \,]$
frame	: passive_volume
IS A	: flow_volume

equations   : [$Q_i = (P_i - P)/R_i$,
                             $Q_o = (P - P_o)/R_o$,
                             $dV/dt = Q_i - Q_o$]
frame   : flow_junction
IS A   : flow_volume
inlet_components   :
outlet_components   :
equations   :

The class hierarchy between the various flow volumes is shown in Figure 12.8.

THE SYSTEM FRAME

It is convenient to consider the PHYSBE model as having two subsystems— INFLOW and OUTFLOW. The INFLOW subsystem controls the flow of de-oxygenated blood from the body to the lungs via the right ventricle while the OUTFLOW subsystem controls the flow of oxygenated blood from the lungs, via the left ventricle, to the body. The INFLOW subsystem, thus, consists of the vena cava, tricuspid valve, right ventricle, pulmonary valve and lungs while the OUTFLOW subsystem consists of the mitral valve, left ventricle, aortic valve, aorta, arms, head, trunk and legs.

This system description is illustrated in the knowledge-base of Figure 12.7(a). The corresponding system hierarchy is shown in Figure 12.9.

SIMULATION OF THE MATHEMATICAL MODEL

Simulation is a useful way of validating the mathematical model. KAM uses an object-oriented method called SIMULATE to convert a mathematical

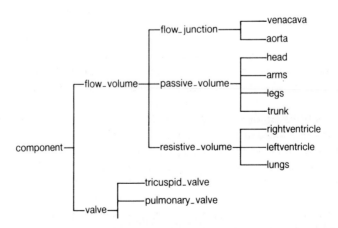

Figure 12.8 *The class hierarchy of the knowledge-base frames.*

Multifaceted knowledge representation and acquisition 377

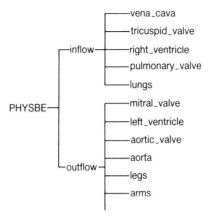

Figure 12.9 *The system hierarchy of the knowledge-base frames.*

model into simulation code for the ESL simulator. For the purpose of the simulation the PHYSBE model was given the nominal resistances and compliances shown in the knowledge-base of Figure 12.7. Some of the simulation results are shown in Figures 12.10 and 12.11. Figure 12.10 shows some pressure curves while Figure 12.11 is a table showing the variation of the resistance of the four heart valves during one heart beat.

12.3.1.2 The Petri net model

The Petri net model describes the sequential operation of the four heart valves during a single heart beat.

The events in the model are denoted by:

$$TV_o, TV_c, PV_o, PV_c, MV_o, MV_c, AV_o \text{ and } AV_c.$$

Where, TV, PV, MV and AV represent the tricuspid, pulmonary, mitral and aortic valves respectively and the subscripts o and c represent the opening and closing of the various valves. Due to the cyclic operation of the heart, it is necessary to define an event X_o to mark the initiation of the cycle.

The transitions in the model are defined by pressure variations in the heart chambers, caused by the compression-relaxation cycle of the heart. There are two main transitions—T_c and T_r, representing the compression and relaxation strokes respectively. Again, the cyclic operation of the heart necessitates the definition of a third transition, T_i, which marks the initiation of the cycle.

The Petri net linking the events and transitions is shown in Figure 12.12, while the FKRL representation is shown in the knowledge-base of Figure 12.7(*a*).

Intelligent Control in Biomedicine

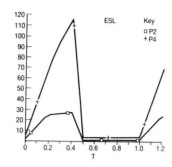

Figure 12.10 *Pressure curves from the ESL simulation.*

T	RI2	RO2	RI4	RO4
0.00000E+00	0.30000E-02	0.10000E+21	0.27500E-01	0.10000E+21
0.10000	0.10000E+21	0.10000E+21	0.10000E+21	0.10000E+21
0.20000	0.10000E+21	0.30000E-02	0.10000E+21	0.10000E+21
0.30000	0.10000E+21	0.30000E-02	0.10000E+21	0.60000E-02
0.40000	0.10000E+21	0.30000E-02	0.10000E+21	0.60000E-02
0.50000	0.30000E-02	0.10000E+21	0.27500E-01	0.10000E+21
0.60000	0.30000E-02	0.10000E+21	0.27500E-01	0.10000E+21
0.70000	0.30000E-02	0.10000E+21	0.27500E-01	0.10000E+21
0.80000	0.30000E-02	0.10000E+21	0.27500E-01	0.10000E+21
0.90000	0.30000E-02	0.10000E+21	0.27500E-01	0.10000E+21
1.0000	0.30000E-02	0.10000E+21	0.27500E-01	0.10000E+21

Figure 12.11 *Table of valve resistances from the ESL simulation.*

The following information can be derived from the Petri net:

(i) The tricuspid and mitral valves are open at the same time. This implies that the left and right ventricles admit blood at precisely the same time in the cycle. This fact is corroborated by the simulation results in Figure 12.11, from which it is seen that the resistances of the tricuspid and mitral valves (R_i2 and R_i4) are low at the same time.

(ii) The pulmonary and aortic valves are open at the same time. This implies that the left and right ventricles pump out blood at precisely the same time in the cycle. Again, this fact is corroborated by Figure 12.11 (R_o2 and R_o4 are low at the same time).

(iii) The tricuspid and pulmonary valves cannot be open at the same time, nor can the mitral and aortic valves. This is also corroborated by Figure 12.11. When R_i2 is low, R_o2 is high and when R_i4 is low, R_o4 is high. Similarly, the pulmonary and mitral valves cannot be open at the same time. Indeed, this must be so, for if the pulmonary and tricuspid valves were open at the same time, deoxygenated blood flowing into the lungs would pass into the left ventricle before it had

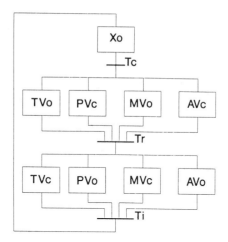

Figure 12.12 *Petri net model of the cardiovascular system.*

been oxygenated. The constraint that two valves at the inlet and outlet of a flow volume cannot be open at the same time is explained by the fact that the opening of the inlet valve is accompanied by a fall in the internal pressure of the volume and such a low pressure cannot drive the outlet valve.

12.3.1.3 The linguistic model

The linguistic model of the cardiovascular system describes such building blocks as the heart and blood vessels (Gregoire, 1992). It also describes the mechanism of blood pressure regulation. This viewpoint is reflected in the process section of the knowledge-base in Figure 12.7(*b*). The top level process, 'blood_circulation', is subdivided into three subprocesses 'heart', 'blood_vessels', and 'blood_pressure'. The heart subprocess is further divided into structure and function subprocesses. The process 'blood_vessels' includes descriptions of the arteries, veins and capillaries. The process hierarchy of the linguistic model is shown in Figure 12.13.

The 'compression-relaxation' subprocess incorporates time in its description. These time-based events are shown in the event diagram of Figure 12.14. The sequence diagram of Figure 12.15 shows the sequential operation of the heart defined by the greater and lesser circulation subprocesses.

12.3.2 Compilation of the knowledge-base

A profile of the Prolog code generated from the compiled knowledge-base is shown in Figure 12.16.

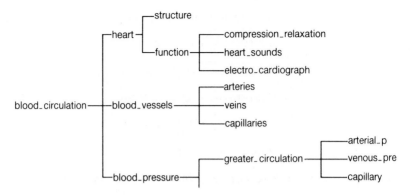

Figure 12.13 *The process hierarchy of the knowledge-base frames.*

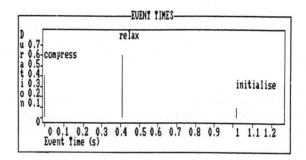

Figure 12.14 *Event diagram generated from the process model.*

12.3.3 Processing of the knowledge-base

Figures 12.13–12.15 and 12.17–12.19 show various kinds of information obtained from processing the knowledge-base. The class and system hierarchies of the PHYSBE model frames are shown in Figures 12.8 and 12.9 respectively. The process hierarchy of the linguistic model is shown in Figure 12.13. All three hierarchies were sketched via the TREE option. The system equations, obtained from the QUERY option, are shown in Figure 12.17. Figures 12.14 and 12.15 show the event and sequence diagrams derived from the process model, while the 'hypertext' facility of the KAM is illustrated by Figure 12.18. The reachability tree, derived from the Petri net model, is shown in Figure 12.19.

12.4 Conclusions

Knowledge-bases describing system models should be able to integrate several types of model, each reflecting a different aspect or viewpoint of the

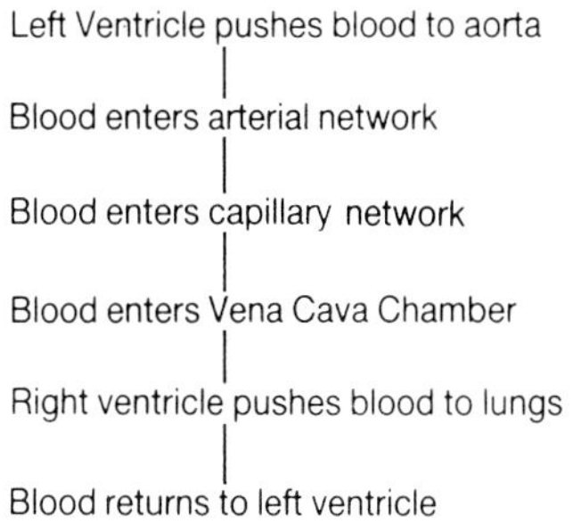

Multifaceted knowledge representation and acquisition 381

```
Left Ventricle pushes blood to aorta
               |
Blood enters arterial network
               |
Blood enters capillary network
               |
Blood enters Vena Cava Chamber
               |
Right ventricle pushes blood to lungs
               |
Blood returns to left ventricle
```

Figure 12.15 *Sequence diagram generated from the process model.*

```
is_a("cardio_vascular","system")
instance_of("cardio_vascular","physbe")
frame("cardio_vascular")
slot("cardio_vascular","views","")
slotvalue("cardio_vascular","views",l(["continuous_time","discrete","linguistic"]))
slotvalue("passive_volume","equations",l(["Qi = Pi-P/Ri","Qo - P_Po/Ro","dV/dt - Qi-Qo"]))
frame("physbe")
node(AVo,["TVo","PVc","MVo","Avc"],["Tr"])
node(AVc,["Xo"],["Tc"])
transition(Tc,["Pi2 gt P2"],[activate("TVo")])
txt(greater_circulation,["The","left","ventricle","pushes","the","blood","under","high","pressure",
"through","the","arteries","to","the","capillaries","." "The","arterial",",venous","and
capillary","pressures","are","maintained ","at","different","levels"])
process(blood_circulation, ["heart","blood_vessels","blood_pressure"],[])
process(blood_vessels, ["arteries","veins","capillaries"],[])
```

Figure 12.16 *A profile of the Prolog code generated from the cardiovascular knowledge-base.*

system. Such a multi-faceted modelling approach requires a hybrid toolkit which supports various knowledge representation paradigms.

One example of such a toolkit is the knowledge acquisition module (KAM) which is a hybrid of four paradigms—frame, object-orientation, Petri net, and process. The frame paradigm facilitates the creation of templates for the components and subsystems which are the building blocks of a mathematical model. The object-oriented paradigm of message-passing enables numerical procedures to be assigned to frames. Such procedures are then automatically invoked by the 'inheritance' mechanism to compute certain parameters of a frame. The Petri net formalism is a convenient way of describing discrete models. The process construct allows the linguistic description of a system to be structured in a way which emphasizes key concepts and entities and allows the description of each entity to be retrieved via a hypertext facility. A process can contain time-based information which is displayed on an event diagram. Similarly sequences described within a process construct are displayed on a sequence diagram.

In addition to the wide range of knowledge representation paradigms,

SHOW EQUATIONS OF PHYSBE

Ri2=Riv2
Ro2=Rov2
Ri4=Riv4
Ro4=Rov4
Pi1 = P1/Ri1+P6/Ro6+P7/Ro7+P8/Ro8+P9/Ro9/1/Ri1+1/Ro6+1/Ro7+1/Ro8+1/Ro9
Po1 = P1*Ri2+P2*Ro1/Ri2+Ro1
dV1/dt = pi1-P1/Ri1-P1-Po1/Ro1+Fe1
Po5 = P5/Ro5+P6/Ri6+P7/Ri7+P8/Ri8+P9/Ri9/1/Ro5+1/Ri6+1/Ri7+1/Ri8+1/Ri9
dV5/dt = pi5-P5/Ri5-P5-Po5/Ro5+Fe5
dV8/dt=pi-P8/Ri8-P8-Po8/Ro8+Fe8
Pi8=Po5
Po8=Pi1
dV9/dt=pi-P9/Ri9-P9-Po9/Ro9+Fe9
Pi9=Po5
Po9=Pi1
Press any key to continue
dV6/dt=pi-P6/Ri6-P6-Po6/Ro6+Fe6
Pi6=Po5
Po6=Pi1
dV7/dt=pi-P7/Ri7-P7-Po7/Ro7+Fe7
Pi7=Po5
Po7=Pi1
Po3=P3*Ri4+P4*Ro3/Ri4+Ro3
dV3/dt=pi-P3/Ri3-P3-Po3/Ro3+Fe3
Po4=P4*Ri5+P5*Ro4/Ri5+Ro4
dV4/dt=pi-P4/Ri4-P4-Po4/Ro4+Fe4
Po2=P2*Ri3+P3*Ro2/Ri3+Ro2
dV2/dt=pi-P2/Ri2-P2-Po2/Ro2+Fe2

Figure 12.17 *Equations of the PHYSBE model generated via KAM's query option.*

The left ventricle pushes the blood under high pressure through the arteries to the capillaries. The arterial, venous and capillary pressures are respectively

Press return to continue

Figure 12.18 *Illustration of the hypertext facility.*

XO———Tc_TVo_PVc_MVo_AVc———Tr_TVc_PVo_MVc_AVo———Ti_Xo

Figure 12.19 *Reachability tree generated from the Petri net model.*

KAM contains various facilities for the acquisition and processing of knowledge-bases. These include a compiler which converts a pseudo-natural language knowledge-base into a more compact form, a Prolog generator which converts the knowledge-base into Prolog code, a tree generator which shows the hierarchical relationships between various knowledge-base elements, and a query handler which retrieves information from frames.

The knowledge representation and acquisition facilities of KAM were demonstrated by applying it to modelling of the human cardiovascular system.

References

Feigenbaum, E.A., 1979, 'Themes and Case studies in Knowledge Engineering', in Michie (Ed.), *Expert Systems in the Microelectronic Age*, pp. 3–25, Edinburgh: Edinburgh University Press.
Forsyth, R., 1984, *An Introduction to Expert Systems*, London: Chapman and Hall.
Gregoire, L., 1992, in Gallagher (Ed.), *Anatomy and Physiology for Health Care Professionals*, Campion Press.
Hayes-Roth, F., 1984, The knowledge-based expert systems: a tutorial, *IEE Computer*, **17**, 87–92.
ISIM Simulation, 1988, *ESL Software User Manual*, Salford: Salford University Business Services Ltd.
Linkens, D.A., 1990, AI in control systems engineering, *The Knowledge Engineering Review*, **5**, 181–214.
Linkens, D.A., Bennett, S., Rahbar, M.R. and Tanyi, E., 1988, 'A Framework for a Knowledge based Modelling and Simulation Environment', presentation at the 12th IMACS World Congress, Paris, July 18–22.
McCleod, J., 1966, PHYSBE: A physiological Simulation Benchmark Experiment, *Simulation*, December.
Minsky, M., 1977, 'Frame-system theory', in Johnson-Laird and Wason (Eds), *Thinking*, pp. 355–76, Cambridge: Cambridge University Press.
Rene, D., 1991, 'Modelling of Dynamic Systems by Petri Nets', presentation at the European Control Conference, Grenoble, July.
Tanyi, E. and Linkens, D.A., 1987, 'A frame-based modelling and simulation environment', presentation at the UKSC '87 Conference, Bangor, September.
Tanyi, E., Linkens, D.A. and Bennett, S., 1990a, 'The Use of a Knowledge Acquisition Module (KAM) for constructing simulation models', presentation at the UKSC '90 Conference, Brighton, September 1990.
Tanyi, E., Linkens, D.A. and Bennett, S., 1990b, 'A Prolog-based driver for the ESL simulation language', presentation at the UKSC '90 Conference, Brighton, September.
Tanyi, E., Linkens, D.A. and Bennett, S., 1991, 'Knowledge acquisition and hierarchical structures for modelling and simulation', presentation at the 13th IMACS World Congress on Computation and Applied Mathematics, Dublin, July.
Tanyi, E., Linkens, D.A., Scott, A. and Bennett, S., 1992, 'Application of AI and model building techniques to software engineering', presentation at the IEE Colloquium on Application of Model Building Techniques to Software, April.
Willson, R.G. and Krogh, B.H., 1990, Petri net tools for the specification and analysis of discrete controllers, *Transactions of Software Engineering*, January.
Zeigler, P.B., 1984, Multifaceted Modelling Methodology, *Behaviour Science*, **29**.

Chapter 13
Automated qualitative model abduction based on bond graphs

S. Xia

13.1 Introduction

A knowledge-based environment for modelling and simulation of dynamic physical systems (KEMS) has been developed and implemented by the Sheffield Intelligent Modelling and Control research group (Linkens *et al.*, 1988). This intelligent environment consists of a graphical interface, an automatic modelling system, a model transformation system, a list of analytical tools, an equation and simulation code generator and a database management system for processing the simulation results (Linkens, 1989). We are incorporating both qualitative reasoning and numerical reasoning so that this environment supports model development, validation, analysis and result evaluation both qualitatively and numerically. Although the current interface between qualitative reasoning and numerical reasoning is still primitive and more work needs to be done, encouraging progress has been achieved in both the individual areas of qualitative reasoning and numerical reasoning. This chapter describes the group's recent progress in automatic modelling and qualitative simulation.

Automatic modelling and qualitative reasoning are closely related since qualitative reasoning is a form of model-based reasoning while modelling is an incremental process of extracting the physical principles governing a physical system, and in this incremental process qualitative reasoning plays a dominant role. As a result of the integration between automatic modelling and qualitative reasoning, models can be produced automatically from system structures, and using these models qualitative analysis can be conducted. So both expert and novice users can qualitatively study physical systems without knowing technical details of system modelling, equation formulation and solving (Linkens et al., 1993).

Although a user's work in system modelling can be reduced, it cannot be omitted. A user plays a vital role in judging whether a model is a 'good' model since the definition of a 'good' model depends on the application. Thus for some applications, a model can be too simple whilst for other applications, the same model can be too complicated. Therefore, a user must make the decision as to what level of model is acceptable.

A model is an approximation of all physical principles inherent in a physical system. In engineering terms, a 'good' model is the simplest and sufficiently complete one for the particular application. A compromise between completeness and simpleness is necessary (Martens and Bell, 1972). Completeness and simpleness are two contradictory requirements: completeness is involved with selection of the main properties of a system, all of which must be accounted for in the model; simpleness is concerned with identification of auxiliary properties of the system, all of which must be neglected in the model. Hence an approach can be taken which uses a simple model, such as an empty model, as a starting model and then augments it gradually until it is complete. This approach requires that a user specifies what properties of a system should be accounted for in the model. This concept has been called 'reticulation' in the field of bond graph methodology.

The main properties of a physical system can often be described only in qualitative terms and not in numerical terms. Hence, numerical methods often do not apply and qualitative methods have to be used. Qualitative reasoning is a form of algebraic manipulation on a structural model using relevant concepts, physical laws and general principles (DeKleer and Brown, 1984; Forbus, 1984; Kuipers, 1986). It can describe and evaluate the behaviour of the system in terms of its major properties. It does not require any numerical information since all cause–effect relations are described in qualitative terms. Therefore when a user specifies a list of main properties of a system in qualitative terms, qualitative reasoning can judge whether a model can explain these properties and thus can conclude if a model is complete.

An assumption is made in this research: non-linear behaviour is limited to the monotonical non-linear relationships. This assumption is reasonable in real-world applications since in the vast majority of cases, the relationships between effort and displacement of a capacitive element, between flow and momentum of an inertial element and between effort and flow of a dissipative element are monotonic functions.

This chapter describes our research work on combined qualitative reasoning and automatic modelling. The second section briefly explains the methodology of bond graph modelling and the third and fourth sections discuss qualitative models, their automatic generation and qualitative reasoning on component and parameter changes. A computer-aided system for automatic modelling is described in Section 13.5 and a case study is presented in Section 13.6. The chapter ends with a discussion of related work and conclusions.

13.2 Bond-graph methodology

In terms of energy changes, the functionality of components can be classified into five categories (Karnopp and Rosenberg, 1983):

(1) a source delivering energy to other components through delivering either a generalized effort (Se), such as force, voltage and pressure or a generalized flow (Sf), such as velocity, current and flowing quantity;
(2) a component receiving and storing energy through storing either a generalized effort (I) or a generalized flow (C);
(3) a component dissipating energy through dissipating either a generalized effort or generalized flow (R);
(4) an energy transforming medium changing energy from one component to another in one energy domain (TF);
(5) an energy transducing medium changing energy from one energy domain to another (GY).

A system is a group of such components connected either in parallel (0) or in series (1). So a system can be described as a function of the nine variables, Se, Sf, I, C, R, TF, GY, 0 and 1.

The dynamics of a physical system can be described by the five elements of bond graphs, which include inertial, capacitive, dissipative, transformative and gyrative elements. The variables associated with these five elements are their effort and flow variables, the momentum variable of inertial elements, and the displacement variable of capacitive elements. These twelve variables are used as primitive variables, through which qualitative reasoning about dynamic systems is conducted.

Three contributions from bond graphs are emphasized in the work presented here: conceptual formulation of physical laws; generalization of a physical nature between systems of different domains (Rosenberg, 1975); and their intermediate role in relating physical structure information and numerical descriptions. As a result, bond graphs contain both structural information and behavioural information, and can be used as a bridge between the two. This makes it possible to derive a behavioural description from a structural description in a systematic manner.

Furthermore, a bond graph builds a one-to-one correspondence between system components and their representations on the graph. This facilitates model modification, since elements and junctions can be added into or deleted from a model (Blundell, 1983; Rosenberg, 1975). This supports the engineering process of model refinement: firstly, an initial, simple model is constructed; secondly, model refinement is made iteratively until a satisfactory model is built.

Having introduced the methodology of bond-graph modelling, we continue to define a qualitative model and build the relationship between a bond graph and a qualitative model.

13.3 Principles of automatic modelling

When a human expert builds a model for a system, many standard procedures are followed. These procedures implicitly reflect what should be considered, what should be ignored and what constraints should be met in building a model. In automatic modelling, these practices have to be explicitly declared as generic modelling principles in order to generate sensible models. Currently, these generic modelling principles include the similar complexity principle, lumped-distributed match principle, modularity principle, order-of-magnitude principle and causality principle. By following these generic modelling principles, the models generated will be sensible models.

The *similar complexity principle* requires that in modelling a system, all components in the system should be modelled in similar detail. It is against this principle if one component is modelled in great depth while another equally important component is modelled at a shallow level.

The *lumped-distributed match principle* explains that components which play equally important roles in a system should all be modelled either in a lumped or in a distributed manner. It does not make any sense if a component is modelled distributively while an equally important component takes a lumped form of description.

The *modularity principle* prescribes that all physical systems have the property that decomposition and reassembly of a physical system should not change the form of the model. This principle has both physical and computational implications. The physical implication is that a physical system remains the same system no matter whether the system is analysed globally or locally. A global analysis is concerned mainly with the input–output relationships of a system, while a local analysis is involved with not only the input–output relationships but also the intermediate relationships between input and output variables. The computational implication is that if all the models of components are modular, then combining them is a simple matter of substitution, which is a tolerable computational problem. Otherwise, combining a model of a component into or with models of different environments may in general require a complete reformulation of all or some of the models, which is a prohibitively complicated computational problem.

According to the *order-of-magnitude principle*, variables which play equally important rules in a system are classified into groups and when one variable is considered in a model, all the other variables belonging to the same order-of-magnitude group must also be considered in the model. Similarly, if one variable is neglected, then all the other relevant variables must also be neglected.

The *causality principle* consists of causal constraints and causality consistency constraints. Causal constraints ensure that a model only describes causal relationships and must not contain any computational relationships which are not physically realizable. For example, a derivative relationship is such a non-causal relationship since its operation depends on future events. Causality consistency constraints express the fact that the descriptions of all components must be causal, and furthermore the input type to a component must be in agreement with the output type of the up-stream neighbouring components, and the output type of a component must be compatible with the input type of down-stream neighbouring components.

The above principles are domain-independent modelling principles and are used to guide the process of model formulation. In addition to these principles, there are many domain-dependent constraints, which are specified by users. The above generic principles are applied to guarantee the validity of a model while the domain-dependent constraints are satisfied to ensure the completeness of the model.

Currently, the following domain-dependent constraints are considered in the automatic modelling expert system: domain (model), effort or flow (causality type), static or dynamic (model type), monotonic or linear (relationship), qualitative or numerical (value), order (model), rigid (component), torsional (component), compressible or incompressible (component), laminar or turbulent (component), elastic or inelastic (component), frictional or frictionless (component) and so on.

13.4 Qualitative simulation

13.4.1 Monotonically increasing and decreasing functions

Monotonically increasing and decreasing functions are used extensively in this section and are defined here briefly: X and Y are two variables, and Y is a function of X. If X increases, decreases or remains unchanged, and Y also increases, decreases or remains unchanged respectively and vice versa, then Y is a monotonically increasing function of X, denoted as $Y = M+(X)$; if X increases, decreases and remains unchanged, and as a result Y decreases, increases and remains unchanged respectively and vice versa, then Y is a monotonically decreasing function of X, notated as $Y = M-(X)$. A detailed discussion of these two types of function can be found in Kuipers (1986).

13.4.2 Simulation model

Bond graphs contain capacitive, inertial and dissipative elements connected via parallel, serial, transformative and gyrative junctions. Capacitive and inertial elements are both involved with integral, derivative and arithmetic operations. Dissipative elements, transformative and gyrative junctions contain only arithmetic operations. Parallel and serial junctions include additive, subtractive, negative and equal operations. Therefore, relationships existing among bond graph elements can all be described using arithmetic, equal, integral and derivative operators. The qualitative descriptions of the above four operators, equal ($=$), negate ($-$), add ($+$), integral (int) and derivative (der) are defined and discussed in the paper by Xia et al. (1992). These operators and the bond graph basic elements constitute a formal language for the description of qualitative relationships.

A qualitative model is defined as a model consisting of a set of physical variables representing the physical properties of a system and a list of the above qualitative operators constraining these physical variables.

13.4.3 Automatic model construction

The qualitative relationship between variables of elements are defined as follows:

$$C: Q = \text{int}(F), E = -Q$$
$$I: M = -\text{int}(E), M = F$$
$$R: E = F$$
1 junction: $E = E(1) + E(2) + \ldots + E(k),$
$F = F(1) = F(2) = \ldots = F(k)$
0 junction: $E = E(1) = E(2) = \ldots = E(k),$
$F = F(1) + F(2) + \ldots + F(k)$
TF junction: $E_{in} = E_{out}, F_{in} = F_{out}$
GY junction: $E_{in} = F_{out}, F_{in} = E_{out}$

where Q, M, E and F stand for displacement, momentum, effort and flow of the relevant element respectively, $E(k)$ representing the effort of an out-going bond k and $F(k)$ the flow of an out-going bond k.

Therefore, if the model of a physical system is described by C, I and R elements connected via serial, parallel, transformative and gyrative junc-

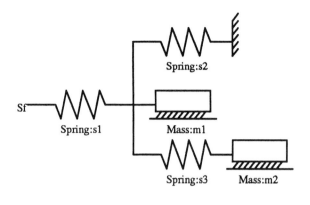

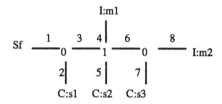

Figure 13.1 *A bond graph modelling example.*

tions, then its qualitative model can be automatically constructed. A physical system and its bond graph are shown in Figure 13.1.

The qualitative model of this system is: $F(1) = F(2) + F(3)$, $E(1) = E(2) = E(3)$, $X(2) = \text{INT}(F(2))$, $X(2) = -E(2)$, $F(3) = F(4) = F(5) = F(6)$, $E(3) = E(4) + E(5) + E(6)$, $X(5) = \text{INT}(F(5))$, $X(5) = -E(5)$, $M(4) = -\text{INT}(E(4))$, $M(4) = F(4)$, $F(6) = F(7) + F(8)$, $E(6) = E(7) + E(8)$, $X(7) = \text{INT}(F(7))$, $X(7) = -E(7)$, $M(8) = -\text{INT}(E(8))$, $M(8) = F(8)$.

13.4.4 Simulation

The qualitative simulation algorithm repeatedly takes a variable(s) with a known state(s) and a qualitative constraint with the above chosen variable(s) and at least one variable with an unknown state. Using the particular qualitative constraint, all possible states of the latter variable are generated. This iterative process continues until the states of all relevant variables are resolved. Filtering out states that violate the consistency constraints, the remaining states describe all the possible behaviours of a physical system. Four types of consistency constraints (local, global, simultaneous and historical constraints) are used and discussed here.

Local constraints refer to constraints used separately and locally. Every constraint in a qualitative model is a local constraint. To satisfy local constraints, a behaviour must at least satisfy some constraints. Local constraints are used mainly to generate states and to construct behaviours.

Global constraints maintain that constraints are dealt with collectively and as a whole. If a variable is involved with several local constraints, it must have a state that satisfies all relevant local constraints.

Simultaneous constraints require that variables related to a power distribution junction all have either boundary qualitative states like 'maximal', 'minimal' and 'zero', or intermediate qualitative states like 'positive' and 'negative'. Furthermore, the qualitative states of these variables change at the same rate.

Historical constraints reflect relationships between current behaviour and past or future behaviour. If the current behaviour is a real behaviour, both its past and future behaviours must satisfy the global constraints.

13.5 Automatic modelling

The knowledge-base, structural description, structural decomposition, model generation and analysis of model simpleness and completeness are explained in this section.

13.5.1 Knowledge-base

A rule-based knowledge-base has been constructed for automatic modelling which contains the descriptions of all the standard components used in the modelling process. These descriptions are called models of components and they are constructed using three standard elements, C, I and R elements and four junctions (serial, parallel, transformative and gyrative junctions). A component can have several models and these models are ordered according to their complexity. The following is a prototype of the knowledge-base:

(1) spring-like components—capacitors and compressible fluids are C elements,
(2) inertial components—inductors and fluid inertia are I elements,
(3) dynamic dampers—static dampers, resistors, frictional effects, valves and electric diodes are R elements,
(4) motors, generators, electromagnetic actuators have several models: GY element, $R + GY$ element, $R + C + GY$ element, $R + C + I + GY$ element (R—coil resistance, C—coil capacitance, I—coil inductance),
(5) gears, electric transformers, levers and pulleys are TF elements,
(6) pumps, slider-cranks, fans, blowers, propellers and compressors have several models: TF element; $R + TF$ element; $R + I + TF$ element; $R + I + C + TF$ element (R—friction, I—mechanical inertia, C—hydraulic compliance),

Automated qualitative model abduction based on bond graphs 393

(7) shafts have several models: a bond (no dynamics); I element; $C+I$ element; $C+I+C+I$ element (C—shaft compliance, I—shaft inertia),
(8) flowing lines (water, oil, gas, air and any other fluid) have several models: a bond (no dynamics); C element; $C+I$ element; $C+I+R$ element (C—flowing capacitance, I—flowing inertia, R—flowing friction).

13.5.2 System structure

In this approach, a system is defined as an ensemble of recognizable components which are interacting. A real machine is split into primary components, each of which realizes only one function. A system can be a primary component or a serial or parallel combination of a primary component and one or more subsystems. In this system of automatic modelling, the description of components and physical connections of components is used as input. This description should be close to a real system so that the structural information can be described completely.

13.5.3 Structural decomposition and model construction

Firstly the structure of a system is decomposed into connections of standard components. If a system does not contain any components, then it is an empty system. If the system contains one standard component, then the component is the output of the system. If the system contains more components, then the system is decomposed into the following two cases: (1) if a point can be found that divides all the system components into two groups of components, then the system is decomposed into two subsystems, which are series connected; (2) if no such point can be found, then the system is decomposed into several subsystems, all of which are connected in parallel. The subsystems thus obtained are analysed iteratively in a similar manner until they contain no more than one component.

Given the basic structure, a model is then constructed. If a system is empty, then its model is empty. If the system contains one primitive component, then the element associated with the component is the model. If the system contains more than one component, then the system is decomposed into primitive components and subsystems and then subsystems are decomposed recursively. Serial connections are modelled by velocity-common junctions and parallel connections by force-common junctions.

13.5.4 Model simpleness and completeness

An empty model is used as an initial model and is then expanded gradually with the addition of more system variables. This addition is performed only when the added variables are essential to the behaviour of a system. So the simpleness of a model is guaranteed.

Before a model can be used to account for the next characteristics of a physical system, it must meet three constraints: the causal constraint, the zero-output-flow constraint and the zero-output-effort constraint. Firstly, an initial model must not contain any causal conflicts. Otherwise, those components relevant to causal conflicts are identified and remodelled with their next highest level models in the knowledge-base with the purpose that these conflicts should be resolved. Secondly, when the output flow is set to zero, the states of all variables must be consistent with intuition and observation. Thirdly, when the output effort is set to zero, the states of all variables also must not be against intuition and observation. In either the second or the third case, if some variables have infinite efforts or flows, which are not as specified, then R elements must be added into the junctions of the variables with infinite values. Some heuristics are articulated as rules for use in this process. For example, a model without any storage elements is a static model and cannot describe any dynamic behaviour; only a second- or higher-order model is capable of modelling an oscillatory phenomenon, an oscillatory phenomenon requires two or more energy stores and at least two of them are of the opposite type; a constant output (flow or effort) means either that the input (flow, effort) is constant or that there is a flywheel-like inertial component; if a dynamic behaviour dies out, then friction, resistance or damping effects should be considered.

This process continues until all the characteristics specified for a particular system can be explained and then this model is produced as the output of the automatic modelling. Therefore the resulting model is both simple and complete. The case study in Section 13.6 demonstrates this process more clearly.

When a simple and complete model is obtained, a user can add C elements to junctions with one or more C elements, I elements to junctions with other I elements and R elements to junctions with other R elements. According to the property of qualitative behaviour aggregation, this addition will not change the qualitative behaviour of the model.

13.6 Case study

This case study consists of two parts, one on the automatic modelling of a motor-pump system and the other on automatic analysis of the qualitative behaviour of the system.

13.6.1 Automatic modelling

Example: A motor is driven by a voltage source (input) and in turn drives a pump through a shaft and then pumps fluid from tank A to tank B (output).

Automated qualitative model abduction based on bond graphs 395

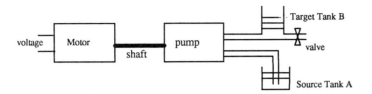

Figure 13.2 *A hydraulic system schematic diagram.*

The structure of this system is a serial connection of a voltage source, motor, shaft, pump, pipe and a flowing fluid output. Its schematic diagram is given in Figure 13.2. A model for this system is required, based on the following specified characterization.

The main properties of the behaviour of this particular physical system are given as follows.

(1) The input is a voltage source and the output is a fluid flow. So the energy form is changed: electronic energy is changed into mechanical energy, which is then changed into hydraulic energy.
(2) When the input voltage is cut off, the output flow does not stop immediately and it changes from normal to zero gradually.
(3) The output of the system is a hydraulic pressure.
(4) When the output flow is blocked, the shaft could be broken.
(5) When tank A is empty of the fluid, the system runs at a very high speed.
(6) When the voltage source is switched off, the system will eventually become static even when the load of the system is negligible.

An empty model is a simple model and it is used initially. This initial model is gradually expanded so that the model can increasingly explain more properties of the system behaviour. If the expanded model can explain all the stated properties, then it is complete and the process of automatic modelling is stopped. The model thus generated is both simple and complete.

(1) An empty model obviously cannot explain the first property and is not complete. The system has five components: source, motor, shaft, pump, pipe, output, and the connection is serial. According to the knowledge-base described in Section 13.5.1, a motor is modelled by a GY element, a shaft by a bond, a pump by a TF element and a pipe by a bond. So Model 1 is constructed, as presented in Figure 13.3.

A GY element can change electronic energy into mechanical energy and a *TF* element changes mechanical energy into hydraulic energy. So Model 1

Model 1 : voltage →|GY|—1→ TF|—2→ —3→ Flow

Figure 13.3 *A static bond graph model for Figure 13.2.*

can account for the first property, that is the changes of energy domains. Furthermore, the causal constraint, zero-output-flow constraint and zero-output-effort constraint can all be satisfied.

(2) Model 1 is not complete as it cannot explain the second property: when the input voltage is switched from normal to zero, the output flow can be any value from normal to zero. This contradiction is identified in the following qualitative reasoning: the qualitative model of Model 1 is: $E1 = F2 = F3$, $F1 = E2 = E3$. If $E1$ equals zero, $F3$ has to be zero and it cannot take any other value.

The fact that there is no energy supply and yet some output flow still exists suggests that the system itself can store energy. A storage element therefore should be considered. According to the knowledge-base described in Section 13.5.1 and using the next highest level models, a motor is modelled as an $R + GY$ element, a shaft by an I element, a pump by an $R + TF$ element and a pipe by a C element. The motor and pump models do not have any storage elements and are not considered. Compared with compressibility of the fluid, the inertance of a shaft mass is more relevant and can explain the second property much better. This is particularly true if a fly-wheel is attached to the shaft. The shaft inertance I_s is modelled next in Model 2 as shown in Figure 13.4.

As a result, the system has two types of behaviour, static behaviour at an equilibrium state and dynamic behaviour at a non-equilibrium state. The second property can be explained by the dynamic property of the new model.

(3) The above model contains a causal conflict in the serial junction after causalities are assigned to Model 2. If the input to a serial junction is flow, all elements attached to the junction must take flow as input. However in Model 2, the shaft mass (I_s) is an inertial element and must take effort as input. This results in a causal conflict.

Going back to the knowledge-base, the next highest level models for a motor, shaft, pump and pipe are respectively an $R + GY$ element, an $I + C$

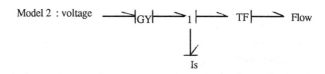

Figure 13.4 *A dynamic bond graph model with causal conflict for Figure 13.2.*

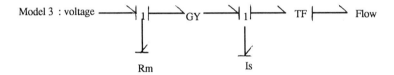

Figure 13.5 *A bond graph satisfying the first two properties for Figure 13.2.*

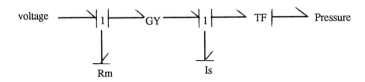

Figure 13.6 *A bond graph containing causal conflicts.*

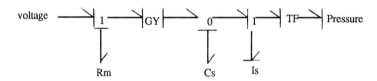

Figure 13.7 *A new bond graph still containing a causal conflict.*

element, an $R + TF$ element and a C element. The new pump and pipe models cannot resolve the above conflict and thus are not accepted. The coil resistance is more likely to be important to the dynamics of the system than the shaft compliance. After the insertion of the coil resistance R_m, Model 3 is generated, as presented in Figure 13.5.

(4) According to the third property, the system produces a pressure on the flowing fluid. So the system has a voltage source as input and a pressure as output. Using these two causal constraints to assign causalities to Model 3, the causal bond graph in Figure 13.6 is obtained.

Another causal conflict appears in the second series junction. This indicates that a system described by Model 3 can only produce a flow. In order to meet this output constraint, the process of automatic modelling continues to examine the next highest level models in the knowledge-base: $R + C + GY$ (motor), $C + I$ (shaft), $R + TF$ (pump) and C (pipe fluid).

Using the new model of the shaft, the causal conflict remains, as shown in the following causal bond graph. Similar analysis also indicates that the above causal conflict cannot be resolved by employing the new motor model or the new pump model, as demonstrated in Figure 13.7.

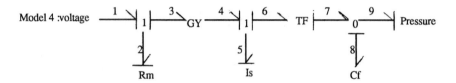

Figure 13.8 *A bond graph satisfying the first three properties for Figure 13.2.*

By modelling the fluid compressibility, the causal conflict is, however, resolved. Therefore, the omission of the fluid compressibility is responsible for the above causal conflict. Accordingly, Model 3 is expanded to include the fluid compressibility, a comparison with Model 4 is shown in Figure 13.8.

(5) The qualitative relationships in this model are: $E1 = E2 + E3$, $F1 = F2 = F3 = E4$, $E3 = F4 = F5 = F6 = F7$, $E4 = E5 + E6$, $E6 = E7 = E8 = E9$, $F7 = F8 + F9$, $E2 = F2$, $F5 = int(E5)$, $E8 = int(F8)$.

If the flowing pipe is blocked, reasoning on the above qualitative relationships results in the behaviour that all variables are stable: $E9 = $ maximal (given), $F9 = $ zero (given), $E1 = $ positive, $E2 = $ maximal, $E3 = $ zero, $E4 = $ maximal, $E5 = $ zero, $E6 = $ maximal, $E7 = $ maximal, $E8 = $ maximal, $F1 = $ maximal, $F2 = $ maximal, $F3 = $ maximal, $F4 = $ zero, $F5 = $ zero, $F6 = $ zero, $F7 = $ zero, $F8 = $ zero.

Thus when the flowing pipe is blocked, a system of the model can still function. The fourth property that the shaft could be broken cannot be predicted by Model 4. The fact that a shaft could be broken suggests that the shaft compliance should be considered. Going back to the knowledge base, the next higher level model of the shaft with compliance is $C + I$. With this new model of the shaft, Model 5 in Figure 13.9 is produced.

(6) The modelling process continues and analysis on Model 5 is conducted to examine whether Model 5 can explain the fifth property of the system behaviour.

It tank A is empty, the flowing entity is air and the resistance and the system output pressure are very small. The qualitative relations extracted from Model 5 are: $E1 = E2 + E3$, $F1 = F2 = F3 = E4 = E5 = E6$, $E3 = F4$, $F4 = F5 + F6$, $E6 = E7 + E8$, $F6 = F7 = F8 = F9$, $E8 = E9 = E10 = E11$, $F9 = F10 + F11$, $E2 = F2$, $E5 = int(F5)$, $F7 = int(E7)$, $E10 = int(F10)$. In this case, $F11$ represents the flow speed of air, not the fluid.

The resistance change of the load is the major change introduced in Model 5 and the system behaviour depends on the effect of this change. Compared with the effect of the resistance change of the load, the effect of the dissipatance change caused by the fluid compressibility change is negligible. So the system behaviour can be decided unambiguously. Using the above qualitative relations, the states of all variables are deduced:

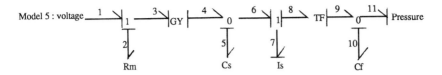

Figure 13.9 *A bond graph model satisying the first five properties for Figure 13.2.*

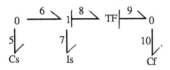

Figure 13.10 *A bond graph model indicating a self-activated system for Figure 13.2.*

$E11$ = very-low (given), $F1$ = very-low, $F2$ = very-low, $F3$ = very-low, $E1$ = positive (constant), $E2$ = very-low, $E3$ = very-high, $E4$ = very-low, $F4$ = very-high, $E5$ = very-low, $F5$ = very-low, $E6$ = very-low, $F6$ = very-high, $E7$ = very-high, $F7$ = very-high, $E8$ = very-low, $F8$ = very-high, $E9$ = very-low, $F9$ = very-high, $E10$ = very-low, $F10$ = very-low, $F11$ = very-high.

This prediction is consistent with the fifth property of the system that when tank A is empty of fluid, the system runs at a very high speed. As a result, the fifth property can be explained and the process of automatic modelling continues without any change to the model.

(7) Consider now the sixth property that when the voltage source is switched off, the system will eventually become static even when the system has no load. This cannot be explained by Model 5. When the voltage source is switched off, the effect of the motor can be neglected. Ignoring the load, Model 5 becomes the following model and the dynamic system of this model, indicating a self-activated system once it has stored energy, as demonstrated in Figure 13.10.

In this case, the computer system adds all possible friction effects into a model: the connection friction between the motor and the shaft, R_{ms}, the connection friction between the shaft and the pump, R_{sp} and the friction between the flowing fluid and pipe R_{fp}. Model 6 is generated, as shown in Figure 13.11.

The process of automatic modelling terminates here because Model 6 meets all the property requirements of the system behaviour. Model 6 does not contain any causal conflict and it meets both the zero-output-flow and the zero-output-effort constraints. Furthermore, it is both simple and complete. Model 6 is the required parsimonious model.

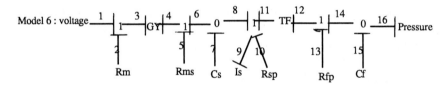

Figure 13.11 *A bond graph model satisfying all six properties for Figure 13.2.*

13.6.2 Automatic analysis

In this section, we use the automatically generated parsimonious model, i.e. Model 6 as described by Figure 13.11 to reason about possible fault scenarios. Compared with the normal situation, we consider what are the qualitative changes to the system behaviour when:

(1) the flowing-out pipe is blocked,
(2) tank A is empty of the fluid,
(3) the coefficient of the motor is changed,
(4) the coefficient of the pump is changed.

The model of the system is that generated in the process of automatic modelling, as described above.

The qualitative model of Model 6 is: $E1 = E2 + E3$, $F1 = F2 = F3 = E4$, $E3 = F4 = F5 = F6$, $E4 = E5 + E6$, $E6 = E7 = E8$, $F6 = F7 + F8$, $E8 = E9 + E10 + E11$, $F8 = F9 = F10 = F11 = F12 = F13 = F14$, $E11 = E12$, $E12 = E13 + E14$, $E14 = E15 = E16$, $F14 = F15 + F16$, $E2 = F2$, $E5 = F5$, $E7 = \mathrm{int}(F7)$, $F9 = \mathrm{int}(E9)$, $E10 = F10$, $E13 = F13$, $E15 = \mathrm{int}(F15)$, $Q7 = E7$, $M9 = F9$, $Q15 = E15$.

We assume that the input voltage is constant. The above fault situations are studied one by one using this qualitative model.

(1) THE FLOWING-OUT PIPE IS BLOCKED
The pipe is blocked, so that $E16 =$ maximal, $F16 =$ zero. The input voltage is constant, so that $E1 =$ positive. Reasoning with the above equations and using the notation $e(1)$ for Equation (1) etc., gives: $E14 = E15 = E16 =$ maximal, $F15 =$ zero, $F14 =$ zero, $F8 = F9 = F10 = F11 = F12 = F13 = F14 =$ zero, $E13 =$ zero, $E12 =$ maximal, $E11 =$ maximal, $E10 =$ zero, $E9 =$ zero, $E8 =$ maximal, $E6 = E7 = E8 =$ maximal, $F7 =$ zero, $F6 =$ zero, $E3 = F4 = F5 = F6 =$ zero, $E5 =$ zero, $E4 =$ maximal, $F1 = F2 = F3 = E4 =$ maximal, $E2 =$ maximal, $E3 =$ zero, $Q7 =$ maximal, $M9 =$ zero, $Q15 =$ maximal.

Therefore, when the inflow is gradually blocked, the current flowing through the motor coil gradually increases, the rotational speed of the shaft decreases, the angle of rotational displacement of the shaft increases, the pump works more slowly and the fluid flowing rate decreases. This process continues until an equilibrium state is reached: the current is maximal, the back emf of the motor is zero, the angular displacement of the shaft is maximal, the shaft and the pump are both static and there is no flow from tank A to tank B.

In this case, if the capacitance (or compliance) of the shaft is too high, the shaft will be broken. This prediction is consistent with the fourth property of the system behaviour specified by the user.

Another interesting conclusion can be deduced from the above qualitative model: there is a limit to the height of tank B to which the fluid from tank A can be pumped. From the above model, if the height of tank B is increased, i.e. $E16$ is increased, the coil current will be increased and the pipe flow $F16$ will decrease. Because there is an upper limit on the current flow in the coil, which is source-voltage/coil-resistance, the height of tank B is also limited. If tank B is positioned higher than this height limit, the whole system will stop working. Furthermore, there is a danger that the shaft will be broken.

(2) TANK A IS EMPTY OF FLUID

The source tank is empty of fluid, so that the quantity flowing through the pipe is air. The pressure and the impedance are both very low, and hence $E16$ = very-low, $R16$ = very-low. Furthermore, the compliance of air is much higher than that of the fluid, so the impedance of air is much lower, $R15$ = very-low.

As far as resistance or impedance is concerned, the resistance or impedance caused by the load is clearly the deciding factor in the system behaviour. The following assumption is reasonable: compared with the resistance caused by the load, the resistance of the motor coil is very low and can be neglected. Therefore the qualitative states of bond 1 and bond 3 are equal: $R1 = R3$. The same argument can be applied to all of the remaining serial junctions, so that $R4 = R6$, $R8 = R11$, $R12 = R14$. On the other hand, the impedance caused by the shaft capacitance is much higher than the impedance caused by the load because the capacitance of the shaft is so low. The capacitance is always connected with the load in parallel and so its impedance can also be ignored. Therefore $R6 = R8$. This leads to the following conclusions:

$R12 = R14$ and $R14$ = very-low: $R12$ = very-low

Applying the transform and dissipation reduction, $R11 = R12$:
$R11$ = very-low
$R8 = R11$: $R8$ = very-low
$R6 = R8$: $R6$ = very-low
$R4 = R6$: $R4$ = very-low

Applying the gyration and dissipation reduction, $R3$ is a reciprocal function of $R4$: $R3$ = very-high
$R1 = R3$: $R1$ = very-high

The voltage source $E1$ is constant: $F1$ = very-low, $F1 = F2 = F3$ = very-low, $E2$ = very-low, $E3$ = very-high

Using the above qualitative model, all the other variables can be assigned a state: $E4$ = very-low, $F4$ = very-high, $E5$ = very-high, $F5$ = very-high, $E6$ = very-low, $F6$ = very-high, $E7$ = very-low, $F7$ = very-low, $Q7$ = very-low, $E8$ = very-low, $F8$ = very-high, $E9$ = very-high, $F9$ = very-high, $M9$ = very-high, $E10$ = very-high, $F10$ = very-high, $E11$ = very low, $F11$ = very-high, $E12$ = very-low, $F12$ = very-high, $E13$ = very-high, $F13$ = very-high, $E14$ = very-low, $F14$ = very-high, $E15$ = very-low, $F15$ = very-low, $Q15$ = very-low, $E16$ = very-low, $F16$ = very-high.

Therefore, when tank A gradually becomes empty of fluid, the current flowing through the motor coil decreases, the angular speed of the shaft increases, the angular displacement of the shaft decreases, the shaft momentum increases and the pump works faster and faster. This change continues until tank A is completely empty of fluid, there is little current flowing through the coil and the shaft and pump work at an extremely high speed.

(3) THE COEFFICIENT OF THE MOTOR IS CHANGED

The impedance of the motor caused by load is a monotonically increasing function of the motor coefficient. Therefore when the coefficient is reduced, the resulting impedance becomes lower under the same load.

Because the coil resistance is constant, the current flowing through the coil becomes higher and the voltage drop across the coil is higher. So the shaft is more powerful but its angular speed is lower.

Based on this analysis, when the motor coefficient is tuned higher, the whole system works faster but less powerfully; however, when the motor coefficient is tuned lower, the system works at a lower speed but is more powerful.

(4) THE COEFFICIENT OF THE PUMP IS CHANGED

When the pump coefficient is reduced, the same shaft speed produces a lower flowrate. The resulting resistance is a monotonically increasing function of the pump coefficient. So under the same load, the resistance is higher.

Based on the above model, when the pump coefficient is tuned higher, the system works at a lower speed but becomes more powerful; when it is tuned lower, the system runs faster but becomes less powerful.

13.7 Related work

Automatic modelling is receiving more and more attention in the qualitative reasoning community. Among several approaches, our work is closest to the 'Compositional Modelling' (CM) work (Falkenhainer and Forbus, 1991) and the 'Graph of Models' (GoM) work (Addanki et al., 1991). In the CM approach, a knowledge-base is implemented before analysis to explicitly declare the relevant conditionalized model fragments. In answering a query, CM firstly identifies an appropriate set of modelling assumptions from this query and uses these modelling assumptions to construct an appropriate model, which is then employed to answer the query. In some ways, CM is not as practical and formalized as our work. Firstly, how to systematically build a set of conditionalized model fragments required for modelling is less clear although a semantics of the concept has been defined. Secondly, it is difficult to check the validity of a model and to detect the consistencies between fragments since fragments are implemented independently and some fragments may be described qualitatively and others quantitatively. Thirdly, generic physical modelling principles which we believe are essential in formulating 'good' models, are currently not considered. In spite of this, CM is still an important first approach in adding assumptions to model representation and formulating different models for different applications and it can be used as a theoretical framework for automatic modelling. In the GoM work, all possible models are directly created and represented as the nodes of a graph and the relationships between different models are denoted as the edges. This graph is called a modelling graph and is implemented by hand before its application. The main difference between our work and GoM is that our work deals with automatic modelling, i.e. models are constructed from low-level submodels of components while GoM are more involved with model selection since all models have already been constructed in advance of analysis. Our work is therefore more flexible than GoM although in some cases when all possible models of a domain are very clear and manageable, GoM could be appropriate and efficient.

Other related work includes DeKleer's multiple representation of knowledge, Davis's multiple levels of structural descriptions for diagnosis, Weld's approximation reformulation, Kuipers' automatic model abduction, Lin's task-driven perspective-taking for qualitative reasoning and Leitch's model commitment. They all show the importance of multiple model representation in analysing physical systems. Our work is different from them in that three levels of model—conceptual, causal and numerical model, are formulated in terms of physical entities of dynamic physical systems. Therefore many qualitative properties, such as oscillation, stability and causality, can be derived in our work while in other work, these physical entities are not modelled and many qualitative properties therefore cannot be examined.

13.8 Conclusions

This chapter has demonstrated the feasibility of integrating qualitative reasoning and automatic modelling. As a result, a bond graph can be generated from a structural description of a physical system. This bond graph is a simple but complete model of a system based on qualitative properties of the system provided by a user. How powerful an automatic modelling tool is depends on how powerful the structure decomposition facility is. The current decomposition facility can deal with serial and parallel interactions. If this decomposition facility can be improved to handle more complex interactions between components, then physical systems with more complicated interactions between components can be modelled automatically. The effectiveness of this automatic modelling tool is determined, of course, by the accuracy of the rules represented in the knowledge-base.

A qualitative model can be formulated from a bond graph systematically, and qualitative analysis can be performed. Two types of qualitative reasoning are conducted, reasoning on states and on parameters. The former refers to the reasoning on relationships between states of variables, and the latter the reasoning on the effects of parameter changes on a system state.

It has been shown by the case study that a user's involvement in this problem-solving process is reduced considerably. The modelling work, which previously had to be done manually by a user, can now be conducted automatically. A user only needs to provide a list of the main properties of a physical system.

This work represents important progress in developing our intelligent KEMS environment. As a result, a model is now more manageable, and a user can examine what has been accounted for and what has been neglected in a model. Furthermore, a model can be validated more easily as it is constructed in an algorithmic manner. The next stage of research will involve expanding the knowledge-base and improving the algorithm for structural decomposition. Plans have been made to apply this work to qualitative fault diagnosis and automatic model validation.

References

Addanki, S., Cremonini, R. and Penberthy, J.S., 1991, Graphs of models, *Artificial Intelligence*, **51**, 145–78.

Blundell, A.J., 1983, *Bond Graph for Modelling Engineering Systems*, New York: Wiley.

Breedveld, P.C., 1987, 'A systematic method to derive bond graph models', in Proceedings of the 2nd European Simulation Congress.

Davis, R., 1984, Diagnostic reasoning based on structure and behaviour, *Artificial Intelligence*, **24**, 347–410.

DeKleer, J., 1977, 'Multiple representations of knowledge in a mechanics problem-solver', in Proceedings of the IJCAI-77, Cambridge, MA, pp. 299–304.
DeKleer, J. and Brown, J.S., 1984, A qualitative physics based on confluences, *Artificial Intelligence*, **24**, 7–83.
Falkenhainer, B. and Forbus, K.D., 1991, Compositional modelling: finding the right model for the job, *Artificial Intelligence*, **51**, 95–143.
Forbus, K.D., 1984, Qualitative process theory, *Artificial Intelligence*, **24**, 85–168.
Franke, D.W. and Dvorak, D.L., 1989, 'Component connection models', presentation at the Workshop on Model-Based Reasoning, IJCAI-89, Detroit, MI, pp. 97–101.
Karnopp, D., 1988, 'Structure in dynamic system models', in Proceedings of 12th IMACS.
Karnopp, D. and Rosenberg, R.C., 1983, *Introduction to Physical System Dynamics*, New York: McGraw-Hill.
Katsuhiko, Ogata, 1990, 'Describing-function analysis of nonlinear control systems', in *Modern Control Engineering*, 2nd Edn, Englewood Cliffs, NJ: Prentice Hall.
Kraan, I., Richards, B. and Kuipers, B., 1991, 'Automatic abduction of qualitative models', presentation at QR-91, Austin, Texas, May, 1991, pp. 295-301.
Kuipers, B.J., 1986, Qualitative simulation, *Artificial Intelligence*, **29**, 289-338.
Leitch, R.R., 1989, 'A review of the approaches to the qualitative modelling of complex systems', in Linkens, D.A. (Ed.) *Trends in Information Technology*, London: Peter Peregrinus.
Leitch, R. and Shen, Q., 1992, 'Being committed to qualitative simulation' presentation at QR-92, Edinburgh, UK, August, 1992, pp. 281-93.
Linkens, D.A., 1989, 'Intelligent modelling and simulation', in Linkens, D.A. (Ed.) *Trends in Information Technology*, London: Peter Peregrinus.
Linkens, D.A., Xia, S. and Bennett, S., 1992, 'Systematic model transformation for analyzing dynamic physical systems at multiple levels', in Proceedings of 1992 European Simulation Multiconference, York, UK, June, 1992.
Linkens, D.A., Xia, S. and Bennett, S., 1993, 'Computer-Aided Qualitative Modelling and Analysis from Unified Principles', in Proceedings of the 1993 International Conference on Bond Graph Modeling and Simulation, Hyatt Regency (La Jolla) San Diego, California, USA, January 17–20, 1993.
Linkens, D.A., Tanyi, E., Rahbar, M.T. and Bennett, S., 1988, 'Artificial intelligence techniques applied to simulation', Proceedings of IEE International Conference CONTROL 88, Oxford, UK.
Liu, Z.Y. and Farley, A.M., 1991, 'Tasks, models, perspectives, dimensions', presentation at QR-91, Austin, Texas, May, 1991, pp. 1–9.
Martens, H.R. and Bell, A.C., 1972, A logical procedure for the construction of bond graphs in systems modelling, *Transactions ASME Journal Dynamic Systems and Measurement Control*, **94**, 183–8.
Oren, T.I., 1979, 'Concepts for advanced computer assisted modelling', in Zeigler, B.P. (Ed.) *Methodology in Systems Modelling and Simulation*, Amsterdam: North-Holland.
Rosenberg, R.C., 1975, The bond graph as a unified data base for engineering system design, *Transactions ASME Journal of the Engineering Industry*, **97**, 1333–7.
Thoma, J.U., 1988, 'Bondgraph philosophy and application', in Proceedings of 12th IMACS.
Weld, D., 1990, 'Approximation reformulation', in Proceedings AAAI-90, Boston, MA.
Xia, S., Linkens, D.A. and Bennett, S., 1992, Integration of qualitative reasoning and bond graphs: an engineering approach, *Journal of IMACS Transactions*, Special Issue on Bond Graphs for Engineers, March, 1992.

Chapter 14
Epilogue

D. A. Linkens

The application of control systems engineering principles in biomedicine encounters difficulties which are greater than those found in industry. Thus, in living organisms it is the norm to find massive non-linearities, parameter uncertainties and even dramatic changes in organizational structures. It is not surprising, therefore, that the simple three-term PID controller which has served industry so well for many decades should not be so successful in biomedical control. For these, and other, reasons on-line feedback control must be carefully considered and designed even when used in an advisory mode with a 'human-in-the-loop'. Not the least of these concerns is the question of safety-critical aspects in the design.

In the very large number of trials undertaken by Sheppard and his co-workers on PI control of blood pressure in intensive therapy units, it became clear that in certain cases the feedback system could become unstable. Whilst clinical surveillance ensured that these conditions were not dangerous, clearly such situations are highly undesirable. At this point, the need for a control strategy which allows for unknown and varying patient parameters becomes obvious. In addition, there is the need for on-line surveillance to give fault diagnosis and mode-switching for different control algorithms (including purely manual regulation). Hence, the advent of the self-tuning parameter-adjusting schemes, typified by generalized predictive control, holds considerable promise in automated drug infusion systems (see Chapter 3). The self-adaptive schemes which have been investigated extensively in industry suffer, however, from requiring a detailed knowledge of the process model structure which usually has to be linear. This has prompted the move towards the intelligent control strategies which form the basis of this book.

Although intelligence is extremely difficult to define, the main considerations relevant to its implementation in biomedical systems are that there must be an adequate and flexible knowledge representation style, a method for reliable and safe inference (i.e. reasoning or control) and the ability to deal with new situations (i.e. adaptation or 'generalization' in the notation of artificial neural networks). Numerous approaches are being made in these areas, and these have been expounded throughout the book in the context of on-line drug infusion schemes for anaesthesia or blood-pressure management. The five paradigms utilized are those of fuzzy logic, expert systems, neural networks, genetic algorithms and qualitative reasoning.

The five topics which have been described in Chapter 1, and occur throughout the book, initially appear to be disparate methodologies, but more detailed studies are beginning to show the common ground shared by the techniques. Further research will illuminate these commonalities more sharply, and in this way it is possible that a synergetic development will take place which will utilize the strengths of the individual ideas to produce robust systems containing concepts of intelligence.

In order to couple together synergetically some of the qualitative intelligent paradigms as well as the established quantitative approaches we shall briefly examine the theme of human control performance and then describe a method of task decomposition based on this framework. In a seminal paper by Rasmussen (1983) it was hypothesized that human behavioural cognition and control can be described by three levels as follows:

(1) *Skill-based behaviour*
Feedforward control
Efficient dynamic internal model
'Man LOOKS'
(2) *Rule-based behaviour*
Goal-oriented feedforward
Cookbook recipe
'Man SEES'
(3) *Knowledge-based behaviour*
Explicit goal-oriented feedback
Functional reasoning
'Man THINKS'

At the lowest level, humans use 'compiled' knowledge in an almost unconscious manner. At the highest level, a 'deep knowledge' model-based approach is invoked where reasoning from fundamentals becomes the behavioural style. This level represents the deepest challenge when we come to the possible implementation of such an architecture in machine format.

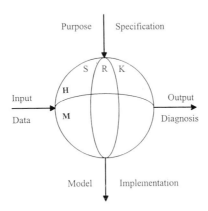

Figure 14.1 Basic task decomposition diagram (TDD).

To incorporate man and machine together in a holistic fashion has long been the aim of cybernetics (a word coined by Norbet Wiener). In order to analyse and (hopefully) design such cooperating intelligent systems we introduce the concept of a 'task decomposition diagram' (TDD) based on the three levels of Rasmussen. Figure 14.1 shows a basic TDD which divides the system boundaries horizontally via a single 'elastic membrane' between human and machine functions. Conversely, there are two vertical membranes dividing each sub-realm into the three regions of skill-based, rule-based and knowledge-based modalities.

Furthermore, the information flow through the plane is represented in two dimensions. The vertical dimension is mainly intended for off-line specification, modelling and design aspects. In contrast, the horizontal dimension signifies on-line features of controller input/output data mapping and higher-level features such as fault diagnosis. The coupling and interaction between these regions in the TDD can be visualized by a set of information trajectories which are specific to particular applications and styles of design. In the following sections some of the Sheffield projects involving intelligent systems in anaesthesia will be subjected to a task decompilation analysis via the TDD approach.

The first examples are based on an intelligent modelling scenario which is used for off-line design studies. An analysis of the tasks and skills involved in the generation of models and simulations for dynamic processes has

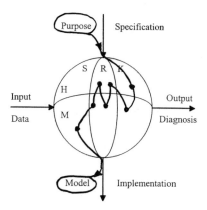

Figure 14.2 *TDD for modelling and simulation.*

suggested the basic requirements for a semi-automated environment for modelling (see Chapter 12). Based on this analysis and the implementation at Sheffield of a prototype knowledge-based environment for modelling and simulation (KEMS) a suggested TDD is shown in Figure 14.2. The main feature in this diagram is the 'stitching' across the human/machine membrane, emphasizing the importance of good human computer interaction (HCI) for intelligent systems. This highlights the need for good communications and interoperability.

In related work done on intelligent abduction of models based on qualitative bond graphs (see Chapter 13) the emphasis has been on the concept of parsimonious models (i.e. the simplest model which satisfies the specified task) and 'granularity' (i.e. the minimum amount of disaggregation required to achieve sufficient distinctiveness). In this case there is constant interchange necessary between human (for monitoring and deep insight) and machine (for routine automation of shallow concepts). The major information flow entails moving through steadily increasing details of model structure, commencing from physical ideas, through concepts and causality, to detailed formal model construction based on bond graphs.

The second application is that of generalized predictive control (GPC) for muscle relaxation anaesthesia (see Chapter 3). This illustrates both dimensions in the TDD of Figure 14.3, in that GPC has several design parameters which require selection via a considerable amount of human heuristic knowledge. Once the design is settled, however, the input–output processing of data is mainly machine-based at the self-regulatory level. One of the key features of this type of computer-controlled drug infusion procedure is the need to administer patient-specific dosage rather than that calculated on the basis of average pharmacokinetics for the population. In this case, the adaptive form of GPC which provides on-line parameter identification is attractive, and this has been implemented successfully in clinical trials in Glasgow and Sheffield.

Epilogue

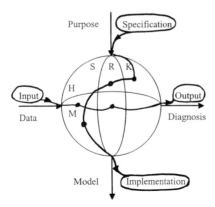

Figure 14.3 *TDD for generalized predictive control (GPC)*.

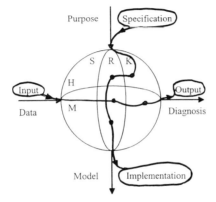

Figure 14.4 *TDD for self-organizing fuzzy logic control (SOFLC)*.

The third project decomposition is based on the use of self-organizing fuzzy logic control (SOFLC) for both medical and industrial applications. In this situation, the whole design and implementation are concentrated entirely in the rule-based and knowledge-based regions of the TDD, as shown in Figure 14.4. The SOFLC scheme is embedded into a multilayered supervisory architecture as described in Chapter 5. The important point to note is that because of the massive patient-to-patient variability in pharmacokinetic parameters it is essential that facilities should be incorporated which make provision for gain estimation and scheduling, and also for controller tuning based on heuristics encoded in a fuzzy logic framework. This project uses a direct form of SOFLC where rules are automatically elicited via an on-line performance-based mechanism.

All of the projects cited so far have been restricted to lower levels of design and control. In the next examples we turn to the field of fault diagnosis and management. Using the fuzzy logic-based paradigm, the TDD of Figure 14.5 again shows a concentration of trajectories away from the skill-based regions. The underlying strategy for fault management is to attempt continually to drive the system into the acceptable behaviour region. Using this architecture the control of muscle relaxation anaesthesia under several scenarios outside normal conditions has been studied (see Chapter 5). This includes changes in patient dynamics during an operation (requiring controller tuning), incipient faults in the relaxation monitoring instrument (requiring set-point adaptation), and actuator failure (requiring shutdown and replacement).

The final illustration of intelligent task decomposition is concerned with an ambitious attempt in another field of engineering to include many of the preceding features in a unified approach utilizing qualitative modelling and control. This involves all of the pathways in the TDD covering modelling (via automated bond-graph abduction), sensor and actuator location, controller tuning and fault detection via a model-based approach. As can be seen from the complicated TDD of Figure 14.6 the trajectories are concentrated, in most phases of this work, away from the classical skill-based regions based on quantitative algorithmic design. This architecture has been validated using an electro-fluid experimental process, and extended to multivariable systems.

Having shown several examples of the way in which a task decomposition diagram can provide a simple visualization of how complex process design can be disaggregated, we pose some questions.

The first question is how should we decompose systems in terms of their structure? Should it be on the basis of hierarchies or networks? The current management fashion seems to despise hierarchy and exalt networking. To me it seems that neither approach alone provides an adequate structure, and that elements of each are requisite. Thus, some form of decentralized control is necessary with partial autonomy, but that ultimate responsibility requires a hierarchical approach.

The second question is more difficult and that is how are we to recompose systems so that they cooperate synergetically rather than destructively? This poses the problem of how to provide knowledge fusion for such aspects as measurement via multi-sensor coordination. It also raises the question of how to 'stitch' across the interacting regions in task decomposition. This reintroduces the concept of the 'permeable membrane' between the regions, and the need for flexible and efficient intercommunication—something which the central nervous system in humans can readily achieve.

The third question is how should intelligence be proportioned between man and machine? The basic principle should surely be that we apportion things in their rightful place. In the realm of intelligent systems engineering this means that machines should augment the facilities which belong to human personality and ability. They should act as 'intelligence amplifiers' or 'tools' rather than replacement parts. At the same time we should

Epilogue

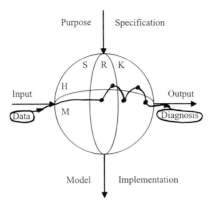

Figure 14.5 *TDD for fuzzy logic fault management.*

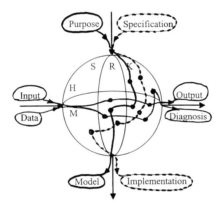

Figure 14.6 *TDD for qualitative control design and fault diagnosis.*

continually recall the Einstein axiom quoted in Chapter 1 that 'Everything should be as simple as possible, and no simpler'.

Finally, we make some remarks on the future of the numerous methods and developments described in the body of the book. It should be clear that we have demonstrated the feasibility of utilizing all of the modern intelligent paradigms within a biomedical engineering context, being that of the limited sphere of anaesthesia. Obviously, there is much scope for widening their sphere of utilization into other areas of medicine.

The question arises, however, as to the appropriateness of the techniques.

At this point let us summarize the different requirements in the production of computer-based control systems. These may be concisely described as:

    Measurement (costly)
+ Signal processing (clever)
+ Signal intepretation (tricky)
+ Control (difficult)
+ Presentation (odd)
+ Persuasion (how?)

In the above comments about task decomposition it has been tacitly assumed that attention should be given to human computer interface (HCI) aspects of the interplay between operator and machine. It is worth reiterating that in the RESAC expert system developed for anaesthesia advice (see Chapter 2), over 50% of the project was devoted to the computer interface aspects of the system.

The question of how to persuade people to employ these intelligence-based computer systems is obviously contentious. Firstly, manufacturers need to be persuaded to market such devices, without fear of litigation and with probability of successful sales. This in turn depends on market-pull from the clinical staff involved in utilizing such devices. At this level, considerable educational aspects are involved in motivating staff and explaining to them both the advantages and basic principles behind these new technologies. It is interesting to note that one of the appeals of fuzzy logic is that it can be understood in its basic concepts very easily by many people. In fact, some researchers have argued that this is its strongest (and even only!) feature, since once inside the machine such paradigms are executed in a non-fuzzy logic fashion. Whatever the merits of that viewpoint, the importance of being able to understand the principles of a technique cannot be overstated.

A further factor to recognize is the reluctance of a market to accept new techniques (particularly in clinical circles where safety-critical aspects are paramount). Returning to the opening theme of Chapter 1, one cannot overstress the danger of too early and exaggerated claims for the merits of a new methodology. Although this may appear to be necessary to obtain research funding, it is highly detrimental to the structured development of technical ideas, since it leads to frequent disillusionment in the market place.

Even from the limited perspective represented in this book it is clear that the field of intelligent systems for modelling and control is currently a very active area of investigation. It clearly impacts heavily on the subject of autonomous systems, for which the AGV (autonomous guided vehicle) is a well-known example, but which has relevance to other transportation systems and social structures, as well as the biomedical situations introduced in this book. We have gone a long way technically from the simple closed-loop regulator, and will need to develop further systems engineering skills to enable these new technologies to be integrated into deeper levels of autonomy.

The overall message appears to be that we should work carefully, patiently and persistently at refining these new intelligent system tools, remembering that it may take 10–30 years before really innovative ideas reach maturity in terms of being embedded into consumer products. Presently, we are at the stage of feasibility and validation of the techniques, ultimately we shall have to move to evaluation and commercial penetration into the market. All of this has resource implications, which are outside the scope of this book, but which must be addressed sooner or later—hopefully the former.

Reference

Rasmussen, J., 1983, Skills, rules, and knowledge; signals, signs and symbols, and other distinctions in human performance models, *IEEE Transactions on Systems, Man, and Cybernetics*, **SMC-13**, 257–66.

Index:

Adaptive ability, 281–3
Alarm-handling 137, 156, 190
Alleles, 326
Analgesia, 37, 291
ANNAD, 297–8, 306–14, 315
Approximate reasoning, 236–41, 265, 286–8
Artificial intelligence (AI), 1, 361–2
Artificial neural networks (ANNs), 11, 294–318
Automated modelling, 385–404

Back-propagation
  algorithm, 261, 295
  neural networks (ANNs), 11–12, 239–41, 259–62
Bayesian inference, 20
Blind searches, 344
Blood pressure control, 128
  depth of anaesthesia, 83, 84–7, 112–13
  fixed control structures, 82
  intensive care, 129
  learning-based fuzzy and neural network, 235–62
  self-organizing fuzzy-neural control, 265–89
  unified fuzzy reasoning, 203–32
Bond graphs, 15–16, 385–404, 410
Bucket brigade algorithm, 346–7, 351

Cardiac output, (CO)
  and blood pressure management, 204, 207, 221–7
  self-organizing fuzzy-neural control, 281
Cardiovascular system (CVS)
  knowledge representation and acquisition, 361–83

Moller's model, 205–8, 219
CARIMA model, 47
CARMA model, 47
Cartesian product, 334
Causal conflicts, 394, 396–7, 398
Causality principle, 389
Cause-effect relations, 386
Centre of area (COA)/centre of gravity (COG), 7, 8, 92, 179–80
  genetic algorithms, 334
  simplified fuzzy control algorithms, 270, 271
  unified fuzzy reasoning, 212–13, 218, 221, 226–7
Chaining
  backwards, 20, 23
  forwards, 23
Chromosomes, 326
Classification problems, 322
Classifier systems, (CSs) 345–7
Clinical signs, unconsciousness, 293–4, 315, 324
Closed-loop control, 292, 293, 298, 306–15, 325
Coarse/fine control, 129, 130
Compartmental models, 43–5, 51–2, 324
Compensation, 213–17
  matrix, 216
Completeness, rule-base, 248
Complexity
  of models, 4
  of rule-base, 249
Compositional modelling (CM), 403
Conceptual model, 403
Conflict resolution, 246–7
Conflicting rules, 177, 179
Consistency, rule-base, 249
Continuous simulations, 3
Continuous-time models, 363, 374

Control
  of anaesthesia, 321–57
  hierarchical, 136–7
Convergency
  learning system, 251
  self-organizing fuzzy-neural control, 284–6
Correctness, rule base, 249
Cost function, 89, 90
Counterpropagation network (CPN), 12
  representation and reasoning by, 271–4
  self-construction of rule-base, 275–7, 279
Credit assignment, 350–5
Crossover operator, 13, 327
Cybernetics, 409

Data fusion, 37
Decay factors, 146
Decentralized control, 211
Decision-making, 322, 333
Defuzzification, 7–8, 92, 138, 179–80
  genetic algorithms, 334, 337
  unified fuzzy reasoning, 211, 218, 223, 226–7
Depth of anaesthesia, 19–20, 37, 82–3, 199–200, 323
  multivariable control, 84–6
  neural network control, 291–318
  RESAC, 20–36
Deterministic systems, 321
Diathermy, 192, 199
Direct adaptive control, 335
Directed graphs, 23
Discrete models, 363, 374
Discrete simulations, 3
Disturbances
  electrical, 192
  generalized predictive control, 64, 73
Domain expert, 5
Drug dynamics
  RESAC, 34
  unified fuzzy reasoning, 207–8
Drugs, muscle relaxant
  depolarizing, 42
  non-depolarizing, 42–3
Dynamic matrix control, 46

Dynamic models, 2
  complexity, 4
  linear, 3
  non-linear, 3

EEG analysis, 84, 292–3
Effect compartment, 45, 83, 324
Electromyogram (EMG), 38, 39
  disturbances, 192
  generalized predictive control, 62–70
Euclidean distance, 269, 281, 284
Evolution, 326, 342–3
Expert systems, 361
  chronology, 9
  features, 9–10
  large-scale, 34
  shell, 20
  see also RESAC

Fault detection isolation and accommodation (FDIA), 74
Faults, 412–13
  detection, 175–200
  diagnosis, 133, 141, 153–6, 167–72
  muscle relaxant control, 134–7
  Relaxograph, 159–63, 164–5, 192, 193, 195
  syringe drive, 163–6, 168–9, 192, 193
Feedback structure, 129, 130
Feedforward structure, 129
Filters
  automatic models, 391
  averaging, 59, 62, 72
  library, 146–7
  median, 147, 158–9
  moving average, 146, 147
  selection, 158–9
  supervisory expert control, 141
Fitness assignment functions, 344–5
Fitness of genotype, 326
FKRL, 369–70, 371
Forgetting factors
  generalized predictive control, 67, 95
  self-organizing fuzzy logic control, 157
  self-organizing fuzzy modelling, 190–2

Frames, 362, 363, 364–5, 370, 381
Functional mapping, 265
Fuzzification, 7, 38
   genetic algorithms, 332, 337
   pseudo-continuous, 140–1
   unified fuzzy reasoning, 211, 212
Fuzzy classifier system (FCS), 347–55, 357
Fuzzy composition, 144
Fuzzy control, 81, 137–41
   genetic algorithms, 13–14, 330–47
   learning-based, 235–62
   and neural networks, 11–12
   self-organizing fuzzy modelling (SOFM), 177–80, 190–2
   self-organizing fuzzy-neural control, 265–89
   simplified, 266–71
   see also self-organizing fuzzy logic control
Fuzzy logic, 6–9
   expert systems, 20
   numeric and symbolic reasoning, 3
   see also defuzzification; fuzzification
Fuzzy modelling, 179–80
   hierarchical, 175–200
   knowledge-based, 176–83
Fuzzy number translation, 240
Fuzzy reasoning, unified, 203–32
Fuzzy rules, 15, 332, 334, 339–40
Fuzzy sets
   interpretation, 239–40
   self-organizing fuzzy logic control, 92, 142
   simplified fuzzy control algorithms, 266

Gain scheduling, 148–9, 167
Gaussian random noise signal (GRNS), 176, 180–3, 184–9, 197, 199
General minimum variance (GMV), 81
Generalized predictive control (GPC), 16, 410–11
   multivariable anaesthesia, 81, 88–90, 128–30
   simulation studies, 95–6, 98–103, 112–19, 126–7
   in operating theatre, 37–41, 73–4
   adaptive controller, 46–50

   atracurium mathematical model, 43–6
   muscle relaxation, 41–3
   performance, 57–73
   simulation studies, 50–7
Genes, 326
Genetic algorithms, (GAs)
   anaesthesia control, 321–57
   chronology, 12
   features, 12–15
   incremental, 344–5, 349
Genetic-based machine learning (GBML), 345–6
Genetic operators, 343
Genetic plans, 339
Genotype, 326
Global constraints, 392
Graph of Models (GoM), 403
Grossberg layer, 272–3, 274–7, 279–80, 281
Grossberg learning rate, 284

Hamming distance, 238, 269, 284
Heart rate
   and blood pressure management, 204, 219
   depth of anaesthesia, 292
Hidden layers, 261, 295
Hierarchical fuzzy modelling, 175–200
Hierarchical self-organizing fuzzy logic control (HSOFLC), 176–200
Hierarchical supervisory self-organizing fuzzy control, 133–72
Hierarchy of control systems, 2
Hill equation, 45–6, 50, 109, 324
Historical constraints, 392
Human computer interface (HCI), 414
   expert systems, 10
   RESAC, 26–30, 35, 414
   hierarchical supervisory self-organizing fuzzy control, 136
   knowledge acquisition module, 370–1
Human operators, 175
Hypertext, 368, 382

IAECE (integral of absolute errors and control effort), 342

Identification of multivariable
    anaesthetic model, 82–8, 323–6
Immune networks, 323
Implication operators, 218, 221
Incremental genetic algorithm (IGA),
    344–5, 349
Indirect adaptive model, 335
Inductive learning, 338
Inference engine
    knowledge acquisition module, 370
    RESAC, 35
Inheritance, 364
Intelligence, 2, 412
Intelligent control, 81–2
Intelligent models, 4
Interactive effects between variables,
    232
Inter-patient variability, anaesthesia,
    108, 128, 192
ISE (integral of squared errors)
    genetic algorithms, 341, 349
    learning-based fuzzy and neural
        control, 250, 253, 257
    multivariable anaesthesia, 112–13,
        126, 219
    self-organizing fuzzy-neural control,
        286, 287
ITAE (integral of time and absolute
    error)
    genetic algorithms, 341
    learning-based fuzzy and neural
        control, 250, 253, 257
    multivariable anaesthesia, 112–13,
        126, 219, 226
    self-organizing fuzzy-neural control,
        286, 287
Iterative learning control, 243

Knowledge-base, 392–3, 395, 396–7
Knowledge-based fuzzy modelling,
    176–83
Knowledge representation and
    acquisition, 361–83
Kohonen layer, 272–3, 274–9, 284

Language, model, 30, 34
Learning, 321–3
    algorithm, 79, 242, 243–4
    automata, 322

error, 243
inductive, 338
machine, 235, 338, 345
    genetic-based (GBML), 345–6
signals 176, 180–3
simulation results, 356
Learning-based fuzzy control, 235–62
Learning-based neural control, 235–62
Limit cycle, 112, 129
Linear mean hybrid (LMH) filters, 147
Linear models, 3
Linear regression patient model (LR-
    PM), 300–1, 306–8, 312, 315
    ventilated (LR-VPM), 303–5, 315
Linguistic labels
    learning-based neural networks, 240
    rule-based fuzzy logic controller,
        138, 145, 151
Linguistic models, 363–4, 375, 379
Local constraints, 391–2
Logical examination, 178
Long-range predictive control, 46
    theory, 48–50
Look-up tables, 288
Lumped–distributed match principle,
    388

Machine learning, 235, 338, 345
    genetic-based (GBML), 345–6
Malfunctioning behaviour, 136
Manual control
    and hierarchical self-organizing fuzzy
        control, 159
    multivariable anaesthesia, 325
Mathematical models, 2
Mean arterial pressure (MAP)
    blood pressure management, 207,
        221–7
    depth of anaesthesia, 85, 292, 325
    self-organizing fuzzy–neural control,
        281, 293
Mean of maximum (MOM), 7, 8, 92,
    179
    genetic algorithms, 334
    unified fuzzy reasoning, 212–13, 218,
        221, 226–7
Median filters, 147, 158–9
Membership function, 331
    genetic algorithms, 334, 336–7, 338

learning-based fuzzy control, 237
self-organizing fuzzy logic control, 92, 140, 145
self-organizing fuzzy modelling, 179, 190
simplified fuzzy control algorithms, 267–8
Memory rules
long-term, 146
short-term, 146
Message-passing, 366
Model-following polynomials, 49, 90, 96, 100–1
Modelling, automatic, 385–404
Models
compartmental, 43–5, 51–2, 324
conceptual, 403
continuous-time, 363, 374
discrete, 363, 374
dynamic, 2, 3, 4
intelligent, 4
language, 30, 34
linguistic, 363–4, 375, 379
mathematical, 2
parsimonious, 406
physical, 2
qualitative, 3
quantitative, 3
static, 2
Modularity principle, 388–9
Monte Carlo simulations
multivariable anaesthesia, 95, 108–13, 114–25, 128
neural network control, 312
Moving average filters, 146, 147
Multilayer perceptron (MLP), 11
Multi-sensor coordination, 412
Multivariable systems, 2, 79–88, 127–30, 204
generalized predictive control, 74, 88–90
genetic algorithms, 323–6
self-organizing fuzzy logic control, 90–5
simulation studies, 95–127
unified fuzzy reasoning, 210–11
Muscle relaxation, 37, 82–3, 291
fixed control structures, 82
generalized predictive control, 50–74

hierarchical fuzzy modelling and fault detection, 175–200
hierarchical supervisory self-organizing fuzzy control, 133–72
measurement, 38, 39
multivariable anaesthesia, 128, 325–6
physiological background, 41–3
Mutation operator, 13, 327

Neural control, learning-based, 235–62
Neural networks, 10–12, 322–3
artificial (ANNs), 11, 294–318
back-propagation (BNNs), 11–12, 239–41, 259–62
Neuromuscular junction, 41
Neurons, 322–3
Noise contamination, 135, 136
artificial neural networks, 294
filtering, 141, 147
learning-based control, 256
percentage, 152
self-organizing fuzzy-neural control, 282
unified fuzzy reasoning, 223
Non-linear models, 3
Non-linear regression (NLR), 295, 298, 306–8
Normalized squared sum of errors (NSSE), 281–2, 284

Objective function, 14
Object-orientation, 362, 363, 366–7, 376, 381
Observer polynomials, 49, 89–90, 96, 102–3
Open-loop control, 292
Operators, 220–1, 227
Optimal gains, 258
Optimization, 2
Order-of-magnitude principle, 389
Oscillatory behaviour, 152, 153

Paralysis control, 128, 158, 323
syringe drive fault, 163
Parameter estimation, 62
Parsimony principle, 4, 406
Patient model artificial neural network (ANN–PM), 298–301, 306–12
ventilated (ANN–VPM), 302–3, 315

Pattern matching, 238, 266, 269–70
Pattern recognition, 322
PD approach, 38, 139
Perceptrons, 11
  multilayer, 11
Performance assessment, 250–1
Performance index, 92, 93, 142–3, 144, 167
Petri nets, 36, 367–8, 381
  cardiovascular system model, 377–9
  discrete simulation, 3
Pharmacodynamics
  generalized predictive control, 40, 43, 44–6, 50
  multivariable anaesthesia, 83–4, 324
  muscle relaxant control, 135
Pharmacokinetics
  generalized predictive control, 43–4, 50
  multivariable anaesthesia, 83, 324
  muscle relaxant control, 135, 156, 166–7
Phenotype 326
Physical models, 2
PI strategies, 407
  blood pressure, 83
  muscle relaxation, 38, 50, 59–60, 63, 70, 183
PID approach, 407
  muscle relaxation, 38, 40, 183
  three-term controller, 139, 144
Plasma concentration
  hierarchical self-organizing fuzzy logic control, 163
  multivariable anaesthesia, 324
Pole-placement, 81, 128
Population, 326
  evolution, 342–3
Possibility theory, 209
Pre-compensators, 204
Process reference model, 93, 143
Pseudo-random binary sequence (PRBS)
  generalized predictive control, 52
  hierarchical fuzzy modelling, 176, 180–3, 184–9, 197, 199
  multivariable anaesthesia, 325

Qualitative models, 3

Qualitative reasoning (QR), 385–404
  chronology, 15
  features, 15–16
Quantitative models, 3

Reachability tree, 368, 371
Receding horizon approach, 48
Recursive Least-Squares (RLS), 50
Reference index set, 225
Reference models, 241–3
Relational matrix
  rule-based fuzzy logic control, 139
  self-organized fuzzy logic control, 92
Relative gain array (RGA), 215, 220, 223
Relaxograph, 159–63, 164–5, 192, 193, 195
Reproducibility, rule-base, 249, 251, 252–9
Reproduction operator, 13, 327
RESAC, 20, 32-6, 293–4
  artificial neural networks, comparisons, 295, 296, 297–8, 315
  clinical experiences, 30–2
  inference process, 23–6
  model representation, 21–3
  user interface, 26–30, 414
Reticulation, 386
Robustness
  algorithms
    generalized predictive control, 54, 55–7, 73–4
    self-organizing fuzzy logic control, 135
  fuzzy controller, 211, 217, 219, 225–31
  knowledge-based fuzzy modelling, 180
  learning-based systems, 262
  self-organizing fuzzy–neural networks, 287
  self-tuning regulators, 80
Rule-base, 203
  acquisition, 265
  formation, 235, 244–9, 251–2
  fuzzy logic control, 138–9, 333
    self-organizing, 97, 126–7, 141–6, 167

genetic algorithms, 340–1
hierarchical fuzzy modelling, 182–3, 199
  learning rules, 176
knowledge acquisition and representation, 362
RESAC, 294
self-construction, 274–81
unified fuzzy reasoning, 208, 210
verification, 248–9
Rule elicitation, 128
Rule modification, 143–5

Safety-critical implications, drug administration, 183
Scaling factor
  genetic algorithms, 338
  learning-based fuzzy and neural control, 245–6
  self-organizing fuzzy logic control, 93, 94–5, 128, 129, 149–50
  modification, 158, 167
  simulation studies, 96–7, 104–7, 127
  steady-state errors, 153
Self-adaptive control, 40, 79–81
  generalized predictive control, 63, 71, 73
  multivariable anaesthesia, 88–90, 95–6, 98–103, 112–19, 126–30
Self-construction of rule-base, 274–81
Self-organizing controller, 236
Self-organizing fuzzy logic control (SOFLC), 4, 9, 81, 411
  hierarchical, 176–200
  indirect, 130
  multivariable anaesthesia, 90–5, 128–30
    simulation studies, 96–108, 110–13, 120–7
  muscle relaxation, 133–72, 190
Self-organizing fuzzy modelling (SOFM), 177–80, 190–2
Self-organizing fuzzy–neural control, 265–89
Sensitivity, patient, 54, 63, 135, 157–9
  changes, 166
  scaling factors, 149–50

Similar complexity principle, 388
Simplified fuzzy control algorithm (SFCA), 266–71
  and counterpropagation network, 273–4
Simulation language, 366
Simulations
  generalized predictive control, 74, 95–6, 98–103
  hierarchical fuzzy modelling, 180–3, 193–9
  learning, 356
  learning-based fuzzy and neural control, 251–62
  Monte Carlo, 95, 108–13, 114–25, 128, 312
  multivariable anaesthesia, 95–127
  qualitative reasoning, 389–92
  self-organizing fuzzy logic control, 96–108, 135–6
  unified fuzzy reasoning, 217–31
Simultaneous constraints, 392
Sine waves, 180–3, 188–9
Single-variable systems, 2
Smith Predictor, 40, 183
Soft matching strategy, 286
Spontaneously breathing patients
  closed-loop control, 306–14
  controllers and models, 295–301
State buffer, 145
Static models, 2
Steady-state errors, 113
  rule-based fuzzy logic controller, 139, 150, 153
Steady-state gains, 207, 211, 217, 219, 223, 231, 232
Steps, 180–3, 188–9
Structural decomposition, 393
Structural mapping, 265
Supervisory level genetic algorithm, 329
Supervisory self-organizing fuzzy control, 133–72
Survival of the fittest, 327
Syringe drive, 163–6, 168–9, 192, 193
System
  bond-graph methodology, 387
  definition, 2
  hierarchical, 133

Systolic arterial pressure (*SAP*), 84–5, 292, 293, 325

Task decomposition, 408–13
Teacher signals, 241, 279–80
Time-delay
  artificial neural networks, 296
  generalized predictive control, 50, 52, 89, 96
  unified fuzzy reasoning, 227
Transputers
  genetic algorithms, 356
  multivariable anaesthesia, 126, 129

Uncertainty
  expert systems, 10
    RESAC, 24
  generalized predictive control, 55
  hierarchical fuzzy modelling, 192

Unconsciousness *see* Depth of anaesthesia
Universes of discourse, 92, 140, 152, 211, 218, 237, 246, 267
Update laws
  learning-based control, 258–9
  self-organizing fuzzy–neural control, 275–6

Venous pressure, 204
Ventilated patients
  closed-loop control, 315
  controllers and models, 301–6

Weighted averaging, 238, 266, 270–1
Winner-take-all scheme, 266, 272

Ziegler-Nichols techniques, 60